The origins of this book stem from [...]
women diagnosed with cancer who w[...]
accessible information about living with cancer. The Women's Cancer
Group was formed and together they chose the themes they felt were
important to them, and scraped together funding from a variety of
sources to employ an interviewer to help each woman record her
story and an editor, Maryon Allbrook, to shape these stories into a
manuscript. Anne Atkinson co-ordinated the project.

Maryon Allbrook is an historian in Aboriginal and Intercultural
Studies at Edith Cowan University and is the author of *Journeys of Hope*
and *The General Langfitt Story*.

Women with Cancer Website
http://cleo.murdoch.edu.au/gen/women-with-cancer/home.html

SONGS OF STRENGTH

WOMEN'S CANCER GROUP

Lynne Alice ◆ Anne Atkinson ◆ Kaye Baxter ◆ Tiny Clephas ◆ Noelle Flatman ◆
Lucille Fisher ◆ Carmen Germann ◆ Anne Kenny ◆ Beth Kingsley ◆ Rae McQueen
Margaret Prince ◆ Mara Sambrailo ◆ Julie Stewart ◆ Ann Taylor
Marinomoana Ward ◆ Margaret Woolley

EDITOR – *Maryon Allbrook*
PROJECT COORDINATOR – *Anne Atkinson*
INTERVIEWER – *Noelene Cooper*
PHOTOGRAPHER – *Mona Neumann*

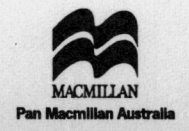

MACMILLAN
Pan Macmillan Australia

First published 1997 in Macmillan by Pan Macmillan Australia Pty Limited
St Martins Tower, 31 Market Street, Sydney

Copyright © Cancer Foundation of WA 1997

All rights reserved. No part of this book may be reproduced or
transmitted in any form or by any means, electronic or mechanical,
including photocopying, recording or by any information storage and
retrieval system, without prior permission in writing from the publisher.

National Library of Australia
cataloguing-in-publication data:

Songs of strength: sixteen women talk about cancer.

ISBN 0 7329 0884 1.

1. Cancer–Patients–Western Australia–Biography.
2. Women–Diseases–Western Australia–Biography.
I. Women's Cancer Group.

362.19699400922

Typeset in Australia in Baskerville 10.5/14 by Midland Typesetters
Printed in Australia by Australian Print Group, Maryborough, Victoria

Front cover: Pablo Picasso, *Girl with a Mandolin* {Fanny Tellier}. Paris, late spring 1910. Oil on canvas,
39½ x 29" (100.3 x 73.6 cm). The Museum of Modern Art, New York. Nelson A. Rockefeller Bequest.
Photograph © 1997 The Museum of Modern Art, New York.

Acknowledgments

THROUGHOUT THE COURSE OF PRODUCING THIS BOOK, WE HAVE BEEN overwhelmed by the assistance given to us by many individuals and organisations. This came to us in various ways; through funding grants and donations, in the provision of services in kind, in volunteering skills, time and energy and in the moral support and encouragement which our families and friends gave us. Without all this assistance, this book would never have been completed.

The Cancer Foundation of Western Australia has been instrumental in assisting us from the inception of this project through to the end. It has given us moral support when our spirits have flagged, written numerous letters on our behalf and handled the funding. In particular, we are grateful to Clive Deverall, Hazel Phillips, John Flint and Anne Tocher who saw the need for this book and encouraged us in producing the manuscript.

Financial assistance for the project came from several government and non-government organisations and from donations made by generous individuals. The Office of Women's Interests in Western Australia provided a grant which enabled us to employ Noelene Cooper, the interviewer. The Lotteries Commission of Western Australia and the Commonwealth Department of Human Services and Health (under the Community Organisations Support Program) awarded grants which allowed us to employ Maryon Allbrook, the editor. Mona Neumann, the photographer, was employed to develop an exhibition of photographs—many of which have been used in this

Songs *of* Strength

book—through funding from Healthway, the Western Australian Health Promotion Foundation. Burswood Resort Casino gave a generous donation which has been used for on-going costs associated with the project. We are truly grateful for the funds raised by one of the members of the Group, Noelle Flatman, her family and friends. Without these grants and donations we would never have been able to realise our vision of this project. Thank you.

We also gratefully acknowledge several individuals and organisations who willingly gave their expertise, provided services, lent equipment or allowed us to use their facilities. Ian Crawford and Blake Dawson Waldron provided legal advice and services. Dr Evan Bayliss read the manuscript and advised us on medical terminology and practices. The secretarial staff, especially Linda Zinni, of the pharmaceutical company Delta West, assisted us in the laborious task of typing the transcripts of the taped interviews onto computer discs. H and R Block of East Victoria Park photocopied endless drafts of the manuscript. Edith Cowan University, Murdoch University and Curtin University, and the Aboriginal Health Centre have contributed towards various aspects and stages of the project through lending equipment and facilities and providing their expertise.

Many, many people have become involved in this project along the way. Whether it has been transcribing interview tapes, delivering letters, researching, helping with grant applications and reports, reading drafts or tackling some of the thousands of little tasks involved in this project, each has given of their time, skills and support. These generous people are:

Addie Mills Senior Citizens Centre	Janette Ballantine
David Allbrook	Mary Rose Baker
Margaret Anderson	Bessie
Julian Atkinson	Peggy Brock
Roger Atkinson	Helen Cattalini
Zoe Atkinson	Anne Delroy
Suzanne Bailey	Margaret Farrell

ACKNOWLEDGMENTS

Geoff Gallop
Rob Ginbey
Margaret Gleeson
Anna Haebich
Gerry Harvey
Naomi Henrickson
Linley Ingram
Eleanor Kapelli
Lesley Lamont
Sonia Lamont
Alison Lee
Fran Lee
Lynley McGrath
Kerry McNamara
Jane O'Dwyer

Anna Poole
Geff Rehn
Sherry Saggers
Andrea Solosy
Carole Spanjich
Leonie Stella
Darryl Ward
Judyth Watson
Kerry Wishart
Mike Woodcock
Helen Wynn

With a special thanks to Mary Anne Jebb.

And to all those who stopped and listened and encouraged us, thank you.

The many aspects of the project have been gathered together and shaped by three empathetic and creative people. Noelene Cooper took our themes, turned them into questions and interviewed each of us, encouraging us to speak frankly and honestly. Maryon Allbrook sorted through the hundreds of thousands of words which had been transcribed from tape and placed on paper. Shaping our spoken words into a readable form while still retaining our individual voices is not an easy task. Maryon has achieved this with incredible skill and sensitivity. Mona Neumann delved into our imaginations and transformed our ideas into photographic images that we could all relate to. Many, many thanks, Noelene, Maryon and Mona for your enthusiasm, commitment and skills.

And finally, our thanks and hugs to our families and friends who have walked the steps with us.

THE WOMEN'S CANCER GROUP

Songs *of* Strength

EDITOR'S ACKNOWLEDGMENTS

I would like to thank all the women in the group for their fortitude in telling their stories, examining transcripts and correcting edited versions of their interviews, and commenting on first drafts of early chapters. Anne Atkinson and Lucille Fisher have earned special thanks: Anne for her support and tireless enthusiasm, and her willingness to talk through all aspects of the writing process; Lucille for her skilful and prompt 'editorial eye'. To my partner, Mike Woodcock, and my family, eternal gratitude for listening to, living through, and encouraging me throughout each stage of writing this book.

MARYON ALLBROOK

CONTENTS

FOREWORD   xi

INTRODUCTION   1

BIOGRAPHIES   5

1. THE DIAGNOSIS   21
   Events leading up to the diagnosis   21
   Being told   33
   Surviving the first weeks   48
   Getting information   56
   Accepting the diagnosis   67

2. MAINTAINING INDIVIDUALITY   77
   Discovering that all cancers are different   77
   Considering choices, making decisions   82
   Myths and stereotypes   97
   Maintaining independence   114

3. STRATEGIES FOR GETTING THROUGH THE SYSTEM   123
   Public and private health care systems   123
   Dealing with staff in the system   131
   The financial cost of cancer   154
   Attending the clinic   161
   Being in the ward   169
   Blood tests, biopsies and scans   176

Songs *of* Strength

4.	**LUCY'S DIARY:**	
	The story of a mastectomy and post-operative recovery	189
5.	**ENCOUNTERS WITH TREATMENT**	205
	Cancers of the stomach and bowel and melanoma	206
	Breast cancer	208
	Cancer of the tongue and neck	214
	Brain tumours	217
	Multiple myeloma	219
	Low-grade lymphoma	221
	Chronic myeloid leukaemia	227
	Cancer of the bowel and ovaries	231
	Cancer of the fallopian tubes	232
	Cancer of the cervix	237
6.	**TRAUMAS OF TREATMENT AND OTHER PAIN**	241
	The trauma of physical and emotional pain	241
	Surviving treatment	256
	Living on drugs	267
	Considering complementary therapies	273
7.	**FAMILY, FRIENDS AND FELLOW TRAVELLERS**	291
	Family—partners, parents and children	291
	Friends—win some, lose some	316
	Fellow travellers—other people with cancer	327
8.	**HOW CANCER CHANGES PERSPECTIVES**	339
	Sexuality	339
	Humour	348
	Working through the issues of dying	356
	Learning to survive	367
	New priorities	386
CONCLUSION		401

Foreword

Songs of Strength relates the very real and personal experiences of a diverse group of women in meeting the challenge of cancer. They are tales of anger, frustration and disappointment but equally of hope, courage and, for most, survival.

This book will help any anyone whose life has been touched by cancer in themselves, a relative or friend. It will help in understanding the stresses it imposes and also in showing what others can do. The diagnosis and management of cancer can be a long and difficult path overshadowed by the threat of recurrence and death. This journey can be travelled with love, hope and dignity with the help of family, an understanding medical profession and access to the appropriate support services. It is the task of us all to make sure these are available.

Professor Richard Fox, BSc(Med) PhD MBBS FRACP
President, Australian Cancer Society

INTRODUCTION

IF YOU HAVE JUST BEEN DIAGNOSED WITH CANCER, OR IF YOU WANT TO help a relative or friend with cancer, or if you are interested in what it is like to experience cancer—it is for you that we have written this book. It is the kind of book that each of us needed when we were first learning to live with cancer: a book that would tell us how other women deal with the diagnosis of cancer—the treatments, the changes to lifestyle and the effect on family, friends and career. Many of us did not want to join a cancer support group, and some of us weren't able to talk to other women with cancer because of geographical or physical isolation and a book such as this would have been an invaluable substitute. We didn't find the book so we formed the Women's Cancer Group to write this one.

The Women's Cancer Group consists of sixteen women of different ages, and from different social and cultural backgrounds. Our cancers and resultant prognoses are just as varied. Some of us have cancers confined to organs such as the tongue, brain, stomach, cervix or the uterus. Others have breast cancer. A few of us have experienced wide-spreading or metastatic[1] disease, while others have blood, lymphatic or bone diseases (leukaemia, lymphoma and myeloma).

---

1. Metastasis—'the transfer of disease from one body site to another: said especially of cancers and infectious diseases. A secondary growth of a malignant tumour at a site separate from which it was derived. It is usually the result of blood-borne or lymphatic spread, although it may occur through the cerebrospinal fluid circulation or along other channels.' (*Illustrated Churchill's Medical Dictionary*, Churchill Livingston: New York, 1989). The word means that cancer has spread to distant parts of the body.

2 Songs *of* Strength

Some of the women were diagnosed as long ago as seventeen years and have fully recovered from the treatments and live normal lives. Others are in remission or undergoing treatment, while three women were in the terminal stage of their illness when this book was written.

The selection of women who could represent a diversity of ages, backgrounds, cancers and prognoses was deliberate because this approach provides a unique focus on the many different aspects of dealing with various types of cancer. This diversity also emphasises the ways in which each of us respond individually to the experience of cancer. Our personal stories, drawn together in a thematic way, provide an array of experiences from which readers can select aspects with which they can identify.

The book covers issues which we agreed were important to each of us as individuals but which we all shared in dealing with cancer, and we have aimed to talk frankly about them. We start with the circumstances which led up to the diagnoses and how we survived those first weeks. We describe our experiences of current treatments (chemotherapy, radiation and surgery), the many diagnostic tests we underwent—which included a range of scans, blood tests and complementary therapies. We also describe our different approaches to maintaining our individuality as we became part of the medical system. We explore the impact our diagnosis had upon our relationships with our families, friends and workmates, and the ways in which it affected our senses of humour, our approaches to death and the re-ordering of priorities in our lives. All are part of learning to survive. Our stories of encounters with modern medical knowledge and other 'experts', our families, friends and ourselves, is what makes this book different and hopefully useful to other 'fellow travellers'.

Throughout the period we have lived with cancer, we have developed strategies for dealing with the many facets of the experience. We want to tell you where we found information, services and, most importantly, the support we needed in its various forms. We want to describe how we gained the confidence to recognise and make known our needs and to take responsibility for decisions which affected our treatment. We want to explain how each of us was able, as far as possible, to take control of our lives within the context of cancer. Finally, we want to tell you of the ways in which cancer reshaped our lives through changes to our personal relationships and the ways in which it has enhanced our independence, individuality and dignity. We hope that the strategies which we have developed will encourage and support you in making decisions and managing your affairs.

The women who contributed to this book, including those who died during its writing, achieved and are achieving optimism and a flair for living with humour and hope. We hope we can inspire and support others in the same way that we have gained inspiration and support from each other.

THE WOMEN'S CANCER GROUP

BIOGRAPHIES

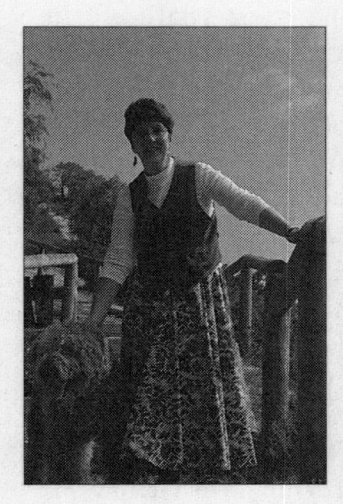

Ann T

MY HUSBAND AND I MIGRATED TO WESTERN Australia from Ireland in June 1974 and we ended up working in a small mining town in the north-west. I got a job running the post office. I was diagnosed with breast cancer in October 1987, when I was only in my mid thirties. I had found a small lump in January 1987 but the doctor couldn't find anything. Over the next nine months I insisted that something was different and finally I got an appointment with a specialist in Perth, which was over eighteen hours drive away. He found cancer and operated immediately. I then had six months of chemotherapy. I went back to work, although I had to convince the townspeople that I wasn't going to die! My doctor had advised me that it was better to do something rather than sit at home doing nothing. I could no longer play squash because the doctors had removed a lymph node from my armpit, so to keep fit I took up swimming and walking.

A year after the operation we moved to Geraldton for four years. Then, after a holiday in Dunsborough when the whole family fell in love with the south-west, I managed to get a transfer to Bunbury. My husband followed five months later. My husband, fifteen-year-old son and I love living in Bunbury: we enjoy walking, swimming and snorkelling and living near the wineries. It's a good healthy lifestyle. In May 1992 we all took a trip back to Ireland to prove to the rest of the family just how well I was doing. We returned there again in time for my mum's birthday during my long service leave in 1996.

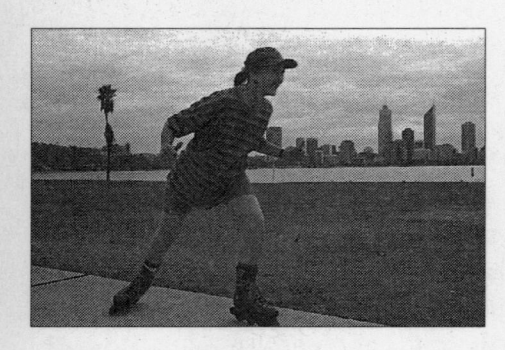

Anne K

I WAS BORN IN IRELAND, THE eldest of a large family and educated by nuns, both of which were good schools in which to hone survival skills. I migrated to Western Australia with my husband and children, where I looked forward to a new and exciting life in 'the lucky country'. But within six weeks of arrival I was diagnosed with leukaemia. From then on life took on a whole new meaning. Survival was the name of the game. It was a long road to travel and there were a few casualties on the way. I lost and I gained, but that's the way life is.

I live with my two teenage boys, work full-time and enjoy what I do. I am fortunate to have good friends and a supportive family. My prime focus has always been my children and that helped to keep me focused. For me, this has been a 'lucky country' in that I live for another day to see my children become adults.

I look forward to the future while enjoying today and will never be able to express enough my love for my brother, whose bone marrow has given me a second chance.

Annie

I WAS FORTY-FIVE WHEN I WAS diagnosed in April 1991 with low-grade lymphoma, an incurable and chronic form of cancer. When I was diagnosed I was working full-time as a university lecturer and completing a PhD thesis. My son, who lived with me, was nineteen and my daughter, who lived with her father, was eighteen. Since my diagnosis I have undergone several different chemotherapy regimens and two courses of radiotherapy. In 1993 I was diagnosed with a form of arthritis which is believed to be associated with lymphoma and for which I am on on-going medication and treatment.

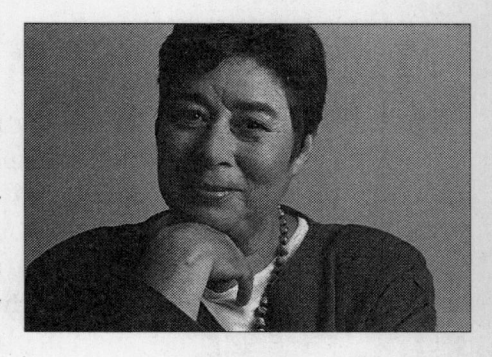

Ironically, it is the arthritis which has limited my activities and has forced me to work part-time. Now I mainly work from home, doing both my university work and coordinating the Women's Cancer Group. Over the last two years I have spent one or two days every week working on the project in a voluntary capacity.

I am passionate about travelling and have gone on several overseas trips since my diagnosis. At the end of 1992, I cashed in my superannuation and took my children on a 'luxury' trip of Canada and the USA. Since then, with financial assistance from my parents, I have made trips to Hong Kong, Singapore, a second trip to the USA and Europe, as well as several trips to the eastern states. Because of frequent periods in which I am unable to be as mobile as I would wish, I have taken up a range of activities which I might never have thought of before diagnosis: tapestry, reading in my spa, admiring my garden (which family and friends now help maintain) and many hours spent drinking coffee with friends.

I am currently recovering from five months of chemotherapy and four weeks in Europe and am returning to the classroom for what I hope will be at least two semesters teaching before the next bout of treatment.

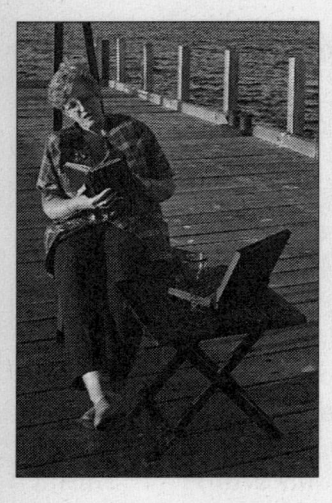

Beth

MY LIFE WAS THROWN INTO TURMOIL WHEN I was diagnosed with both ovarian cancer and malignant bowel cancer that had already spread to my abdomen. The physician gave me four to six months to live and about a five per cent chance of survival. Well, I'm still here and I'm planning to stay for some time yet.

After surgery and before starting chemotherapy I wanted to get back to being as 'normal' as I could. So with the help of family and the support of colleagues I returned to work as a nursing lecturer and, although I can't always work at full pace, it is important to me to be working and to have some useful contribution to make.

Facing the crisis of a life-threatening disease changed my life and I now have new priorities and a new enjoyment of living each day at a time. Three things are central to my experience with cancer: my Christian faith; my family—John, Simon, Stuart, David and Gwyneth; and the friends and colleagues who have loved and supported me through the good and bad times.

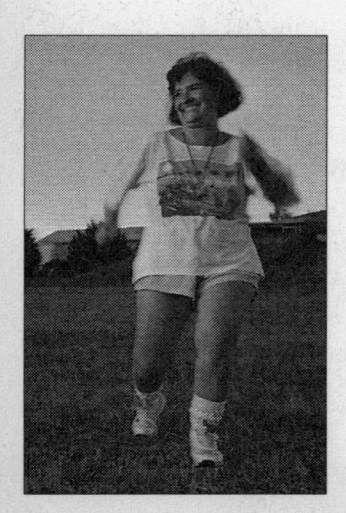

Carmen

IN MAY 1982 I EMIGRATED FROM SOUTH AFRICA to Australia with my husband and two children. At the age of forty-six, on 5 January 1994, I was diagnosed with breast cancer. On 25 January 1994 I had a lumpectomy and six months' chemotherapy plus thirty-two treatments of radiotherapy. After being a year off chemotherapy I was diagnosed with secondary cancer in three of my ribs. These have also been treated with chemotherapy. During treatment I continued to work as a secretary at Edith Cowan University, taking various weeks of sick leave for the operation and treatment.

My life has not changed much since being diagnosed with cancer except that I am much slower. Formerly I was leading a normal healthy life doing aerobics and eating moderately, so I intend to carry on the same way as soon as my ribs get back to normal. In 1996 I intend to do further study to either improve my job situation or change over to something else so that I can enjoy the rest of my life to the fullest. Having cancer has made me more aware of the meaning of life and I intend to make the most of it.

Julie

I WAS DIAGNOSED WITH A RARE FALLOPIAN tube cancer in April 1991, after having gone to hospital to have a hysterectomy to remove a 'non-cancerous fibroid'. Three weeks after the hysterectomy I was told that I would need further major surgery to remove the omentum[1] and some lymph nodes in case further cancerous cells were present. When I was diagnosed I was working full-time as a public servant, my daughter was going for her TEE, my seventy-two-year-old mother had just been diagnosed with lymphoma and my husband was seeing a doctor because of severe blood noses—probably caused by stress.

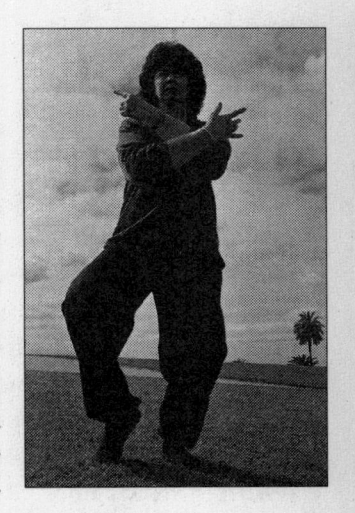

Since being diagnosed I have undergone fourteen months of chemotherapy, eight months intravenously and six months on tablets. The treatment actually extended over eighteen months because sometimes my white blood cell count was too low to permit treatment. After 'chemo' I was violently ill for one week in every month and was

---

1. Membrane linking the stomach to other abdominal organs.

not able to go to work. My major goal was to resume work as soon as possible after the second operation. I hoped to get back to work after six weeks. I made it in eight weeks! Once I made it back to work I think my recovery went full speed ahead. Being busy with people was certainly the best medicine. I also decided to try a few things I have never done before. I went abseiling at the Gosnells Quarry and also parasailing while I was on holiday in Phuket.

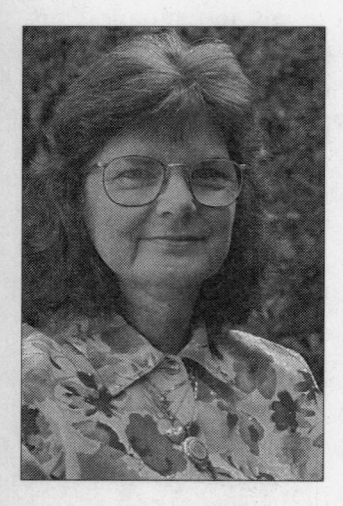

Kaye

I WAS DIAGNOSED WITH CANCER OF THE mouth and neck in 1980. At the time of the diagnosis, I was part owner of a shop, married with two small children, a boy aged six and a girl aged four.

Ever since my teens, my tongue had been covered with a white coating. Now and then it would turn red and sore, but it would clear up. I went to numerous doctors and had been given different diagnoses. Their remedies didn't work so I learned to live with the discomfort. In 1980 an ulcer formed on my tongue and became very sore. It would not heal and I became worried so my doctor sent me to a specialist who did a biopsy. I was then told I had cancer. Part of my tongue was removed and, when the cancer returned in my neck, I had to have my lymph glands removed. This was followed by radiotherapy.

Since then I have had some needle biopsies on some lumps but they have all been clear. Now I only need to see my specialist if I become worried about anything. In the years since then we moved, owned another shop and moved again. I feel lucky that I have been able to have these years with my family and I am now hoping to enrol in some courses at TAFE.

Lucille

I AM A MOTHER AND A DAUGHTER. My children and my parents are the constants in my world, giving my life perspective and purpose. I was born in 1946 and spent my early years on a farm in rural Western Australia. My family moved to Perth, where my sister and brother and I attended school. I then went to the University of WA and later travelled overseas for two years. After a succession of jobs, I joined the *West Australian* as a cadet journalist, and have been making a living from journalism ever since. Apart from three years living in the Victorian Dandenongs in the late 1980s, I have spent my adult life in Perth. My children were born in Perth; Soren in 1974, Miriam in 1978 and Lawrence in 1980. They are beautiful and healthy children who become more interesting every year.

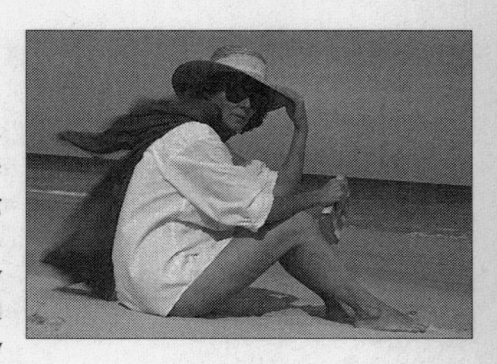

We live near the city in a house that was built about the time I was born. For four years we have been working on it, stripping paint, uncovering floorboards and re-creating a garden to make it what we want. We also have a much-loved dog, Emmy. Domestic life suits me.

I was diagnosed with breast cancer in 1989 and, except for the first few years after my mastectomy where I worried about its re-emergence, I have put the experience behind me and continue to have a comfortable lifestyle. As well as my family, house and garden and Emmy I find pleasure in swimming in the sea, reading, sitting with friends over cups of coffee and taking long walks beside the river. I choose a simple life and avoid situations which are likely to cause stress. For me, this is the way to live.

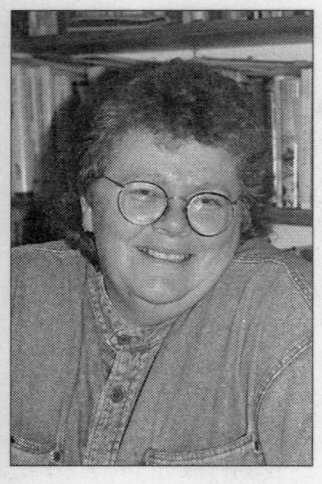

Lynne

AS A LONGTIME SCIENCE FICTION ENTHUSIAST there is little that gives more tingling pleasure than the words 'Make it so!' (spoken with confident authority on the bridge of the starship *Enterprise*, with an imperious gesture towards the cosmos as the ship begins to hurtle into the unknown). I often watch *Star Trek* with my three teenagers and we discuss the ideas and technology involved in these stories of the far frontiers of space.

Ideas and analysis are central pleasures in my life. For example, when I was first diagnosed with advanced cervical cancer in 1992 I was writing my doctoral thesis about the plasticity of gender. My work analysed the ways in which popular use of the concept and academic use by feminists and other social theorists reveal many interesting and sometimes inadvertent discrepancies. I wrote about how difficult it is to achieve social equity when there are so many different ideas about what being female and male is, and could be about, in our everyday world. At the same time I read lots of science fiction by adventurous minds exploring other views of these taken-for-granted ideas.

In a sense this eccentricity, and my community work with sexual abuse survivors and people with HIV/AIDS shaped how I approached my diagnosis and treatment. I was diagnosed and first admitted all in one alarming day in July. By early summer after weeks of radiation, I felt as though I was living in someone else's body. I've learnt to live with that strangeness. The treatment has been successful and I've moved to New Zealand where I am now the director of a flourishing Women's Studies program. My encounter with cervical cancer was frightening and changed my life and that of my children in basic ways. The treatment helped me survive but it is my children, close friends and passion to question everything and take nothing for granted that enriches my life.

Mara

I WAS BORN IN CROATIA SIXTY-four years ago and arrived in Australia in 1959 with my husband and two daughters, who were just six and three years old. I often used to walk in the gardens of the University of Western Australia with my young daughters and dreamed that one day I would have a chance to study. In 1980, after twenty years raising my family and helping my husband in his boat-building business in Fremantle, I decided to enrol at Murdoch University. It took me seven years to complete an Arts degree, majoring in History, and I then decided to continue studying for a post graduate degree in Public History.

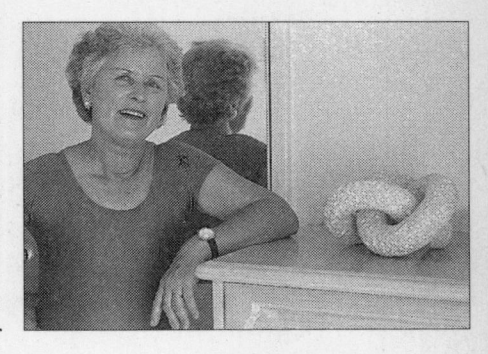

My family history was such that all women on my mother's side, for at least three generations, had breast cancer and in mid-1990 it was discovered that I had it too. That stopped my post graduate study because I had to have a bilateral mastectomy[2]. I spent my sixtieth birthday in hospital recovering from the operation. My post-operative treatment was fitting artificial breasts and buying a swimming suit with pockets to fit my prostheses. I also take one tamoxifen tablet every day to suppress the oestrogen hormones which are thought to be a culprit in causing some breast cancers.

Presently I am secretary of a charitable organisation, Care Croatia, raising funds to help war orphans in my homeland. My husband and I will be travelling to Croatia in that capacity in 1996. Our two daughters succeeded in producing six grandchildren between them. Having my grandchildren around was the best therapy.

---

2. Removal of both breasts.

14 Songs *of* Strength

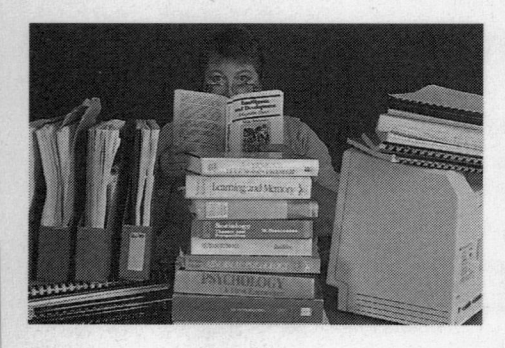

Margaret P

I CAME HERE FROM YORKSHIRE IN 1975 with my husband and three children. We lived in country WA and had a tree growing business when, in October 1988, I was diagnosed with low-grade lymphoma. I had never heard of it but it is also known as chronic lymphocytic leukaemia. I didn't want to die 'being nothing' so I studied for my Year twelve Tertiary Entrance Examination and then went to Curtin University of Technology where I studied for my psychology degree. Apart from my divorce, things went along reasonably until in 1993 when my disease became more aggressive. Since then my health has been very up and down, but inexorably gets worse. I do expect to see my fiftieth birthday in October 1996 because my cancer is slow growing, but I can only hope to see the year 2000. I shall try.

I am very slow and tired now. I can do little physically, even walking, but I do a lot of voluntary health consumer work and I give talks on the patients' perspective to groups such as medical students and nurses. And, of course, I am part of the Women's Cancer Group, writing this book and working on our photographic exhibition.

I wasn't always as slow as I am now. I used to be quite a 'mad sod', always rushing around, swimming, dancing (especially rock 'n' roll), partying, cycling and walking for miles. At age sixteen I won a twisting competition which 2000 people attended. I adore my kids and was often just as mad in my efforts to entertain them and have fun. This included several occasions when I got pushed overboard fully dressed, one occasion being when I was wearing a long dress and a hat! I loved it.

But the kids are all grown now and settled although they don't always cope well with my being ill. They will have to cope when I die—I won't! I'm going to be so angry when I do finally die but whatever happens in the meantime, I still have a lot of fun. Whilst I can still laugh and joke with others, whilst I can think, argue, read and understand, then life is sweet.

Margaret W

MARGARET WAS EIGHTY-FOUR YEARS OLD WHEN she died. Her only son remembers her fondly as a 'real lady' who was 'not only a very good woman but the nicest person I've ever known'.

Born in Yorkshire, Margaret migrated to Australia when she was thirty-nine years of age. She was very active in a women's association and won awards as a writer, poet and playwright. Her life story *Mother's Little Snowflake* and many of her poems give a clue to her humour, her willingness to help others and her strong, independent personality—a woman who would never give in and never let life get on top of her. Margaret lived for some years with cancer of the stomach but maintained her independence, her positive outlook on life, her belief in 'the power of the good', and her philosophy that living within that power is the only way to go. She was a firm believer in 'sharing that great experience of love which is true culture and which is the answer to the sickness of the world'.

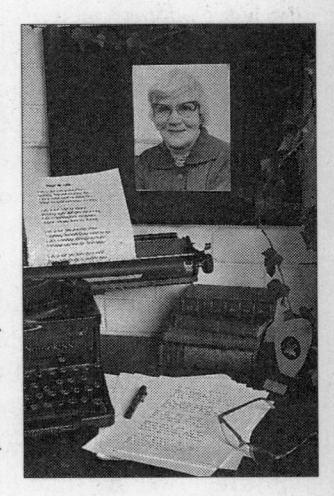

Marinomoana

I AM A NEW ZEALANDER OF MAORI descent. My life has always been very physically active, with sport and a lot of family activities.

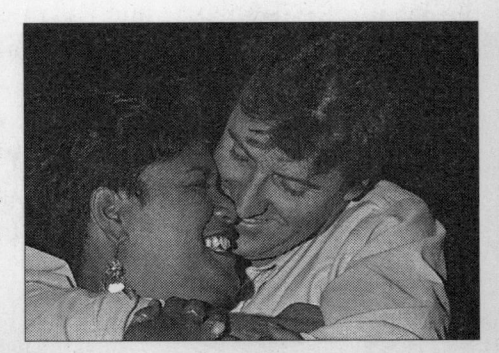

Before I married I was an owner/driver of a seven-ton truck. I was a bottle-o, with a run around Wellington city. I married a West Australian and we moved to Western Australia sixteen years ago. My husband and children are a very important part of my life but I felt a long way from my own family when I first noticed things weren't going too well. I was only twenty-six years old when I was first diagnosed with a brain tumour. My eldest child was four years old and my youngest was only two.

At first, the doctors didn't know what was wrong with me. During the treatment—chemotherapy and radiotherapy—I went through some very rough times. Sometimes I felt so sick and so very tired I could hardly look after my own children. But when that was over, I decided to get some more education. I enrolled at university and have recently completed a bachelor of arts. As my kids say, I am currently involved with saving the world from itself! I am interested in human rights issues, care of the environment and keeping my nose in my now-teenaged sons' lives . . . and annoying my husband! Money permitting, we are planning a six-week trip to the United States of America, to visit friends. I am in excellent health and life looks wonderful.

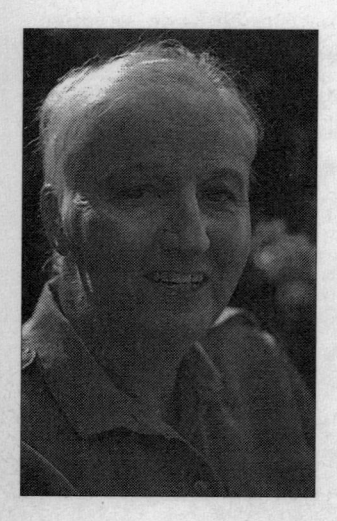

Noelle

MY DAUGHTER NOELLE WAS FIRST DIAGNOSED with melanoma between her toes in 1992 at age forty-four. The doctor removed a section and a skin graft was done. Noelle went back to work as a social trainer and kept living her life to the fullest. In March 1993 she and her partner Robert left for a trip around Australia. While in Queensland they did a scuba diving course. She loved the water and was a strong swimmer. While away, a lump came up in her groin but then subsided. On arriving home it returned. She had a biopsy done which proved to be positive so a block dissection involving major surgery was done on her groin and leg. A large number of glands were removed and tested but these came back negative. This was a relief to all, but no-one, especially Noelle, could be sure of the future.

Noelle had a wonderful positive attitude, got all her affairs in order and got on with living. She went on a special diet, meditated and tried alternative medicine. We were asked to respect all her decisions. Christmas 1993 a lump came up on her face. This was removed and she continued work. In April 1994 Noelle and Robert went to Coral Bay to swim with the whale sharks. This was the highlight of her life. She felt an urgent need to cram so much living into a short space of time and she did that in so many ways.

More lumps kept appearing all over her body and face and these were removed. She started a course of vitamin C injections and although some lumps subsided she developed a flu virus in October. Her lumps got larger, she lost her appetite, was very lethargic and in great pain. She was too ill to have more surgery. She entered hospital, was put on morphine and was sent home but was back in hospital a few days later. She started a course of interferon[3] but had such a violent reaction to it that it had to be stopped. A CT scan[4] on her head showed ten or more tumours on her brain. This was devastating news for Noelle and her loved ones. She was given three months to live. Radium treatment was suggested, along with steroids to take the pressure off her brain. In a few days she looked so bright and was eating well again.

Noelle went into the Cottage Hospice at the end of December 1994 as her growths were much larger and she had severe pains, especially in her head. She had lost most of her hair and had the rest shaved off. Her brother painted on her scalp. This was a great talking point. Soon she was confined to bed, very confused, with the pain

3. Interferon is a treatment used to stimulate the body's immune reactions.
4. A CT Scan is an X-ray procedure that uses a computer to produce a detailed picture of a cross-section of the body.

much worse. Noelle had wonderful love and support from Robert and her family and many caring friends. She passed away on 15 March 1995, aged forty-seven years, her brother and his wife at her bedside. Noelle left behind precious gifts for all of us to share; her love in abundance, her caring and concern for others, her wonderful crazy sense of humour and beautiful laughter and, last but not least, her amazing courage. We are all so much richer and wiser for having her in our lives.

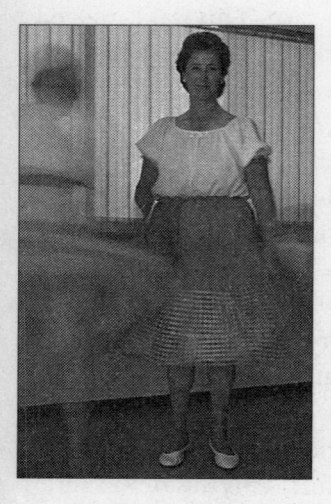

Rae

I HAVE BEEN MARRIED FOR THIRTY-EIGHT YEARS and have three children: two daughters aged thirty-six and thirty-one and a son aged thirty-four. I have seven beautiful grandchildren. I was fifty-six years old when I was first diagnosed with cancer. The first diagnosis was a melanoma, in 1991. Then in 1993, I was diagnosed with bowel cancer and in 1995 another melanoma was found. In each case I was very fortunate as the cancers were found in their early stages and were caught before they spread.

My hobbies have been numerous over the years but my main interest was tennis. Now I have taken up square dancing and, last year, I became a member of the Prime Movers—an exercise group for the over fifty-fives. I have found great joy in being with my children and grandchildren. One daughter and my son live in the country so my time with them is very special. My other daughter and her children live close by. Before my husband Ian died suddenly in September 1996 we enjoyed our life in the retirement village and led a busy life. We went camping whenever time allowed. My health has been good and my last colonoscopy was 'all clear'. Life is very precious.

Tiny

TINY AND HER HUSBAND CLEO, son Harry and daughter Anja arrived in Western Australia in 1985. They came from Holland, where they ran a nursery. The family established themselves in the hills outside Perth, buying a two hectare property, extending the small house and setting up an orchard. The property produces fruit, grapes, berries and flowers. Until she became ill with multiple myeloma in 1993, Tiny played a big part in building up and running the garden. She also enjoyed reading and was always ready to offer help where it was needed. In 1995 she returned to Holland to visit her family. She died in December 1995.

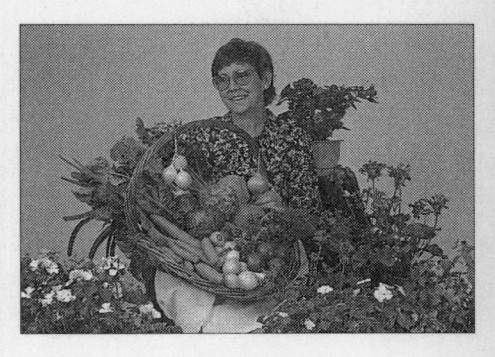

1
THE DIAGNOSIS

THE WHOLE PROCESS OF DIAGNOSIS, FROM THAT FIRST VISIT TO THE GP through to confirmation of a particular form of cancer, revolves around waiting and uncertainty, accompanied by a kaleidoscope of emotions: shock, disbelief, panic, anger, fear. Amidst this turbulence, the doctors who conveyed the news of cancer played a huge role. Some did so with great skill and sensitivity, others only added to the predicament.

EVENTS LEADING UP TO THE DIAGNOSIS
Aches and pains, blemishes on the skin, the appearance of lumps, the odd discharge, increasing tiredness and decreasing energy levels: there are few people who have not experienced some or all of these symptoms. Often, such complaints are explained away as temporary abnormalities, physical signs of stress which will pass with a rest, a change of lifestyle, or simply by ignoring them.

What took the sixteen women in this book to their doctors in the first place? When and why did they make a decision to seek medical advice? Each woman has a different story to tell, for their lives have all been shaped by unique circumstances.

Some women delayed their first visit to the doctor because of prior commitments and other more personal stresses. For example, Lynne was a university lecturer in sociology when she was diagnosed with cervical cancer in 1992.

I'd had this niggle about a discharge I was having which had gone on for several weeks. I put it down to maybe having an early menopause or that I was under incredible stress. My mother had died six months earlier from cancer that had started in her pancreas and spread really quickly. I was also having hassles at work, hassles finishing my thesis and hassles with a couple of my relationships. All these were really unsettling me. I figured that my cervix was probably the most primal part of me so if anything was going to stress out, it was that.

I wasn't really taking much notice until I went to three conferences in a row during one semester break and the discharge never stopped. By the time I got to the third conference I realised that something was chronically wrong and, on the last day, I dreamt that I had cancer. For me, that was that because dreams are an important part of my life. I just knew I had cancer. So I came back and the first thing I did was phone the doctor at the university where I worked.

Sometimes making a decision to go to the doctor about a particular problem was delayed for several related reasons. Margaret P, a mother of three with three young grandchildren, was forty-two years old when she was diagnosed with a low-grade lymphoma in October 1988. When she began having bad sweats at night four years earlier, her doctor told her she was going through the change of life. After eighteen months of hormone replacement therapy she was feeling increasingly tired, but thought this earlier diagnosis probably accounted for her decreasing sense of wellbeing.

I was fat and thought that was the reason I was tired. Then in March 1988, I found a lump on the side of my neck. I'd had the car window open because it was hot, and I felt an insect on my neck, so I thought I'd been bitten. The lump didn't go away, so a couple of weeks later I went to the doctor, and he said it probably was this insect that had caused a local allergy, and to come back in three months. When I went back it was still there, rock hard. He said, 'It's not cancer, it's nothing like cancer. It feels different from cancer. Come back in three months.' By the third visit in August, my jaw went straight into my shoulder and I didn't have a neck! I was hardly in the door before he said, 'Goodness! We will have to do something about that.' He was still telling me it wasn't cancer, and that there were six different possibilities, all equally obscure.

Individual knowledge about health issues can also delay seeking medical advice. Just before Christmas 1992, Noelle was diagnosed with a melanoma that had metastasised. She had put off going to the doctor for the simple reason that she thought there was nothing serious about her first symptoms.

My partner always massages my feet and one night he commented that there was something between my toes. It was quite fleshy and looked like a blood blister. I couldn't figure out why I would have a blood blister between my toes because I hadn't kicked my toe or dropped anything on it. Straight away he said I should go and get it seen to but I thought, 'It's only a blood blister. It will go away'. Of course it didn't. Three months later it had got larger, hardened and gone quite dark, so I took myself off to the doctor.

Other women got to the doctor fairly fast, but were assured that there was nothing abnormal to be found, despite their symptoms. In some cases, such as the diagnosis of Marinomoana's brain tumours, this false reassurance was given for sound medical reasons: there was no clear indication of what was causing certain symptoms. Eleven years ago, when she was only twenty-five, she started dropping things. She had just given birth to her second son.

> *If I wanted to put my baby son down, I would have to get down on the floor, feel the floor, put him down to make sure it was there cos I didn't know how far away the floor was. I have a bad left eye and thought it was that because I have been told since I was a little child that one day my eye would go blind. I went to the doctor and I told him, 'I'm dropping things. I mean completely missing. My judgement has gone all haywire.' He checked me and checked my eye. Nothing. The same wonky eye.*
>
> *Maybe five months later, I started walking into things. I couldn't see. My perception and reflexes had gone completely haywire. I stopped driving because I couldn't tell distances. I couldn't feel pain either. In the first year before I was diagnosed I burnt all the prints off my fingers on the stove. We had electric hotplates and I kept putting my hand on to see if it was hot. I didn't know and it'd be my partner saying, 'Honey! You're cooking!' I thought this is wrong and my doctor was getting a bit worried so I went to have a neurologist look at me. I had all these neuro tests—a whole heap of stuff. Things started coming good again and I didn't hear anything from them for nearly two years.*

Beth went straight to her GP in 1993, when she began getting pains in her bowel.

> *I'd get this sharp pain in the lower left hand side and I'd be sick at the same time. I didn't know what to do first, race up to the toilet or be sick. I couldn't go to the toilet for a month. That's why I put on so much weight. I went to the doctor about two years ago and he said, 'You've got irritable bowel syndrome, go away for three months on a boat cruise,*

preferably with a man of your choice.' He did some tests for worms and things to see if I had anything else. He kept telling me that because I was putting on weight, at least we knew it couldn't be cancer. So I went away.

Anne K, who was diagnosed with chronic myeloid leukaemia in February 1986, had a similar experience when she first took herself to a local GP, barely six weeks after migrating to Western Australia from Ireland.

I had become very thin. I slowed down and had no energy. I felt as if I was walking against a very strong wind. I had been very busy finishing up a business and madly finishing off a house to sell to get enough money to get out here and set us up. I put everything down to being over-tired and in a new climate. The doctor agreed and told me to go home and get some rest. I should have seen the warning signs because he was very dismissive and treated me like another neurotic female. I thought perhaps he was right! A couple of days later I got this really bad pain in my side. I nursed it for about three weeks and when I went back to him it was very bad, particularly when I lay down at night. I had night sweats.

When I went back to him I had visibly deteriorated in three weeks. It was really strange because he never touched me. He never examined me. He sat one side of the desk and I sat the other. He said, 'Do you think you could be pregnant?' My husband had had a vasectomy fourteen weeks to the day so it was very unlikely. Eventually he came round and took my pulse and blood pressure but he still said, 'I really don't see anything wrong with you. Like I said to you three weeks ago, you are just over-worked and over-tired.' It was a five minute consultation and he had me out the door before I knew where I was. I got really annoyed because I thought, 'This man is not listening to me. There is something really wrong.' But I let him intimidate me.

Two days later the pain was a lot worse so I rang him up and said, 'I am coming up to you and I'm not leaving until you give me a thorough physical and a blood test.' He was very cold and dismissive and I said, 'I am not leaving. There is something radically wrong with me. You will have to find out what it is. If you don't come up with anything I am going to get a second opinion.' He said of course I was entitled to a second opinion but got very hoity toity.

Medical encounters such as this can be extremely daunting and require a person to draw on powers of assertiveness that do not always sit easily with unexplained declining health. Even when you are feeling well, the attitude of the doctor can have an enormous influence on the choices you make. Ann T, who also born in Ireland, was thirty-five years old and living in a mining town in the north-west of the state, when she had to make her first decisions about what to do about a lump in her breast.

We'd come down to Perth for Christmas 1986. I'm not one to examine my breasts every month or anything but in January 1987 I felt there was something there, a tiny abnormality. There were times when I could feel it more than others and I think that's what led the doctor to believe it was only hormonal activity when I went to see him. When my doctor finally found it in March, he decided to do an aspiration on it. The results came back and he said everything was fine. Then it started to get bigger. Even though my aunt had a mastectomy and my sister had had a benign lump removed, it never entered my head that it was cancer. When April came I thought I'd go to the doctor again because I didn't like the idea of it there.

I was referred to a doctor in another town, which was about two hours overland, forty-six kilometres of which was a *dirt road. It had been raining and we'd left about seven o'clock in the morning for the appointment at about twelve but we drove over a nail that went into two wheels! By the time I got to the doctor I was all stressed and he was livid because I was late. From the start there was a clash. He examined me and I felt like he was examining a cow. Then he said, 'I'll do an aspiration' and I said, 'No, you won't! It's all right!' Then in front of me he actually dictated a letter to my GP saying that there was nothing sinister with that lump. So again I thought, 'Fair enough'. But I didn't like that man so I asked my doctor for a referral to someone in Perth because I was going there later in the year. I said, 'I really want to have this cyst removed because I want to get pregnant.' I was looking at it as a cyst. He gave me a referral and a letter to have a mammogram.*

Even when a doctor comes up with a plausible diagnosis, it can be essential to persevere if the symptoms persist and refuse to respond to initial treatment. In her forties, Julie discovered this before her symptoms were finally tracked down to a rare cancer of the fallopian tubes. In January 1991, she was working full-time as a customer service officer in a government department when she started to feel an appendix-type pain in the right side of her abdomen. For about five weeks, the doctors she saw in the evenings after work maintained that she had a urinary tract infection. Finally she was referred to a gynaecologist, who, upon examination, informed her that he could feel a large fibroid in her abdomen.

He said it was nothing to worry about. It wasn't cancerous, but he would perform a complete hysterectomy. I was stunned. I wanted to keep all my bits and pieces together, so I came home shattered. My mum had been diagnosed with lymphoma six weeks before so I thought, 'I can't get sick. Mum needs me! My family needs me.' I went to hospital and underwent the

> *operation. I didn't seem to recover terribly well from the anaesthetic, which normally I do. For three days I lay there. I couldn't lift my head, and I couldn't eat. I felt dizzy but I'd just started wearing glasses so I began to think it's because I can't focus and I was too ill to put my glasses on or my contact lenses in anyway. I put it down to that.*

For others, that first visit to a GP led to a rapid escalation in events, often with little time to dwell on the significance of a quick referral to a specialist. In April 1991, forty-five-year-old Annie was diagnosed as having a low grade lymphoma. Her first symptoms appeared just after she had started her first lecturing job at one of Perth's universities, so it had not been long since she'd had a complete medical examination.

> *I was standing in the driveway talking to my next door neighbour and I put my hand up to my neck and felt a lump. During the week it got bigger and bigger. It didn't hurt but I thought that since it was semester break I'd go along to the doctor. She thought it was a blocked lymph node and it was rather large, so she sent me off to a surgeon to have a look. He took one look at it and I got a whole list of questions about who in my family had cancer. I still didn't twig and then he said, 'I'll do a needle aspiration.' One of my friends who had breast cancer had told me that if it's just a cyst then it's easy to draw back the needle but if you've got cancer then it's gonna be hard. So the surgeon put the needle in and he had a job getting anything out of it. That was when I first twigged that there may be something difficult here. Then he had me up on the couch and he did this examination for an hour, including a rectal exam. I thought, 'Hang on, this node, this lump, is in my neck!' I started to get a bit panicky but it still didn't really dawn on me.*

THE DIAGNOSIS

Similarly, in 1991, Rae, who is now sixty, wasted no time in getting to a doctor because she was concerned about a mole on her stomach. She has had to contend with three different diagnoses of cancer in the last five years, two melanomas and one bowel cancer, but memories of her first encounters with cancer remain.

I was concerned about the mole on my stomach. I'd also had a little freckle on the corner of my eyebrow which had been growing. I wasn't too worried about it, thinking it was just one of those little spots. When I went to the doctor, he didn't worry about the thing on my tummy. That was just a mole with a crust on it. He was worried about the freckle on my eyebrow. He sent me off to a plastic surgeon and I had it out straight away. It was a malignant melanoma in the second stage out of five. The surgeon got it all out.

Thirty-three-year-old Kaye had always had a 'funny tongue' with a white coating. Periodically it would get red and sore.

I'd been to a few doctors through the years and they'd all given me different diagnoses, some with funny names. I smoked quite heavily and was told by all of them to stop smoking, but I didn't listen because my tongue would clear up periodically. In 1980 we bought a takeaway food shop. Some time later, I noticed a sore on my tongue, like an ulcer, which wouldn't go away. Some foods, drinks, even smoking hurt, as they came in contact with this sore. Thinking I was just feeling run down from the new business I went to our local GP. He didn't like the look of it so he referred me to a specialist. I kept asking him, 'You don't think it is cancer, do you?' All he would say was, 'Let the specialist see you.' So I went to the specialist who said he'd have to do a biopsy on my tongue. I even asked him: 'Do you think it is cancer?' He said, 'What makes you think it is cancer? Don't think along lines like that. We'll put you in for a biopsy.' That gave me the impression he must know—maybe it wasn't cancer. How wrong I was.

Eighty-year-old Margaret W was an English immigrant, a poet and active member of a women's association. She had 'never had a day's illness' in her life until 1992, when she was diagnosed with stomach cancer.

I had been one hundred percent fit. I was very active but I started to get a lot of discomfort in my stomach. There was no pain to make me think it might be anything serious and the doctor I was seeing thought this discomfort was due to an infection. He stuffed me up with antibiotics but I never got any better. In the end I went to my son's doctor. Straight away he got on to X-rays and discovered that it was cancer, and quite advanced. I had the operation not very long before Christmas 1992.

Although Tiny had never been sick before, her doctors believe she may have been developing the bone marrow disease, myeloma, as long as ten years before she was diagnosed.

We did everything together, me and my husband, but maybe a half year before I went sick in 1993 I did not feel like doing anything. I wasn't feeling sick, I just didn't really feel like helping any more. I did my normal work, the cooking and everything, but I started getting tired quicker. I wanted to sleep all the time and soon I couldn't do the cooking in one go. I'd have to have rests in between. Then I got a pain in my back. That's why I went to the doctor. He sent me to the local hospital for X-rays.

Four, five days later the doctor says, 'It is something in your back. We've got tablets for it. Should take only a couple of weeks and then it's OK.' But after a week I went back because

THE DIAGNOSIS

the pain goes to the front. Then he says, 'Better we do a blood test.' They found me to be anaemic and wanted to find out the cause so I was referred to a specialist at one of the big public hospitals.

Getting to the GP and being referred to a specialist or sent to a clinic for tests isn't always a guarantee of rapid diagnosis, as sixty-year-old Mara discovered. Her family had a history of breast cancer. In her home town in Croatia, both her grandmother and mother had had unilaterial mastectomies[1] when they were in their seventies, while her aunt, who lived in New Zealand, had a bilateral mastectomy when she was forty-five. So Mara was very conscientious about having a mammogram every two years, and wasted no time getting to her GP when she first noticed a change in her left breast.

My second last mammogram they said: 'Fine. Nothing wrong.' Probably a year later, I noticed that on one of my nipples there is a clear fluid coming out. I ask my GP and she said, 'It's probably nothing to worry about but because of your family history you better go for another mammogram.' I went in and they did discover that there is something suspicious on my right side while that fluid was coming on my left side. That worried me and my doctor sent me to the specialist, who sent me to a clinic to have a fine needle aspiration on my right side. My specialist was away for a holiday so he didn't see the results for a whole month. That was when I was finally diagnosed.[2]

Reflecting on the events leading up to her diagnosis of breast cancer in January 1994, when she was forty-six, Carmen says that although she tried examining her breasts, she didn't really have the knowledge to check herself properly.

1. Removal of one breast.
2. See 'Being told', p. 33.

> Women should ask their doctor to show them. It's all written in books but people don't read books. I didn't. Even though I saw it in diagrams, I didn't know what I was looking for and I got confused when I used to check myself. I used to think 'It's all lumpy! How do you know what is a lump and what isn't?' The books says it feels like a pea. When I think of a pea, I think of a frozen pea that is all soft and fleshy. But my lump felt rounded and hard, like a marble. It's not the same as the soft lump, it's a hard lump. If that point had been stressed I think I would have checked a little more. Also, I didn't know that you had to check yourself after every period. Nobody ever stressed that. I checked myself every three months, because I didn't think it was possible a cancer could grow fast between one month and the other.

While she was enjoying the last week of her holidays, Carmen 'bumped into' her lump while she was having a shower. It was a little painful but her first thought was that, being the middle of the month, it was her period. 'I just have swollen breasts.' But it was a 'different pain', not quite like the normal monthly ache.

> Had I not hit myself it could have been growing and I wouldn't have known. It could have got worse without even knowing. The doctor looked at it, told me to put my arms up and felt under my arms. I said: 'Oops! That's sore' and he said: 'That's not so good.' Instantly I knew there's something wrong.
> I had to go for a mammogram, six on that side where the lump was and two on the other. It was really extremely painful because they knew the lump was there and they really zoomed in. I swore I would never have another mammogram again. They sent the results to the doctor the next day. He phoned me up and said they never found a thing on the mammogram even though they taped the lump. I said, 'All that pain for

nothing.' That was my first impression of a mammogram. I never wanted one and because breast cancer wasn't in my family I thought I'd never get it. That was my attitude. I was an ostrich. I put my head in the sand. I never wanted to hear about it. I also thought that the minute you heard the word cancer, it was death. That was how I felt. Here I was with these symptoms but nothing showing on my mammogram. The doctor said that I'd have to go for a needle biopsy. I still didn't panic because I thought: 'I'm not going to get it.'

BEING TOLD

The very word 'cancer' strikes horror into the hearts and minds of most people, so it is not surprising that doctors sometimes experience difficulty informing their clients of such a feared diagnosis. But, given the psychological impact of cancer, the first indications of its existence and the subsequent confirmation of a diagnosis need to be told with sensitivity. While some women were able to look back on the process of 'being told' with a remarkable degree of humour, the situations they recounted indicate how important the manner of disclosure could be to the subsequent development of survival strategies.

Of course, the ways a person—doctor or client—responds to the first evidence of cancer are highly individual. Noelle recalled that when she went to her doctor she

was soundly rounded on and made to feel like a small child. 'You stupid woman! How long have you had that?' When I said about three months, he sent me straight off to the surgeon. I got the same treatment from the surgeon. He said straight away that it appeared to be a melanoma and they wouldn't know until they had removed it whether it was benign or malignant. I really didn't know what to feel when I was told. It was sort of, 'OK. Should I throw myself on the floor? Should

I go screaming out into the streets?' If anything I *was feeling very calm about it.*

Lynne had a 'shock-horror' response when her GP did an internal examination to explore the cause of vaginal discharge.

He freaked. There's no other word for it. He said it was the worst thing he'd seen in a long time and that it was beyond his expertise. Whereupon I said, 'What does it look like?' I'm a very visual person and I wanted to know. There he was, peering up my bum, and I wanted to know. So he described it: my cervix was bleeding continuously; it had bobbly bits on it and when he touched them, they just broke away and bled some more. That sounded pretty horrendous. He got on the phone after finding out that I didn't have private health insurance and started making phone calls and said he'd phone me at work within the hour. So I came back to work. I felt totally frozen, totally numb. I knew I had an hour so I went to the library and read everything I could lay my hands on about cancers of the reproductive system. By then I had figured out it was either cervical cancer or ovarian cancer.

When Lynne's doctor phoned back, she was instructed to go straight to one of Perth's major hospitals where there seemed to be

. . . a mandatory four hour wait, in a room where everyone was totally stressed out and looked absolutely ghastly. There was one examination where they said, 'Don't worry about it. It probably isn't cancer. It looks more like herpes. You must not assume the worst.' Of course I already had.

I had an interview with a medical student. Now I think it was a hoot but at the time it really stressed me out. There's something about having to recount your medical history in extreme detail over several pages of case notes. When it ended

up with a question, 'When was the last time you had sex?', I just burst out laughing. She was really taken aback. I said, 'I haven't had sex with a man for years. I've lived with a woman for the last seven years.' That really floored her because there is no category for relationships between same sex people and she dutifully wrote down 'lesbian'. I had never uttered that word once in the whole diagnosis session but it remained ringed in red ink on my notes. It's probably still there. I think the whole diagnosis process is one in which you get put into little boxes progressively. All the aspects of your diagnosis get categorised and catalogued like that and there's nothing that's private.

Lynne had to go back to the hospital two days later for blood tests and a laparoscopy,[3] and remembers this as

... an extraordinary experience. I came out of it feeling as though I had died and come back to life again—I remember this unearthly chill in the waiting room. At some stage I had a discussion with the house surgeon who had done the laparoscopy and she had told me her mind. About three hours later, the cancer boys swept into the ward and I was taken to a room to be told what had happened. There must have been about six or eight of them, all dressed in suits with white shirts and either black, red or blue ties, and shiny black shoes. These experts said that the house surgeon was possibly right, it was quite possibly cancer of the cervix in an advanced state, but I wasn't to worry about it until the pathology reports came back. Needless to say, this didn't allay my fears one little bit. My partner had been waiting all day to find out what was going on and they'd been fobbing her off so the boys could tell me what was wrong. On our way out, the ward sister said, 'Go home and drink a bottle of whisky.' I said, 'They've just told me in no uncertain terms to not drink alcohol because I have

---

3. Internal abdominal examination by means of a tube with a light and camera attached.

> to come back for tests.' She said, 'Don't worry about it!' I went
> home and was just a total mess. I had three kids waiting for
> me and a student living in the house. Everyone was extremely
> anxious and I had the sense that I couldn't let it all out.
> Despite the fact that the decision about the cancer had been
> deferred to the pathology boys, I knew that I had cancer.

Margaret P was living in a country town. Her GP sent her to see the local surgeon who told her she had blocked parotid glands[4] on both sides and that she would need to see an ear, nose and throat specialist in Perth. The first appointment she could get was three weeks later.

> He examined my neck and said straight off that it was either a
> malignant or benign tumour of the parotid or I had
> lymphoma. On the spot, just from his hands, he gave me two
> out of three chances it was cancer. I had an hour's drive home
> after that appointment and I found that very difficult. I had
> been visiting my doctor for six or seven months at this stage
> and now this guy wants to move fast. He was going away on
> two weeks' holiday and he didn't want me to wait that long,
> so he referred me straight away to another surgeon in Perth to
> do a needle aspiration.
>   If things are clear they may not go any further but for
> people who have cancer they do further tests. I was told during
> the week that I'd have to come in on the following Monday for
> a biopsy.
>   The anaesthetist came to see me the night before my biopsy
> and had a go at me about my weight. Before anybody had told
> me that they thought they knew what was wrong, he told me
> that with my health I would be having lots more anaesthetics
> and eventually one of them would kill me. And the day after
> that he's knocking me out! Of course, I bawled half the night.
>   Tuesday morning, after the biopsy on Monday, the resident

---

4. Salivary glands situated in front of each ear.

doctor of the ward comes around and I said, 'What did you find? When am I going to find out?' He said, 'Oh, well,' smiling gently at me, 'we already know, dear.' He was going to go off without telling me, so I asked him again and he said, 'Actually, dear, you've got lymphoma. You'll be needing CT scans and a bone marrow biopsy before we decide on treatment.' I just stared at him, and as he was turning to go I said to him, 'Is there anybody who can help me? Can I have some information? Can somebody talk to me?' He just said, 'The resident will come back and talk to you,' and left. That was it. Two minutes flat, and I had been told I had cancer.

This feeling that you've been tossed around, turned upside down, and then left to find your own direction is shared by many people when first diagnosed. Annie now likens the early days of diagnosis to

. . . being thrown into a clump of prickle bushes and then told to wriggle out. You have to find your way to where you were before without a road map, without a compass, without any sort of guide at all.

A few days before Annie was due to have the lump in her neck removed under general anaesthetic, her surgeon got the results of the needle aspiration back from the laboratory and phoned her at home.

I'll never forget it. He said, in two sentences, on the phone, 'We've got the results from the lab. It looks as though it's malignant lymphoma so I'll see you for the operation Friday.' I put down the phone and sat in a daze for about an hour thinking, 'What the hell does malignant mean? What does lymphoma mean? What does this mean?' That's when I started to panic. Apparently the results of the first biopsy were so clear that it was just a matter of removing the node and having a really good look.

The surgeon was absolutely certain but I was still uncertain: for me the panic and the wait came with the lab results from the removal of the lymph node. I was really packing it, waiting for those results. He again rang me and said, 'We've confirmed that it's malignant lymphoma and I've arranged for you to see an oncologist tomorrow morning.' No 'Is there anybody you'd like to see?' Just 'You will go to this hospital tomorrow to see this oncologist.' I sat in the chair again and thought, 'What the hell is an oncologist?' All these terms that you know go out of your head!

Annie was not the only woman to be given her diagnosis over the telephone. Five out of these sixteen women received their first diagnosis over the telephone, although in some cases personal choice, which seemed logical at the time, left the doctors with little alternative.

After putting up with pains in her side for several months, Beth returned to her GP, to be told again that it was probably irritable bowel syndrome. This time she insisted that it was a different kind of pain, so her doctor did a blood test.

Within a couple of days he got back to me and said, 'There is something drastically wrong here.' He sent me down to a physician who said it might be a dermoid cyst[5] so I went to have an ultrasound. That showed a seven inch lump around my ovaries. I was in pain because it was pushing all the organs out of the way. They pushed me in for a CT scan and then I went back for a biopsy. I'd taken a couple of days' leave to go and see my sister in Brisbane. We had been there one day when we got the telephone message, it's malignant. It's funny how you don't listen. He didn't say secondaries so I thought I'm OK—until I sat down and thought through what he had

---

5. A cyst containing hair and sebaceous glands.

said. Then I just kept saying: 'I don't want to die.' So we had to rush back to Perth very quickly because I had to go and see the specialist the next day.

The doctor gave me five or six months and said, 'I seriously doubt that this is curable or treatable.' That's what he put on the report because they found two separate primaries, one in the bowel and one in the ovaries. I went back to my GP and he got me an appointment with a general surgeon fairly quickly. My GP rang me that night to see how I got on with the surgeon. I said, 'I'm really very angry with you. Don't you dare ever, ever tell another person that because they're putting on weight it can't be cancer.' I went to him because I knew he was good with people, good with women's issues and he had done a lot for people in the hospice. I wanted to stay with him, but I just wanted to make that clear. That's not like me to speak out like that. Normally I just get upset and sit and stew on it.

Anne K also received her initial diagnosis over the telephone after she had asked her doctor to ring her with the results as soon as they came through from the laboratory.

He had said they would be back by Wednesday. He rang me Thursday evening at six o'clock and said, 'Is there anybody there with you at the moment?' I said, 'Yes. My two kids and my husband is just on his way out the door.' He said, 'Would you ask him to hold on because I have got good and bad news for you. The good news is that you are not pregnant.' I said, 'What is the bad news?' 'Well, you have a form of leukaemia.' I said, 'Pardon?' He said, 'You have a mild form of leukaemia.'

To me, there was no such thing as a 'mild form' of leukaemia. You either have it or you don't. So, it took me almost six weeks to find out what the problem was. I had to really push to find out and then it was delivered to me over the phone. Once he finally got jolted into doing something, he set the wheels into motion very quickly and passed me on to the appropriate areas. I went from there.

Things also moved very quickly for eighty-one-year-old Margaret W when she suddenly became ill again almost eighteen months after her first operation for stomach cancer. She received the news over the telephone one afternoon when she was sitting quietly with her son.

I suddenly felt as though I could vomit up my entire stomach. I didn't but I felt as though I would like to. My son rang the surgeon who quite cheerfully said, 'Oh she's probably got cancer on the liver. Tell her to come and see me.' That was that. I wanted to see our GP before going to the surgeon and he suggested I have a CT scan and barium meals. These quite definitely showed cancer so I did make an appointment with the surgeon and then he hurried it through. Within a fortnight the second operation was all over. I didn't really have time to think about it.

Marinomoana's diagnosis was rather drawn out. Two years after first going to the doctor because of her deteriorating reflexes, she was told to go to hospital for another CT scan. Her neurologist told her they would let her know the results but she was totally unprepared for the way in which the news was given.

I was home one day and I got a phone call and he says, 'Do you want the good news or bad news?' I says, 'Oh, I'll have the good news.' He said, 'Well, it's not your eye.' I thought, that is good and then he said, 'You've got cancer.' He did say that we need to go and talk to him. I thought, 'Where have I got cancer? You can't just say that over the phone!' He rattled off this big name: something sarcoma, something cranial, something opticum. I still don't know the name. It's too long! I said, 'Thank you.' It's funny how polite you are! It was a bit hard and quite a shock because I was home by myself with my youngest son. He was two by this stage so it was two years before they let me know what they were doing! I couldn't believe it. When my husband came home, I said: 'We've got to go and talk to the doctor. I've got camcer.' He says, 'Where?' I says, 'I don't know.' See! I still didn't understand where because I didn't understand the medical language!'

Our GP was wonderful. He explained that when they did the first CT scan there were two dark areas in the back part of my brain, about the size of a pin head. At first they didn't know what it was. Then when they did the second CT scan there were four small areas showing cancerous cells. Then we went to see the specialist. We were there for about an hour and I know I was in shock but my husband just sat there and listened. Then my husband asked: 'How long?' and the specialist said, 'At the rate it's multiplying, between two and five years, maximum.' I got angry, really angry! I said, 'You're not God. How can you sit there and tell someone when they're going to die? You don't know what kind of person I am.' And he said, 'Things will start ... and blah blah blah ...' I said, 'I don't care. You help me get better. How dare you tell me I've got two to five years. That's a death sentence! No!'

That was nine years ago!

Carmen's recollections of the days between first seeing her GP and finally getting a diagnosis of breast cancer highlight the confusion felt by many women—the desire to put it out of your mind coupled with constant fear and uncertainty. A week after she first saw her GP about the lump in her breast, Carmen had an appointment at one of Perth's major hospitals.

I found the worst experience was waiting for the results. If they could only do it quicker it would take away a lot of the anxiety and suspense of knowing and not knowing.

The first doctor who saw me said it was a cyst. The second doctor said it was a cyst but that they would needle it anyway so I went to the ultrasound department. That was a Friday and the woman there said she'd let me know by the Tuesday. I was quite complacent about the whole thing and I didn't think seriously about it. I just got it out of my mind totally until Tuesday evening when they phoned me. I was still at work and I was so upset because they wouldn't tell me the results over the phone. I had to go and see them. That was my most stressful point. I was getting clammy hands and I worried. I had to go into the hospital the next day, Wednesday. I did break down a bit because I didn't know what to think. As they called me in the nurse put her arm around me and I thought, 'No! I don't like this.' I don't like being pampered. I could see it was serious by the look on the doctor's face when he saw me. He just said, 'It's cancer.' At least the wait was over. It wasn't long in time span, only about eight days from first seeing the doctor to being told, but it was that waiting over the weekend from Friday morning when they did the needle biopsy to telling me Tuesday night that they couldn't tell me.

Tiny had to go to one of Perth's major public hospitals for bone marrow tests. These revealed that she had multiple myeloma of the bone marrow.

The doctor said, 'It's not a cancer and it can be cured.' That made it sound a lot better because it can be classified as a cancer. Initially the shock was softened by that. My husband was on holidays in Holland at that time. He knew I was sick but when we spoke on the telephone I just told him we would have to visit the doctor when he got back—otherwise he would just take off. I didn't want that because he cannot do much about it and we had still to wait for the results from the doctor.

It was a week between the diagnosis and the date my husband got back and then we both went to the doctor and were told there was only one cure, and that was chemotherapy. That was a shock because you don't know much about it. All you know is that everyone loses hair and all these things. They did a CT scan that day, and I had to stay in the hospital straight away. I couldn't walk. I was paralysed from the waist down because there was myeloma tissue on my spine. I did not feel good at all.

Julie was in hospital after a hysterectomy when she was informed that her diagnosis was worse than first thought.

On the afternoon of the third day the specialist came. He said, 'We've found a nasty. We've found cancer.' I immediately thought, 'You're wrong! Whatever was in that jar the pathologists examined—you glued the wrong name on that jar. It definitely wasn't bits and pieces out of my stomach.' I couldn't absorb it at first.

Kaye was also in hospital when she received her first diagnosis of cancer. She had been admitted to one of Perth's large public hospitals to have biopsies on her tongue to determine the cause of her problem, which the doctors initially thought was a form of leukoplakia,[6] which had 'gone bad'.

One of the doctors said that type of thing usually happened in people in their sixties, so I was a novelty and everyone wanted a look. They even took photos. Anyway, they took little bits off the top of my tongue. The day my husband was coming to take me home, the registrar came in and said, 'The tests have come back and you've got first stage cancer.' It wasn't even my

---

6. Abnormal thickening and whitening of the epithelium of the mucous membrane.

specialist who told me! Everything just fell apart then. I said, 'What's going to happen?' He said, 'We'll have to do a very big operation on your tongue to try to catch it.' I think the operation was called a glossectomy.

Over the next weeks, her surgeon excised the cancerous cells from her tongue and the skin graft needed to reconstruct her tongue healed well, if slowly. Several weeks later, back at work in the shop, one stitch in her tongue got infected and she returned to hospital to have it removed. Around the same time, she noticed a small lump, 'almost like a pimple', under her chin. It started to grow, so when she went back to her doctor for a check-up, she asked him about it. Initially it was explained as a consequence of the operation upsetting her lymph system, but it kept getting bigger. By the time it reached the 'size of a small bead' which could be rolled around under the skin, Kaye knew things were not right.

I went up for my next check-up and said, 'That lump under my chin is still there.' The surgeon said, 'Yes, it has become bigger. We'll just pop you across to the clinic for a needle biopsy.' It was the first needle of several biopsies and I hated them. The pathologist explained the procedure, which was to insert a needle into the lump and remove some fluid. There was a slight stinging sensation. He went away and I was told to wait. When he returned he told me I had better go back and see my doctor. I asked why and he said, 'We've found some cancerous cells.' It was unbelievable. My husband was waiting for me outside and I could hardly tell him the results because I was crying so much.

When initial tests to determine the causes of Rae's tiredness found nothing, she was sent off for a colonoscopy,[7] but she couldn't figure out why and 'had no idea what was about to happen.'

---

7. Internal examination of the entire colon using a flexible illuminated fibreoptic or video-camera instrument.

That was the Friday I had that done. The doctor who had done the colonoscopy had said, 'We've found something there in the upper bowel. It'll be surgery for you, but don't worry too much about it. It should be all right.' So he gave us the warning, even before the biopsy had been done. When my own doctor saw me the next morning, he virtually repeated what the first doctor had said. My doctor couldn't look me in the eye when he told me—but then, he's one of those doctors that looks down at his books all the time.

That diagnosis was traumatic for me because it was so unexpected. I thought there was something wrong with my throat and never realised it would be in the bowel. It was from one extreme to the other! My doctor explained that the lack of iron had made my tongue all smooth. Usually it's furry, and it feels any hot or cold, but if your tongue is smooth it can't tell you the difference. That's when they know you are anaemic. Also, my bowel motions hadn't changed and the doctor explained that they had found the cancer in the upper bowel, at the highest point in the large bowel. There was no blood coming through because by that time it probably got all mixed up. I would never have noticed it.

Within a week of seeing her local doctor, Rae was in hospital having surgery. As she commented, 'It was all very quick so we didn't have time to be shocked.' Mara had a much longer wait for test results while her specialist was away on holiday. She recalls being 'fairly calm' because she knew all the relevant tests had been done and had assumed that if there had been any doubts she would have been contacted.

When the specialist came back from holiday I went to see him and he said: 'You have cancer on your right breast. But I would like to do a fine needle aspiration of your left breast.' That upset me terribly. I said 'If there was already the suspicion because of the fluid, why didn't they do it straight away?' I had to wait for another week for the appointment and then a week for the results. I already wasted a whole month and I started thinking if I have a cancer on my right side, the cancer is just progressing and I am sitting and waiting and nothing is done. If I'd had that fine needle aspiration on both my breasts at the same time I would have all the results and I could make a proper decision.

I started asking him questions and he just wouldn't communicate. He gave very short answers, just yes or no, without explanation, just like he was scared if he tells me everything he is supposed to that he will have a hysterical woman on his hands. I also got the feeling that because I have an accent, he was not elaborating on my problems thinking probably that I can't follow because I come from a non-English speaking background. That has happened to me on other occasions: you meet people and when they hear your accent they raise the voice or treat you like a child. They don't want to explain or just ignore what you're saying!

An intelligent person wants to know everything possible that concerns their own body! I got so upset. I was driving and crying all the way home because I have cancer and I have to remove my breast. I was close to my sixtieth birthday and I felt so proud of my body. I had kept in shape and nothing hurt me. Why should I do such a drastic thing when I don't have a lump or any pain and the doctor wouldn't tell me what sort of cancer is it? He just gave me a booklet to go home and read.

I got home and the house was empty. My husband wasn't there and I didn't have anybody to pour my heart out to. Luckily my son-in-law is a doctor who specialised in industrial medicine so I rang him and really blasted my head off to him. I said, 'I am upset. OK I have to have the mastectomy but now it's dragging and that waiting period is terrible. I don't know what to do but I'm so furious because doctor didn't do the examination on both breasts straight away. I have to wait another two weeks.' He said, 'I know the people at the clinic. I'll ring them and try to push you in straight away.' He rang the clinic and rang me straight back and said, 'Would you be able to come this afternoon?' Of course I went. They did a fine needle aspiration on my left breast and the results went straight on to the specialist. When my husband got home I told him and he said, 'As long as you're OK I don't mind having you without a breast.' He was really good but he was scared stiff. I could see how scared he was. I was more calm than him.

Ann T, on the other hand, did not feel at all calm when she finally found out that the lump in her breast was malignant. Although she was convinced that the lump was only a cyst, she had decided to have a mammogram next time she was in Perth. In October 1987, six months after her first tests had come back negative, she did so. Two days later, she visited the specialist.

The results were supposed to be down to his office by then but he hadn't seen them. But as he was examining me he said: 'I'll just mark these and I want you to go to have an aspiration.' At that time there was another lump on my right hand breast, near the nipple, but it was so sore. I got off the table, got dressed and went in and he said, 'Ann. It's cancer.' I just looked at him. I felt a strange freezing. It started from the top of my head and I could literally feel it going right the way down. I just looked at him and said, 'But it's only a cyst!' He said, 'No. I'm afraid it's cancer.' He was straight and so grim-faced. 'I haven't got the results of your mammogram here as yet, but I've just phoned the clinic and they have confirmed it is cancer. I want you to have an aspiration because I won't do anything until I know exactly what it is, what size it is, where it is. Ring me.' From then till the Tuesday is a little bit of a haze.

I went to the hospital for the needle aspiration and that put the wind up me because that place is awesome. It's so big. And, oh Jesus, did that needle aspiration hurt. I kept asking the chap questions. He couldn't answer. There were so many questions going on in my head. I wanted them answered and not enough people knew what to say or what to do. That was the way it was all along.

I stayed on tenterhooks for the next twenty-four hours. In the end I couldn't handle it. I got on the phone and the specialist said, 'Yes. It is cancer.' I said, 'Whatever it takes, keep me alive. I just want to live, please, please, do what you want.' Afterwards I thought, God! How bloody dramatic!

When he said it over the phone, I just went to pieces. My husband brought me down to the doctor. He gave me Mogadon to sleep, and Serepax. Our friends, my husband and son tried to get me out of myself and outside but I kept thinking, 'Here I am—whole today, half of me gone tomorrow.' Then I'd see old people on the street and I'd say to myself, 'I didn't want to grow old anyway.' I didn't give up but I think it was the unknown factor—not knowing how bad it was.

SURVIVING THE FIRST WEEKS

Irrespective of the form of cancer, the first weeks after being told are a testing time. The shock of diagnosis combines with these 'unknown factors' to produce a range of reactions—fear, disbelief, numbness, resignation, sorrow, pity, anxiety, anger, determination, pragmatism. How a person wades through this turmoil is highly idiosyncratic.

There are no rights and wrongs of surviving the first few weeks. Each person does their best under circumstances which vary so widely that any attempt to categorise and label 'stages of acceptance' becomes a theoretical exercise. The ways in which a person survives the first weeks after diagnosis are affected by personality, faith or philosophy, the nature of family relationships, work or other commitments, the kind of cancer and, of course, the initial prognosis.

Many localised cancers are curable if they are identified early enough, so the anxiety of the first weeks may hinge on the uncertainties of not knowing whether the disease has progressed beyond a certain stage and fears about the outcome of radical treatments. An answer to those questions may be months or even years away. As Lynne observed, if cancer of the cervix is caught in time, it is generally responsive to treatment, so 'the first few weeks are it in terms of the treatment, although the threat and certainly the fear of cancer goes on and on'.

The first few weeks were really about coming to terms with how I was going to live with the fact that I didn't have a choice but to go through the medical technology of this disease. I really felt as though I didn't have a choice. I thought that if I didn't have children, an unfinished PhD and a whole lot of plans stretching out in front of me that I would try to do something alternative, like herbs or meditation—something different. Then I thought, 'This is ridiculous. Either I want to live or I'm going to die. I have to make the decision about what is going to happen really quickly.' In terms of the medical profession, there was no decision to be made. It was a matter of, 'You will have radiation. We cannot do surgery. It's too advanced. It's too dangerous.' For me to have said, 'I'm going to use herbs' would have been riotous!

Mara found that her longest period of worry came during the week before her operation. The operation itself did not worry her because she knew it was necessary: her specialist had shown her the X-rays, drawn diagrams and 'explained every detail'. Her left breast appeared to be clear so she and her specialist made a decision to proceed with a mastectomy of her right breast. That was in a consultation on a Monday but as he usually operated on Tuesdays, he recommended postponing the operation till the following week because he thought it was 'a little bit late to organise the operation'.

> *That week was the longest week in my life. All the time I was thinking, 'Why didn't I force that doctor to operate on me that Tuesday? My whole body is being overtaken with cancer. It's late and I've already wasted two months doing all the tests and nothing was done really constructively to remove the cancer.' Ah, that was the longest week of my life.*

Noelle went through a different process altogether because of the nature of malignant melanoma. There were eighteen months between the diagnosis of a malignancy in her toe and the appearance of secondaries which indicated the cancer had reached her lymph system.

> *With my toe, I don't really think I took it all in. At that point I did not really know what melanoma was all about. I was quite ignorant so when I was told that the surgeon had got it all, I totally accepted that. He told me that he'd operated on melanomas before and people were still functioning twenty years down the track. My surgeon's quite a character and his words were, 'Go home and sin no more.' I told him I didn't want to sin in the first place! I just got on with my life and totally blocked it out although I was still going to the surgeon for three monthly check-ups. Every time I went to him he checked all the major lymph areas: around the back of my ears, throat, under the armpits, the groin. I was checking those areas myself but I was definitely in total denial.*

Julie had no opportunity to block out her diagnosis of cancer of the fallopian tubes, perhaps because she was in a hospital ward surrounded by concerned medical people, although she found that in itself was trying. She recalls lying in her hospital bed the night she was told feeling extremely frightened about going to sleep.

> *That continued for the whole period I was in the hospital. I didn't want to close my eyes although I was very tired. I was still very weak from the hysterectomy and I would think, 'I need my strength. I need my rest. I'm going to get better.' Then I'd think, 'My God! I've got cancer!' and my eyes would spring open again. I'd lie there looking around thinking, 'I've got to close my eyes.' The nursing staff would come in, look at the medical chart at the end of the bed and then they'd look at me. I've got a fairly good sense of humour, and I'd just chatter on. They'd say, 'How are you?' And I'd say, 'I'm good! Yeah, good!' (meaning I was ratshit!) and they'd look at me and say, 'Has the doctor seen you?' But it was like they were really saying: 'You shouldn't be smiling . . .' The next shift would come on and they'd go to the chart and say, 'Did you want to talk about anything?' I'd say, 'No!' They avoided the word cancer completely. It was like, 'Have you been told? Why aren't you crying and doing your bit? Why are you just sitting there exactly the same as I saw you yesterday? You should be different.' I got this feeling that they wanted me to be a little bit different to make it easier for them. It was pretty scary because I began to realise that you really are alone in this world. Here I am. I've got a husband. I've got a daughter. They can't really do anything. I'm on my own. I've got to battle this myself. This is my fight. I'm not a religious person insofar as I go to church a lot but I've got a lot of religious beliefs and I do pray. I've got a lot of strength out of religion so I guess that got me through too.*

Beth remembers being 'matter of fact' after her surgeon explained the different stages and possible prognoses of bowel cancer, and the likelihood that it had already spread to the ovaries. She had about five days to wait for an exploratory operation.

> *The physician said, 'Tell people. Let people know. They've probably been wondering anyway. Telling people will also concrete it in your mind, for your acceptance.' By this stage, I could just crawl into work, and out again. I couldn't stand up to give a lecture and I couldn't get up the stairs. I was huff and puff and obviously quite ill. When I left him that day, I went out and bought nighties to go to hospital, and went back to work. I went to my friend's office. She wasn't there, so I told her secretary, got in the car and came home. I got this phone call: 'Were you joking?' I rang work, and told the boss. I went in to work a couple of times that week and cleaned up my room. I couldn't believe it: people came into my office, and started putting dibs on my books. I said, 'I am not dead yet! Don't you dare touch my books!'*
>
> *My GP had said: 'We need to make some decisions and some choices now. You'll have a time of clarity, and that will be our window of opportunity to discuss it and make some decisions. If you get worried and upset later, or if you're not too good, you might not think clearly.' I went and saw my friend. She is a social worker. I was being fairly superficial and she said: 'Don't insult me. You tell me. Don't exclude me from all this.' She was great. She brought an acquaintance up who was a counsellor, a minister. I wrote a new will and they witnessed that and I sorted my stuff out.*

The first few weeks after a diagnosis of cancer are turbulent enough even if you are told that it is technically curable. But if you are told that there is no known cure, the first few weeks, and in some cases, the first years, are likely to be dominated by attempts to come to grips with the implications. The practical and emotional difficulties of dealing with a diagnosis of incurable cancer are hard to summarise, more so because constant changes in medical treatments mean that an initial prognosis might prove to be wildly off the mark. After the neurologist had given her a 'death sentence', Marinomoana and her husband got through the first month by keeping the news to themselves and going into 'really nice to each other' mode.

> *During the days we were like everyone else but night times, when we had pillow talks—those were usually crying times. Actually the night times were lovely because we'd just hold each other and cry, feeling terribly sorry for each other. I think that's what got us through it. It got to a point that we couldn't even watch tellie 'cos for some reason at that time there were a whole heap of trauma stories of people dying of cancer. It was too hurting, too sensitive to what we were going through. We had chosen not to tell his parents straight away. We wanted it to ourselves. We didn't want people pitying. When you've got a family like mine, they just surround you so that you don't think about it. They do it out of love, but you* need *time to think about it.*
>
> *It was about a month before we had gotten stronger and felt we were able to cope. Then we told people who needed to know why I wasn't around. I remember being angry at everyone but not really wanting to be and then really feeling sorry for myself. After being so angry and putting this face forward at hospital with the doctors I went into 'I don't care' mode. I felt this sadness all the time. It was very sombre. I basically went into quite a deep depression. I still can if I think about it too much and it's very horrible for everyone living with me.*

Anne K remembers holding herself together until she could find a neighbour to look after her two young sons for a while.

> *I think I came unglued at that point because I have no memory of the next two days, until I was ferried down to Fremantle to see a specialist in that area. I decided very quickly that there were two things that I could do: I could absolutely fall apart and then there would be no-one to look after the kids, or I could deal with it myself. We were new to WA, so we had to keep working. My husband made it quite clear that while it was a terrible thing to happen to me, and that when it came to the crunch of me having a transplant he would be there for me but in the meantime I would just have to cope the best I could. Which is precisely what I did. I tried to keep everything in perspective.*

Margaret P recalls going into shock for 'quite a while' after her diagnosis, especially after CT scans revealed that she was already at stage four, which she understood to be 'getting towards terminal' for lymphoma.

> *At the time you're just in it. It don't matter what they tell you. You've got cancer—that's it. You think you're going to die. Obviously it must be different for different people but I really thought I would either live or die shortly. We had a business and my husband wanted to sell up and go around the world. I remember saying: 'No. What if I live? We'll have nothing to live on when we come back.' I realised later that it was important to carry on as normal. I didn't want my life to change and I had a big enough change that had slapped me right in the teeth. I didn't want any more. It's like a mental hibernation. You want to hide away and pretend nothing has happened. If you've got your normal routine, you just do what you're used to doing and you don't need to think about it. In a way you are trying to convince yourself nothing's changed. I suppose it is a part of denial but it's also comforting: a feeling that life is still continuing.*

THE DIAGNOSIS

For Annie, survival during the first few weeks was dominated by her first encounters with an oncologist and her attempts to get accurate information about low-grade lymphoma. She recalls that first month as an 'horrendous procedure'. By the time she first visited an oncologist she had already discovered that her form of lymphoma was incurable. She knew that there was no set pattern and that 'some people live for fifteen years, some people for two'. To add to her sense of confusion, she 'got off on a really bad footing' with the first oncologist she was sent to see.

> *It was as though I had nothing wrong with me. I had a pad and a pencil to take notes but this doctor clearly didn't approve of the patient writing things down. I was told that I was overweight. I was sixty-five kilos at the time and I was actually normal weight for my height and age. I was told I had to give up smoking. This lymphoma wasn't caused by smoking! I was treated as if I was a naughty child for doing something wrong. It was so unsettling and underlying all this was this doctor's sense of: 'I really can't see what the concern is? You just go ahead and lead a normal life! What's the fuss?'*
>
> *I really turned into a victim. I thought it must be my fault that this person was behaving like this so I took a friend in with me to my second appointment.*
>
> *I could never have built up a relationship of trust with this oncologist. Each of my visits was forty minutes long, and this oncologist never did a physical examination. I was told that my CT scan was perfectly normal when it wasn't—there were two masses of tumours under my arms at that stage. There was much time spent listening to private and professional telephone calls, even arranging tennis at lunchtime. It never occurred to me that a professional person would act so unprofessionally!*
>
> *I was asking a lot of questions about lymphoma. I mean, it's not something you come across every day. This doctor*

decided that I was being over anxious and promptly arranged for me to see a psychiatrist. I never went because I couldn't figure out why a psychiatrist would know more about lymphoma than an oncologist. All I wanted were some answers to questions like, 'How long does one live with this disease?' The answer was, 'If you're sixty-five it doesn't matter but you are not, are you? You are forty-five!' It's those little responses that keep in your head.

A month after she was first diagnosed, Annie flew to Melbourne where she had a two-and-a-half-hour consultation with a specialist. Despite the depressing news that the physical examination revealed she had 'lumps coming up everywhere', this oncologist was prepared to answer her questions and discuss her treatment options.

It was like being released from a cage because someone actually recognised that I've got a disease which is going to kill me, and that I have every right to be anxious about this. I mean, it's life changing stuff!

GETTING INFORMATION

As with other aspects of receiving a diagnosis of cancer, there are no rights or wrongs about an individual's particular need for information. Some people want as much information as possible right from the start; others require specific kinds of information at different times. Still others have little inclination to know anything, preferring to leave themselves in the hands of the experts. For example, Kaye doesn't remember being given much information about her throat and neck cancer.

I had a lot of large words thrown at me but it was almost as if the less I knew, the less I had to worry about. The more they wanted to keep talking about it, the more it upset me. I was given tablets for my nerves. I found out afterwards they were anti-depressant tablets. No wonder I was sleeping most of the time! But I found it was good while I was asleep. I didn't have to think about it. For me it was like, 'You've told me it's cancer and that you're going to operate. All right, get it over and done with. Just get it out of me.'

Carmen hated anything medical and had minimal interest in finding out more at the time of her diagnosis. She found that her doctor gave her little information and, reflecting back, believes she would have let her doctor do whatever he thought necessary.

I was just like a Grade One child: I'll do what I'm told. That was my attitude. I wasn't assertive. I think I was just terrified, without knowing that I was. A lady at work had frightened the hell out of me. She had told me her friend had breast cancer and she went into the operation not knowing that they were going to remove her breast and when she came out it was all gone. I was too much in shock to ask any questions. As soon as they saw it was cancer the doctor just said to me: 'We'll do a lumpectomy.' He didn't explain why I wasn't having a mastectomy or why the glands under my arms had to come out: I had to ask a chemistry teacher that. They didn't tell me anything in a really clear way. Everything I needed to know I felt I needed to ask. I did ask them the size of the lump because I feel it's part of me. They should tell you and give it to you in writing because you forget when you're in shock. I still feel quite unknowledgeable about the whole thing. The person who gave me the most information was a woman from the Cancer Foundation who came to the ward. I didn't expect anybody to come and that visit was really a wonderful thing because I needed to speak to somebody in the same predicament as me.

Similarly, Julie recalled that it was difficult to get information after her hysterectomy, particularly in the three weeks after her operation while her doctors debated whether chemotherapy or radiotherapy was the most appropriate treatment for her fallopian cancer.

I was given a couple of pamphlets on chemotherapy and how to cope with cancer. When I came home I didn't want to read them. I put them in the drawer. I don't really know how to explain it, but the more time I spent at home, the more I was feeling that I was going to get over this. I wanted to know how I could help myself. I wanted to seek alternative medicines. I wanted to know what diet was best. I wanted to know whether I should exercise. I felt so tired, and I wanted to know whether I should rest. These were issues to me, but you couldn't ring your doctor up every five minutes. You just have to do what you feel you can do. It's really left to you. Then I felt that I did want to learn more about chemotherapy and it was then that I pulled the drawer open where I'd thrown the pamphlets.

Noelle also wanted information about how to help herself and much of her early information came from books that 'dropped in her lap'. She found Dr Ruth Cilento's *Heal Cancer: Choose Your Own Survival Plan* particularly helpful because it fitted in with her own ideas of self-healing and personal dignity. She did not go out of her way to find specific information about melanoma because she was 'frightened enough' as it was and understood her own 'information tolerance' levels.

Sometimes too much knowledge can cause your mind to run off in different directions. Sometimes a basic knowledge is a blessing. I felt better able to deal with things as they came along because you take on board as much as you can handle at the time. I realised that unless I knew the questions to ask I was not going to get the answer: and sometimes when you ask a question, you have to be prepared to hear the answer and the answer isn't always going to be what you want to hear. It might be your worst fears and then you have to deal with those.

The confidence that doctors are pursuing the most appropriate and up-to-date treatment is crucial. Tiny's haematologist suggested that she did not try to seek information from libraries because the books would be out of date and would say things like 'there is no cure' and 'you have only got two years to live'.

He said, 'We'll tell you any information. Write down a list of questions, in three days come back, bring me the list and I'll answer them on paper for you.' That was a good scheme. For those few days, all we did was think about questions and write them down. He answered them all on paper so that when we got home we could read and re-read everything. That doctor was very open and very concerned about the whole family.

Anne K found her specialists equally forthcoming and believes it is possible to build a good relationship with the professionals if you are certain of your rights and persist. While she considered herself very fortunate, she admitted that:

I'm not the sort of person to sit back and I probably presented better than I actually felt at the time. I asked and I wouldn't let anything go that I didn't understand. I just kept pounding away for information. If there was something I didn't understand, I was damned if I was going to apologise because I was living with the damned thing. There was no aspect of the disease that I didn't understand. I knew exactly where I was going at all times, exactly what the next step would be. Everything was very, very clear and nobody ever tried to fob me off or dismiss me. People were always very positive and probably it was because I was positive myself. But I think it's the luck of the draw. I think it's who you get. My haematologist was a gorgeous man, a real humanitarian. He would say, 'Is there anything else that I can do for you? What can we do for you?' I never had to fight with him, or with anybody.

Like Anne, Margaret P believes that 'information is power' and that one of the biggest problems confronting people when they are first diagnosed is lack of power. She speaks from her own experience because, until she changed doctors and hospitals three years after she was diagnosed, she had 'a job getting information'. Several hours after she was told she had lymphoma, the resident doctor came and spoke to her. He sent a social worker to talk with her and a 'clinical nurse from haematology came with a leaflet, a short piece with bugger-all on it'. Although she understood that there was no cure for lymphoma and she would need treatment on and off all her life, she had no idea lymphoma would shorten her life span. She thought she had 'a chronic illness, like diabetes', and it was six months before she was told by a registrar that 'in ten to fifteen years you will be dead'. After that, she got more information about low grade lymphoma from a book by the American Cancer Society which she found in her town library. She also got a relative to go to the Medical Library at the University of Western Australia.[8]

There are different levels of information that you need for different stages in your illness. If you've got everything given to you at the beginning, it would frighten the pants off you. People need more information at some times than they do at others. Individual personalities come into play as well. Some people don't want to know as much as others. My specialist

---

8. All members of the general public may use the Medical Library at the University of Western Australia, although borrowing is restricted to members of the public who become special borrowers at a cost of $75/six-month period. Photocopies of material held in the library are available at normal rates.

answers everything when I ask it. He doesn't force anybody to have knowledge that they don't want, that makes them uncomfortable, but if they start asking, he tells them. He volunteers stuff to me because he knows I always want to know the far end of everything.

Like Margaret P, many other women resorted to local libraries and bookshops in the search for information about cancer in general, as well as their particular form of cancer. As Annie explained—

Finding information is part of my job so that's the initial thing I did because if there is something you don't know, you find out about it. So I went to a bookshop and bought every book on the shelf about cancer. One, by Trish Reynolds,[9] *was really good because in the introduction it said something like: just because you have cancer doesn't mean you're not an adult. You have rights. You have choices. You need a lot of information. You need to be able to equip yourself to deal with it and it is* your right *to find out if you want to. That was just what I needed after my first oncologist. These books kept me going for almost a year and then I went to the Cancer Foundation and got some more material. Then I discovered Medline at the university library and I've been using that ever since. I've built up a collection of material and articles on my particular lymphoma.*

Marinomoana recalled the difficulty of 'trying to find out how you can do things for yourself, what you should do and what the doctors are doing to you'. It was particularly hard 'getting information out of the medicos', although she found her GP was good at explaining things which the specialist couldn't. She remembers that some nurses would 'look at you with "oh dear me" eyes, or else they

---

9. Trish Reynolds (1987). *Your Cancer, Your Life.* Greenhouse Publications, Richmond Victoria. For clear descriptions of various cancers see Ray Lowenthal (1990). *Cancer: What to Do About It.* Lothian Publishing Company, Sydney.

would explain things to you in baby terms'. The Cancer Foundation people 'were wonderful' but she also went to bookshops and borrowed medical books from friends in the nursing profession to supplement the information in the pamphlets she was given.

> *I spent a lot of time at the Medical Library at UWA but I spent more time with a medical dictionary to find out what they were damn well talking about. I couldn't always understand the language, and the books and the literature tend to generalise so much about cancer that it was irrelevant. I felt like they were talking about someone else. You can pick up some things: 'That's kind of like me, but no, that's not what I've got!' That's hard work, and you don't want to go through all of that.*

Information could also be acquired from unexpected sources, as Marinomoana discovered when she visited her family chemist to get her many scripts filled.

> *He is a lovely man so one day I asked him, 'What is this stuff? I'd like to know what I'm shoving into my body.' It was oral chemotherapy. He said, 'It will take me a day or so but I can do you an exact breakdown of everything that you've taken right to the milligram.' That was a help. I'd sit up there for about an hour and we'd go through everything: he'd tell me what it was and what it was for. That's how I got information about drugs.*

Rae got information from an old Reader's Digest medical book which described 'the symptoms and how you could get bowel cancer'. She contacted a friend in their retirement village, a doctor who 'explained a little about what was going to happen'. She also rang another woman in the village who had an advanced bowel cancer.

That was really helpful because she put me in the picture. I felt easier then, because I knew what was going to happen. She told me lots of little things, like after the operation you eat ice for four days without anything else. I thought I can't believe this, but when I was admitted to hospital the nursing staff gave me the same sort of information and told me why. It makes a big difference in the recovery if people tell you what's going to happen.

Mara also found that it was helpful to talk with someone who had been through a similar experience of breast cancer because even the smallest bits of information could be useful. She was visited by a woman from the Cancer Foundation a few days before she had her operation.

I asked her a few questions and she gave me a few good points and said how she survived. She also said if I had nighties with buttons up the front or pyjamas it would be easier because then I could take the top off while my doctor examines me while the normal round necked nighties are awkward. That was a really helpful hint. I always think of that now when I talk to other people and remind them to do that. She said she would come and visit me in hospital. I only can praise the lady who came to see me in hospital but the funny thing is, I never rang her, she always rang me. I purposely avoided going to a cancer support group because I felt that I would be put in the league of sick people if I did. But that's my own personal feeling. A lot of ladies probably feel isolated in their own misery but I only felt terrible during the waiting period before the operation. After that I was on the way up. I have a daughter who's a psychologist and another who is a microbiologist, and a son-in-law who is a doctor, so I felt I had enough help at hand. I found that what my doctor gave me was very informative and precise, and my daughters both sent me articles that they picked up from medical magazines and medical journals. Some were technical and some were about the psychological effects of breast cancer. I wanted to read them because they really give you insight into things from all different perspectives.

Ann T found it much harder to get information about breast cancer.

I was very surprised the nurses in the hospital weren't able to help. In the end I felt it was me who was giving them the information. When I was in hospital I insisted on somebody from the Cancer Foundation coming to see me. I was only thirty-five so I said, 'Please don't send me somebody who is old because I won't be able to relate to them.' They sent me somebody who was forty and who had had a double mastectomy when she was thirty-two. She gave me a lot of information. When I got back home, I took all the books I could with me. The girls in the medical centre there helped but I had to go and look for most of it myself. I wanted anything I could get on the subject.

Lynne had already looked up as much information about cervical cancer as she could find in her university library by the time she went to see the specialists, and many of her first questions concerned the physical and emotional consequences of the treatment.

They diagnose you as having this life-threatening disease but then they can't talk about the emotional issues. That's not part of the medical profession and it's a terrible, terrible thing. If you're dealing with something like cervical cancer, you've got to deal with people in the hospital or outworkers who can at least talk to you about your life. No-one would talk to me about the effects of radiation on my sex life, perhaps because I wasn't a heterosexual person. It's probably a lack of knowledge but I imagine it would be difficult for women generally to have a conversation with their doctor about the fact that they've had these bloody radiation rods stuck up their bum and it's going to affect their sex life for the rest of their lives. What does that mean in practical terms? The only information you can get is from pamphlets where it's said in such circumspect language that it's very difficult to know what they're talking about. And it's got to be different for everyone: not everyone's heterosexual and not every heterosexual has the same sort of sex life.

I got really upset about the literature that was given to me in the hospital when they described the radiation treatment. The pamphlet talked about the possibility of the vagina closing up, shortening or narrowing as a result of radiation treatment. Later on, when I talked with the doctor at the Cancer Foundation, I found out that it's a remote possibility but you wouldn't think so from the literature so I did this enormous freak out. One week you go from being a normal stereotypical woman with three kids and a supposedly healthy, functioning cervix to being a woman with no cervix, with an unsupportive gynaecologist who has all the information and the hint that your vagina is going to close up. It's like a horror movie. It was only bit by bit that I discovered it's not as extreme as that for most women unless they go on to have recurrences of cancer. But there is this massive gap in the information you need and it's all mediated by stereotypes, by the schedule of the hospitals on any given day, and by most doctors' inability to talk about day-to-day things, let alone talk about something as intimate as sex.

Beth couldn't seek specific information about her cancer until after her first operation because she didn't have much time and the doctors weren't sure 'what the extent of the problem was'. As she worked in the nursing field, she had plenty of textbooks she could refer to, but they were mostly 'horrible pragmatic things about nursing dying people'. She took them to hospital with her but didn't even open them. She found a book on meditation and relaxation far more appropriate.

> *I got information after the operation. I asked the staff at the hospital about Hormone Replacement Therapy. The pharmacist brought me up some articles and I took some brochures which had been placed on a big board in the cancer ward. After I came out of hospital I had trouble finding out whether I could or should go on Hormone Replacement Therapy so I phoned the Cancer Foundation and spoke to their doctor. They said there was very little to say with ovaries. It depended on whether it's oestrogen receptive. She sent me just a photocopy of the only thing they had which said there wasn't much research on it. She gave my name to an outreach[10] nurse who brought me some tapes for relaxation, some books on diet and more brochures to read. I also rang the menopause people, and a lady brought me over a video and some stuff on Hormone Replacement Therapy. So I got the information I wanted, but I got it partly because I knew where to go.*

INTERNET INFO

* *For those who have access to the Internet, the World Wide Web has sites offering information about cancer. Information helps you learn what to expect from the system, and what you can realistically demand. A few useful and general addresses are:*
http://oncolink.upenn.edu/
(general Cancer Site)
and

---

10. Outreach is a service providing counselling, support and practical help run by the Cancer Foundation of WA.

http://oncolink.upenn.edu/faq
(Frequently asked questions about cancer)
and
http://www.arc.com/cancernet.html
and
To get Help from a Human write to:
hem-onc-request@sjuvm.stjohns.edu

ACCEPTING THE DIAGNOSIS

What does it mean to accept a diagnosis of cancer? The whole notion of acceptance depends upon an individual's unique circumstances and the nature of the cancer they have been diagnosed with. Paradoxically, acceptance covers a range of possibilities which can include acknowledging one's own mortality, refusal to accept a death sentence, total submission to a stated prognosis, comprehension of the implications of the diagnosis and reconciliation to the process of treatment. Acceptance can also mean refusing further treatment, as eighty-two-year-old Margaret W explains:

> *I'm pleased I had those operations for my stomach cancer but I don't think I'll have another. The second one has been a lot harder to get over than the first one. Strangely enough, these diagnoses didn't really affect me and I have absolutely no recollection whatsoever of either operation, not even coming out of the theatre. I wasn't used to being ill—perhaps that was it. I can't remember being unduly worried and I don't remember getting a shock. My son had a bigger shock than I did. I've heard of people being absolutely devastated when cancer has been diagnosed but I don't remember any undue worry about whether I was going to die. I just carry on from day to day. It must be much more difficult for younger people to cope with the fact that they've got cancer. I have had a good, healthy, active*

> life and I haven't got many more years left anyway. Of course, I would rather manage to live the rest of my life without cancer, but if I can't, so be it.

Tiny found that she had little choice but to accept her diagnosis because her health deteriorated so rapidly once myeloma had been identified.

> I could do nothing—not in the house, not outdoors—so I had no problems accepting the diagnosis. But it was not easy. I used to work outside the whole day in the nursery but then I lost so much weight I wasn't allowed to walk. Then I had to stay in the hospital for five weeks for radiotherapy. That burnt my insides so I couldn't eat. After five weeks my husband said, 'We're taking her home. She's not going to get better in hospital.' We set up a bed in the living room so I could lie down and receive visitors. I could only eat little amounts of food because everything was coming up. I didn't like it, but still I eat it because my husband says, 'Otherwise you have to go back to the hospital.' He was very hard, very strict, and that was good—afterwards but not at that time. All the family was very supportive and it was not that bad.

In the case of incurable cancers, accepting a diagnosis could be a particularly contrary process, as Margaret P explained:

> I haven't had any trouble accepting the diagnosis. I think my trouble is fighting it. Now there's a conundrum for you: accept and fight? How can you do both? When people talk about accepting the diagnosis, it's basically death they're talking about, and I cannot accept that without a fight, although I know that is what I have to look forward to. I think it was a case of: 'Oh dear, poor me.' I never had the 'why me?' If I ever I thought that it was always 'why not me?' I'd been a nurse

when I was young, and seen a lot of people die of cancer. It was one thing I'd always been frightened of getting. So I've been through depression and acceptance at various times, and a bit of bargaining, especially after I'd had chemo again for thirteen or fourteen months, then I had a year with none. That was when I remember doing the bargaining in my own mind: just let me have so long off and I'll accept it, I won't mind. Bull! When the lumps and the sweats came back it was like being diagnosed all over again. I'd been so fit and belting around. By time that I was in second year at uni, and I was getting good results. Then everything just fell apart. With my diagnosis, I've got no hope, never have had.

The nature of acceptance can also change as a cancer progresses, especially if there is no treatment. For eighteen months after melanoma appeared, Noelle was able to get on with her healthy, happy life. Then, a lump in her groin had to be removed. Six months later, another lump appeared in her parotid glands. This one proved to be malignant, and it was then that she realised that the cancer had reached her lymph system and moved into her bloodstream. After that, lumps kept appearing.

It's only recently that I've accepted I have a very aggressive cancer. It's one of the few so-called incurable cancers. While a lot of the other cancers are treatable, mine does not respond to treatment. The response rate they do get is very minimal and the side-effects of the treatment sometimes outweigh the response. In that respect it's quite scary stuff. It's frightening in one way but I'm relieved in another way. I don't have to face the treatment. I don't have to make that decision at this point in time and it's a decision that I've been very reluctant to make. No treatment has been offered. The hardest part about this is not so much the disease itself, it's the waiting in between. Every time another lump comes up, it's the waiting to get to see the doctor. Then it's the waiting to go to the hospital. I don't worry about the test results any more. I know what the test results are going to be. This last time I didn't even bother to ask him what the test results were because it's a foregone conclusion. But prior to that, I'd be hanging on the time to get back to the doctor to find out what the results were. That waiting to find out was hard.

In contrast, Rae had no doubts about the possible severity of melanoma. Her greatest difficulties came with the unexpected diagnosis of bowel cancer almost two years later. Her strong faith and her belief that 'When God calls me, I will be ready to go home' helped her come to an acceptance of her diagnosis, although it was 'still a big ordeal'.

My dad had melanoma and I knew what he went through, so when my doctor said I had a melanoma, I was expecting the worst. Thirty-three years ago there was no chemotherapy and Dad's melanoma wasn't picked up until a very late stage. Although he did survive for two years after that, he was in a lot of pain so I psyched myself up when I had to go and have my first melanoma removed. I didn't tell anyone in the family, except my husband, that I was going to have it done because I wasn't even in hospital overnight. I told them once the results came through and everything was fine. It was so quick it wasn't a big trauma.

The diagnosis of melanoma didn't get to me, whereas the bowel cancer did after a while. I kept saying to myself, 'I'm going to think positive whatever the result. I am thinking positive. Whatever happens, I'm going to beat it.' I have seen friends over the years who have died from different cancers but my dad was the greatest example of all. He was in so much pain and yet he always had time for all of us. I had a very strong relationship with Dad, a psychic thing, and even today, when I'm having problems, Dad comes to me strongly. I feel his strength there all the time. I felt that he'll look after me, no matter what. I have always felt that way. There's someone up there with a greater power who will always look after us, no matter what happens.

A strong faith in God, prayer and the knowledge that others were praying for her also helped Carmen through a period of 'total confusion' as she grappled with the fact that she had breast cancer.

I would say that my first three months has been a period of denial. It's not to say that I don't accept it, or that I don't want to know I've got cancer. It's that I can't believe that I can have it and that I don't feel it. I don't have pain. It's been a shock to me because breast cancer is not in my family and I didn't show any symptoms. I was at my peak of fitness. I'm the only one around here who did aerobics. I don't drink, I don't smoke and I'm forever chiding people, 'Don't smoke. You'll get cancer.' Now I'm embarrassed because I'm the one with the cancer! What do you tell them? I just hide in a corner and I'm glad I'm in this little dungeon of an office now! I don't know that it's psychologically good but it is a good hiding place from people. This whole experience has shown me that anybody can get cancer from one day to the next. Now that I've finished all my radiotherapy and I'm half-way through the chemotherapy, I've accepted that I've got breast cancer whereas before I'd say, 'They took the cancer out: it's gone.' At this stage I'm still surprised. Up till now I haven't really accepted that I've got cancer, although I am starting to.

For other people, the whole notion of acceptance was tantamount to a form of submission. In that case, acceptance meant not being willing to accept that cancer equals death, and that even if it does, there is a whole lot of living to do before that point. For Annie, initially the implications of having an incurable cancer were incomprehensible.

> *My friends tell me that I didn't know what incurable meant for about four or five months. I do, however, remember being given a definite prognosis. It is something that I've never asked for and I don't believe anyone can tell you specifically anyway. But I did ask my second oncologist what the average prognosis was because the first one wouldn't tell me. I was under the impression that it would be ten to twenty years but he just looked at me and said two to six years. It was an amazing feeling because I went instantly cold. Then I took the extreme end of the average—six years—and made that my total minimum.*
>
> *It took me two years to realise that I tend to take averages and look at them as the minimum and it wasn't until about a year ago that I started to think, it's not a minimum, it's an average. Fifty per cent of people have a good chance of dying before six years and the other fifty per cent have got a chance of going beyond six years. Then it started to make sense. For everything I had read about lymphoma, I had turned the average into the minimum. It was a protective mechanism. I still don't think I know what incurable really means, and I'm not going to accept what it means. I don't think that is such a bad thing. I go blithely along doing my own thing. That's the way I deal with it and I really can't see whether it's anybody else's business whether someone with cancer accepts it or not! For me anyway, it's better if I don't sit around wallowing in the fact that I've got cancer.*

Julie had similar views on the issue of acceptance, and refused to talk at length about her disease or accept an introduction to any cancer support groups after her operation. Watching her mother's struggle to understand the implications of her own prognosis at the same time merely consolidated Julie's aversion to the idea that a person must accept their diagnosis.

> *After my operation I was confused. I would say to my doctor: 'Can I ask one more time? I haven't got cancer now because you've removed that bit?' 'Yes.' 'So I haven't got cancer now?' 'No.' 'And this chemotherapy is to kill off any cells that might be there?' 'Yes.' I must have asked them a hundred times to reassure myself. They didn't seem to mind. It's expected. You go through a great shock. Everybody deals with their disease in their own way. I preferred to have had my own little fantasy battle and think: 'I'm winning!' A lot of people say you must accept cancer when you're diagnosed, but I still don't think that I have accepted it and I don't want to ever accept it because I think that once I accept it I might throw in the towel and not do anything about it. I was determined that I was going to get better and I thought: This is ridiculous! I'm not accepting this! I feel very strongly about that. But the doctors and the nurses say: 'She's got to accept it. Time will tell. Just give her time.' The staff are trained and perhaps they're channelled through one tunnel vision: this is the way you must tell a person and this is the way the patient must deal with it. Rubbish! There's no way I'm going to accept it and I really think that I've got through by not accepting it.*

Like Julie, Anne K refused to accept the possibility that leukaemia might prove to be terminal. Unlike Julie, she developed this conviction by accepting her diagnosis 'totally'.

> *I never for one minute allowed for the fact that I might not make it, never. It just wasn't in my round of thinking. Maybe I projected that, I don't know. I know that most people I came in contact with responded quite positively to me. I found them*

great. It's your disease and it's up to you to take ownership of it. You've got to control it, not let it control you. I think that what happens to a lot of people is they become overwhelmed by it. Never ever allow yourself to become a victim. I made sure I knew exactly what my diagnosis was because when you're on your own and you're faced with something like this, and you've got kids to bring up, and you've got other responsibilities, you can't fall in a heap because there is just no-one there to pick you up.

Not long after an intensive round of chemotherapy, Beth's views on acceptance help to show the fluctuating feelings that can accompany the daily reality of an uncertain prognosis.

It is a year since I was diagnosed and they gave me a pretty tight time frame as a prognosis. I think that is wrong. I think that if death is imminent, people probably need to know so that they can get their affairs, their mind, their family, in order. But I think it can become a self-fulfilling prophecy. If I give you six months, you'll be dead in six months, just to prove I'm right. I don't think people should put figures and dates on things. It's very stressful. I was down at the hospital the other day for a CT scan and it shows that there is no new growth at the moment. I am really thrilled to bits but the doctor said, 'It will most probably come back.' I said, 'What do we do if it comes back?' He said, 'If it's a long time, we can use the same chemos again', because I've had two sorts for both cancers. They don't work as well the second time. I sat there thinking that a long time means five or ten years but I asked him what he thought a long time was. He said, 'A year.' I don't want to think of that. Sometimes I just forget about cancer and do other things. I have come to the conclusion that, for me, that is fairly healthy. I suppose it's a sort of denial. Not denial that it is there, because I don't think you can have chemo every week and think it's not there. But if I sat and thought about it all the time, I would get morbid and I don't want to do that.

When people talk of accepting a diagnosis of cancer, there is no simple rule, no prescribed behaviour, no right or wrong way. Perhaps, as Lynne suggested:

The most important place to start when you've had a cancer diagnosis is that you're actually alive. You have to keep affirming it all the way along. If you have cancer, it's not about wrapping things up and preparing to die. It's actually about understanding you're going to live for a period of time. It might be a few weeks, it might be a year or two, or it might be twenty years, but it doesn't matter how long it is. It's important that we are able to talk about how people survive with these diseases. I'm not prepared to accept the diagnosis that cancer equals death.

2
MAINTAINING INDIVIDUALITY

WITH HIGHSIGHT, THE WOMEN ALL AGREED THAT A REFUSAL TO ACCEPT 'the diagnosis that cancer equals death' would have been a good place to pick themselves up after their initial diagnosis. However, many of them discovered that it took some time before they could get to that point. Most had to go through a complicated process of discovering that their experience of cancer was different from everyone else's before they could learn how to make the best decisions for themselves. Many found that they had to learn how to deal with the good intentions of other people who had little understanding of their situation. Recognition of stereotypes of cancer made it easier for the women to maintain, or regain, control after their world had been turned upside down. That feeling of control was crucial to their sense of individuality and to knowing that they were doing the best they could under the most distressing of circumstances. Noelle summed up this situation.

> *Whatever way you feel is the right way because we are all individuals and we all come from different backgrounds and lifestyles. There is no right or wrong way.*

DISCOVERING THAT ALL CANCERS ARE DIFFERENT
The difficulty many women experienced getting information about their particular form of cancer and treatments left them feeling very

much on their own. Many were left to discover that all cancers are different by themselves. As a consequence, it could take some time to realise that no two cases are the same. The kind of cancer, the speed of diagnosis, the fact that even the same kinds of cancer and their treatments affect individuals differently, and the differences between technically curable and incurable cancers were all factors which highlight the individuality of the cancer experience.

Unfortunately, the need to acquire this knowledge came immediately after diagnosis or in the initial stages of treatment, when most women were in a state of shock and fear. For some, this presented no problem at all. For example, Anne K coped with her diagnosis of leukaemia by 'pounding away' at her specialists for the information she needed. In the process, she realised very quickly that

> ... *obviously cancers are all different. Some people suffer a lot more than others, depending on the type of cancer that they have. I think that most people are aware there are very different types and treatments.*

In contrast, Margaret W hadn't actively sought information about stomach cancer, and although she was well read, she didn't 'know much about cancer medically'. She was, however, struck by the ease with which she could get access to information about breast cancer.

> *There seems to be a lot of discussion on breast cancer, in the newspapers and in the information letters that I had from the Cancer Foundation. But it isn't only breast cancer that affects women. There's a lot of other cancers too, so I don't really understand why most of the help and discussion seems to be going to women with breast cancer.*

Marinomoana, who found she couldn't always understand the terminology used by her specialists, read anything she could find 'that had the big "C" on it, anything that had stories of people who had cancer' in her attempt to understand the cancer process. As she did she

> ... started realising a lot of their experiences weren't mine. A lot of the information that I was finding was irrelevant to me but it helped me realise that there were different cancers and how they affected people.

Lynne also read everything she could lay her hands on in her quest to understand cervical cancer, but she found that

> ... being in oncology wards was an impressive experience in terms of realising that everyone is different. Sometimes nobody is observably the same as you are. I mean there's a sense in which there's a camaraderie which is about beating the disease, or learning to live with the disease, or just coping, but there's a sense in which nobody is the same.

Rae understood that there were different kinds and degrees of cancer because she had known several people who had died of cancer, including her father. When she was diagnosed with melanoma, she found it helpful to talk with a friend who'd had a melanoma removed.

> He was in stage three, so because his melanoma was a little more advanced than mine, he had to have more cut away. But he was progressing so well that I found it was interesting to be able to talk on the same wavelength and share our fears and positive thoughts.

For Kaye it wasn't until after her first operation that she realised that there were many different kinds of cancer and that a similar diagnosis could have different outcomes.

> Sitting in the clinic waiting room I saw people with different cancers but there was one woman who had cancer similar to mine. Overhearing her conversation with the doctor I heard that the surgeon had to remove her jaw, and lymph glands right down her side and under her arm, besides the ones in her neck. When I saw the doctor he mentioned our case similarity and pointed out the differences in the surgeries. I thought then that as bad as mine was, that lady's was worse.

While understanding that all cancers are different was important, it had particular significance for women who were diagnosed with an incurable cancer. It was immensely difficult to comprehend the implications that there was no known cure for your cancer. Annie recalled how when she was first diagnosed she

> ... was told there is nothing they could do about it, 'We can give you palliative care but we can't actually treat the cancer itself.' That had never occurred to me. I had always thought that cancer was something that if you got it early, then you were right. If you left it late or it was tricky cancer, like pancreatic cancer, then it wasn't too good but at least you had a bit of a chance.
>
> It was finding out that there are only five cancers that are totally incurable that left me really objecting to being dumped in the whole pool of cancer. For two thirds of the lymphomas there is now a good chance of cure but there's a couple of leukaemias, a couple of lymphomas and a couple of other cancers that, from the outset, the doctors say, 'There is nothing we can do to actually get rid of it.' One third of the lymphomas are totally incurable and I have got one of them. Once I knew that, I looked at other cancers with a bit of envy because they at least had a chance of cure.

Most people try to find a cause for their cancer in the attempt to understand how they came to have it in the first place. Annie knew that some cancers are caused by lifestyle.

On the other hand, there are many cancers that aren't caused by lifestyle and nobody knows how they are caused. Low-grade lymphoma is one of those and therefore lifestyle changes will have no effect on my cancer at all.

For Margaret P, understanding of the nature of her incurable cancer came with trying to make sense of the survival odds of people diagnosed with low-grade lymphoma. In the process she read anything she could find about treatment.

When I read the survival odds it seemed that things are improving all the time. Nowadays, with most cancers they say that if you survive the first five years, you're counted as cured, and although that doesn't apply for your low-grade lymphoma, it is really important to realise how fast things are changing. Improvements in drugs, in particular. One book that I read said that you don't necessarily need a cure. What you need to keep going is an improvement in the medication. Improvement may be in its efficacy, whether a drug works or not, or how well it can be tolerated. I have read that twenty-five per cent of people with low grade lymphoma die from treatment-related effects. If you've had one drug treatment after another, you get too tired and your heart gives up, so it is really important to know how drugs are tolerated.

At least there are refinements coming out all the time and some of them are more effective. The other thing to remember is that what works for one person won't work for another and vice versa, and the response rate will vary in each case.

Improvements and changes in treatments have proved to be particularly significant to Margaret P because she believes that her life has been saved at least three times in the last three years by new combinations of chemotherapy treatment.

CONSIDERING CHOICES, MAKING DECISIONS
Margaret P maintains that for any woman confronting cancer, the ability to consider choices and make decisions is largely contingent upon

> ... *information, knowledge, and a lot of it, because knowledge is power. That's your control, that's your choices. Knowledge is everything.*

However, obtaining the knowledge relevant to decision making takes time and effort. Finding a doctor who will give information freely and listen to your choices is the first step in acquiring information and control. Beth tells the story of a friend who, when she first arrived in Perth, made appointments with a range of doctors and then arrived to interview them.

> *She actually got them to fill in an application—a form of what they believed and what they thought about working with and caring for people with cancer—before she chose her doctor. One doctor said, 'I've never been interviewed by a patient before, but why not?' Indeed, why shouldn't we interview our doctor?*

But in reality, the women in the group found that after a diagnosis of cancer events moved too swiftly to allow much time and thought before they got caught in a vortex of activity, of which they were the centre. Suddenly nearly all areas of their lives became possible targets for some form of intervention. Life was rapidly inundated with professional people who had a huge say in what happened to them. It was a confusing time, and difficult to maintain a sense of autonomy. In most cases, their lives were literally in the hands of the medical profession, so it was easy to get lost in decision-making about things which affected every aspect of their existence. Disbelief and uncertainty about the accuracy of an initial diagnosis and the recommended treatment only made this worse.

A diagnosis of cancer hit as a crisis, so it was quite normal to feel that there was neither the time nor the presence of mind to step back and calculate the next move. These women found that the ways in which they created or re-created a sense of command in the situation depended on many factors, some beyond their control. For many, the knowledge that they were entitled to a second opinion provided time to consider choices and make decisions and enhanced their sense of independence.

Ann T was aware of the importance of a second opinion after having to go to Perth for an accurate diagnosis of breast cancer. When she returned to the north-west after her operation she found that

> ... me having a breast cancer which wasn't diagnosed till I went to Perth scared every woman in town. A rush of people rang me up: 'I've got a lump, Ann. What am I going to do?' I told them what I did. 'Go to Perth. Don't stay around here. Whatever you do, get a second opinion.' I've always stuck to that and I think that it's very important.

Even though it is every person's right to seek a second opinion, it can be a difficult decision to make and act upon, especially if you believe the problem of poor communication with your specialist lies with you. Margaret P struggled through three-and-a-half years of discontent with her first specialist and felt 'cowered into submission' by his manner. She believes that the first thing she learnt after getting cancer was that she was no longer in control of her own body, and that she did not have the knowledge or experience to choose her treatment, its regularity, its timing or its strength. She considers that most women are in the same position and that they 'can develop learned helplessness—just like a prisoner getting tortured'. She is certain that the stress this sense of helplessness caused made it much harder to cope with the disease process.

My first specialist did the positive bit that much that he didn't make the situation plain. He was oily-creepish with this professional smooth manner which was real artificial. He could insult you with a smile on his face but there were words coming from behind him. He gave me really negative vibes right from the beginning but I thought I must be in shock and not responding very well. My husband told me it was me.

I couldn't talk to my oncologist so I tried writing to him. I had a heap of questions—I can't remember them all now but I wanted to know how I could help myself, I wanted to know the survival odds, and I wanted to know if lymphoma ran in families because my mother was diagnosed with the same thing a month after me. At the same time, one of my daughters had two lumps come up on her jaw. Maybe three weeks after, I got a letter back. He would not give me any statistics on survival rates but there was an enormous paragraph where he crapped on about the tale of the four statisticians who drowned in an average of six inches of water! Then he says the way to help myself was to lose weight. He told me flat in the letter that I was in more danger from my weight than I was from my illness.

I wrote to him another time because I was putting more weight on with the steroids. I was totally out of condition, couldn't walk any more, and I was getting worried about things: could he refer me to the physiotherapist and the dietitian at the hospital? I was divorced by this time so I told him that I was living on an invalid pension and had no income to go anywhere private. He writes back and tells me that the physiotherapist at the hospital was only for therapeutic purposes! What would you call somebody who'd been on chemotherapy a long while and had got more and more out of condition? He told me to join a gym, and to go to some private place for physiotherapy. I'd already said to him I was living on a few bob a week pension! It was all stupid and it got worse.

The specialist battered me into the ground psychologically for three-and-a-half years, to the point that I didn't know I had a choice and that public patients could change hospitals and doctors. When I found out, I was frightened to move and it was a few weeks before I got around to doing anything. After I did change hospitals, I got angry at the previous treatment.

In comparison, Marinomoana, who was under a team of specialists, had no problems deciding to find another haematologist. She was 'very comfortable' with her oncologist and 'adored' her neurosurgeon, so her relationship with the haematologist stood out in stark contrast.

I couldn't stand his manner. He was condescending, an absolute arsehole and I reckon he was racist. His role was to keep an eye on my anaemia but all he seemed to do was prod me and poke me and make me hurt. I used to think that sometimes he wished he could put on gloves so he didn't have to touch me. I couldn't stand him and as far as I was concerned it was wasted money. That was one of the really bad choices I made. I was told he was the best and when you are paying for private you go to the best. Well, the best in what? Making you feel like shit? That's what I told him when I heard about someone else and changed. He was very upset but I thought, 'So what? My money. I'll ask for who I want.'

Annie also elected to change specialists very soon after diagnosis because she could not communicate with and did not trust her first oncologist.[1] Without trust, she lacked confidence in the treatment she was being offered, and without confidence in her treatment, she felt unable to make decisions about how she wanted to proceed. Even when she found an oncologist she trusted, making decisions about her own treatment took a while.

> *It came through knowing that this is my body: I know what it's doing and I'm able to communicate that to my oncologist. Being able to make decisions about my treatment also came through empowering myself with knowledge, being aware of what's going on in research and what new treatments are being developed.*
>
> *Although I'm not an expert, I read whatever I can find on the latest treatments for low-grade lymphoma. For example, I read about some English research into the successful use of bone marrow transplant for a small number of people with low-grade lymphoma. I haven't any siblings, and I'm too old to go on the register to get bone marrow. That's fair enough. So I thought that if my bone marrow was clear then it made sense to have my own bone marrow taken and stored. When I first presented this argument to my oncologist I was told it doesn't work but I was able to say, 'According to some research in England it is working to some degree, and even if it is only twenty per cent successful, I've got a twenty per cent chance. It's no skin off my nose that my bone marrow is taken. Okay, it will be sore. There is a financial cost to the hospital to do it, but I'm prepared to do it privately if need be because it's giving me a twenty per cent chance.'*

Although, like Annie, some women found immersing themselves in knowledge about their form of cancer and current treatments was the most effective way of considering their choices, decision-making about specific medical treatments could be relatively easy once they

---

1. See chapter 1.

had faith in the professionals who were caring for them. Even so, for the women whose cancer required on-going treatment, the need for information and control was greater than those who had immediate surgery followed by an intense course of follow-up treatment. In these cases, decisions frequently seemed to be made for the women. This was quite satisfactory if, like Julie, they accepted the notion that their 'life was in the doctor's hands' and trusted that they would be given all the information they needed.

> *I don't think I was in any state to make any form of decision and I didn't know a lot about it anyway. The doctors must decide for you and I accepted that. I felt comfortable with both my gynaecologist and oncologist. They seemed to give the information out fairly well and they would always say, 'Are there any questions?'*

However, without information, it could be very difficult to ask relevant questions. For some women, this did not matter. Rae found that a diagnosis of bowel cancer and the surgery which followed were

> *... over and done with so quickly that most of the decisions and choices were actually taken out of my hands. The doctors stepped in and said this is what we are going to do. To my way of thinking, the quicker the better. Except for one relieving doctor not telling us the results for four days[2] there was nothing I would have wanted more control over.*

Similarly, Tiny found that in her case

> *... there weren't any choices about treatment. I had to take the chemotherapy because otherwise I don't know what happens. However my family did make a choice to bring me home while I was on treatment, and the doctor agreed with us because in hospital I couldn't keep the food down. It would come up with*

---
2. See chapter 3.

all the tablets and everything so I was on the drip and intravenous fluids for one week. I was getting sicker and sicker, and the doctor agreed that I'd be better at home. That was a good decision for me.

Although Marinomoana believed that she 'wasn't given any opportunity to make choices about treatment', and that she was told 'this is how it will be', she found ways to make decisions about how her treatment proceeded.

The only control I felt I had was over my medication, what I actually put in my body, and that was only through default. Most people in oncology get all their medication from the hospital and then go home but I couldn't be bothered sitting there and waiting because they really make you wait. I asked them to give me the list of drugs and told them I would get my own. They didn't like doing that but it meant I was out of the hospital and could ask my family chemist what these various drugs were.[3] I guess that was a decision in itself.

Despite her medical team's insistence that they could not make a clear diagnosis, nor understand the growth of her tumours, without exploratory brain surgery, Marinomoana has refused to 'allow them to go in and have a look'.

I realise they probably need to see what is actually going on because they can't always tell by the CT scans but it's my choice to leave it. I'm very vain and they said they'd have to shave my head. Sometimes I have my hair so short they may as well shave it, but I don't mind them not knowing because it keeps them guessing. In 1988 they had a big neurosurgeon over from a famous American medical centre. He wanted to meet me. My first reaction was, 'Get lost! I'm not your guinea pig!' but I was so curious I had to go down. He was a nice

---

3. See chapter 1.

man but after looking at all my files even he couldn't put a name to my cancer. So they've given me a general sarcoma label and that annoys me. Why don't they know? They say, 'We would know if we could have a look.' I say, 'You can have a big look and poke around when I'm dead, but leave my face nice! Promise?' I had to sign a book and agree to an autopsy. I don't mind that, but while I'm alive, no thank you. I'll let them know when I'm sick. It all comes down to choice.

As the years go by, Marinomoana has become more confident in her own ability to 'read her body' and in her dealings with the medical system. She has begun to make crucial choices about her treatment and the amount of intervention.

Now I only go back once a year for check-ups and a CT scan every twenty-four months. That's because I put my foot down. I told them, 'Each time something has gone wrong, I'm the one who has informed you in the first place. Let's go with that.' I hate CT scans but if I feel that something is awry I book myself back in for one. The thing is, I'm a lot nicer patient now. I've been told that by a lot of the staff and they're right because I'm only going in because I am sick and I want their help to get better. It is definitely empowering for me because I am making the decisions and they are listening. That's another big change that I've noticed. More doctors in oncology are listening and it's about time; we're the ones who realise that there's something wrong—or at least I do. I know what I'm like. I am a clumsy person. I tend to walk into things but that's because I'm usually talking and looking the other way! I know the difference between my normal clumsiness and something else. Over the last nine years, I've been the one that's twigged to something not being right.

It does not necessarily take years to 'read' your own needs and translate them for your medical team. Beth recalled the speed and ease with which she made decisions about her preferred treatment after diagnosis, but she also recalled the shock she felt the first time she encountered the possibility that someone might not accept the treatments on offer.

> *The surgeon gave me the different alternatives. It wasn't so much asking me which I wanted. Rather it was telling me all the different things they could do. I wanted surgery. I wanted that cancer cut out. As for chemo, at first he said that he didn't know whether it was worth doing. I said: 'I want it. There's part of me that wants to be doing something.' He said that it was the conclusion he'd come to, so we agreed and there was no big decision to make. I think he would have abided by what I wanted if I'd made a different decision. I remember we were at the hospital for my first chemo treatment. Another young lady, who looked quite healthy, was having chemo in the same room and she said how she hated Tuesdays. My husband said, 'Yes, but you wouldn't not come would you?' She said: 'If I have to have any more after this lot, I won't come.' I thought: Wow! I'd never even considered that. Someone asked me one time, at what point would I consider saying no more treatment. I can't think of that. If I was on my death bed there might be a point at which I say so much, and no more. But I can't envisage when that would be, so not having treatment isn't something that I've considered.*

The need to make decisions about treatment could occur at unexpected times and, as Mara found, it was important and productive that she let her specialist know how she felt about her preferred options.

> *At the same time as they removed the right breast they did a biopsy on my left breast. The third day after that the doctor*

came to visit me with the results of my left breast. He said, 'In your left breast there are some dormant cells. We call that carcinoma in situ. *I would advise you to go home think about it and then in few months time you come back and we'll remove your other breast. There is no hurry. You can wait six months and it won't make any difference.' Oh God! I knew very well how hard the waiting period was for me the first time. It was the most difficult period waiting for the operation. I thought of going home with Christmas coming up and going back again for the second breast operation after New Year. I knew how calm I felt because I was in hospital and the waiting was over. Before the operation my doctor said I could have a problem with lifting my arm, combing my hair, buttoning my bra and washing myself because he might have to remove lymph nodes from my armpit. But after the first operation I felt good. I could move my arms and I had a shower the next day, as soon as I got off that drip. So I said, 'Listen, doctor. For my mental state it will make such a difference. If you think that I can survive, go through two anaesthetics, two operations in a short span of time, I would rather wait in hospital for you to do the second operation straight away.' He said, 'You seem positive enough in every way. Just try to walk around as much as you can for this week and next week I will do it.' That's what happened. I stayed in hospital another week and had my other breast removed.*

Noelle was also confronted with a range of choices despite the fact that the treatment of melanoma is currently restricted to surgical intervention because it does not respond well to chemotherapy or radiotherapy. Surgery was, in fact, better suited to Noelle's views on diet and lifestyle and she chose to supplement her treatment with dietary advice from a naturopath.[4] Despite the limited choices regarding medical treatment, she made a decision to change her oncologist and asserted her right to be consulted about the progress of surgical

---

4. See chapter 6.

intervention. This decision-making process was made easier because she developed a 'good relationship' with her surgeon.

> *My surgeon didn't want to operate on these last six lumps I had and wanted me back to the oncologist for a review. He kept saying, 'We've got to try something else,' despite the fact that I didn't want chemotherapy even if it was offered. In the end we compromised: he operated and when he took out the sutures[5] I told him I wasn't impressed with the oncologist he had sent me to. After two visits to this oncologist I felt like I'd been fobbed off. I know he's a busy man, but he was very off-handed and didn't seem interested in me as a patient, perhaps because he couldn't treat me. When I finally told my surgeon he said, 'Fine. Go and see someone else.'*

Noelle also had to decide whether to participate in research into the effectiveness of the drug Interferon in the treatment on melanoma.

> *The oncologist said that if I'd like to participate he could get me on the list as a guinea pig but he added that it was still too early to know what the response of melanomas were to Interferon, and that the side-effects of the drug was quite horrendous. It meant I would have to go to Sydney and find accommodation. Plus there was no guarantee that I would receive the drug. I may receive the placebo. The oncologist didn't appear to be positive about the results and I thought that as he's the expert in this field, he should know if he's on the ball. Beyond that, the whole idea of taking myself off to Sydney for an undetermined period of time on my own was unappealing. Financially I really couldn't afford to and I'm not interested in experimenting with different things. If it was tried and true, then I'd take it on, but I don't intend to subject my body to harmful substances that are going to cause*

---

5. Stitches.

it to be weakened. If I can keep my body as healthy as I possibly can, I can try to fight the cancer with my own immune system. From what I have read and heard about chemotherapy and radiation treatment, the cancer only responds up to a certain point and after that you don't get a response. Then they have to increase the amounts and it is doing more and more damage to the healthy part of your body as well. I can't see why I should. My body is already under attack! It doesn't need to be attacked any further.

While decisions about medical specialists and the treatment they recommend were among the most important these women were confronted with, other issues arose which could make a difference to the quality of care. Margaret W had no problems accepting her doctor's recommendations regarding two operations to inhibit the growth of her stomach cancer. She did, however, assert her right to choose where she would be treated because this impinged upon her son's ability to visit her, and hence her peace of mind.

My specialist wanted to send me to one of the big teaching hospitals because they had more facilities for intensive care. But those great big hospitals are a bit impersonal and I didn't want to go so far from home. My son was very upset and I knew it was handier for him, so I said, 'If I can't have it done at the district hospital, I'm not going to have it done at all.' They let me have the operation in the local hospital and my son could just pop in.

There were many little ways in which the women took control and made choices about their physical and emotional needs, even if those decisions were frowned upon by the medical establishment. Marinomoana started smoking to help her cope with anxiety when she found out that she had to have treatment for her brain tumour.

A lot of the time I would feel numb, nothing but oh dear, oh dear, oh dear. *Then I found that if I sat there and 'oh deared' with a cigarette, I didn't 'oh dear' so much! I remember a nurse coming up and telling me that smoking was going to kill me. I couldn't believe it. I looked at the silly cow and said: 'This is going to kill me? In how many years?' She says, 'You've got to look at the long-term effects in twenty years.' I said, 'I'll take the risk and the twenty years!' Gosh! Some people are so stupid. They ought to mind their own business.*

Unfortunately, many people did not mind their own business and learning to manage the interventions of well-meaning friends or acquaintances was an important part of maintaining individuality and autonomy. Anne K ensured that people would not interfere by not telling many that she had leukaemia. She told people only when she had no choice because her treatment entailed a prolonged stay in hospital. Thus, she only

. . . came across do-gooders at the end of the day, after I came home from having the bone marrow transplant. It was very traumatic because I realised that on top of this my marriage was breaking down. One well-meaning friend told me my problem was that I was too serious and I needed to lighten up. That was akin to telling someone who is having a nervous breakdown to pull yourself together! At this stage, I got plenty of good advice from people who gave me the good advice, said all the wrong things, then walked out the door and kept going. Everybody was very vocal, and there it ended. There was nothing after that.

Annie, on the other hand, had no objection to people knowing she had been diagnosed with an incurable cancer but was stunned by the

> ... amazing number of people who had never had cancer, who had never had much to do with cancer, who would come up to me and say, 'Now, you must think positively.' I used to go stark raving mad. What bloody right has anyone else got to tell me to feel or think positively? They are not facing what I'm facing. Bugger them! It took a few times and then I cottoned on to the most effective retort, 'I will think or feel positive when I want to. There are times when I don't want to! When I don't want to, I won't and I will think and feel negatively. It's none of your business!' I suppose that they were shell-shocked because they thought they were doing the nice thing but you can't think positively a hundred per cent of the time.
>
> I find it very annoying, and offensive, when people try to impose their ideas of cancer on me without allowing me to say how I deal with it. I went through a brief couple of weeks when I looked into some of the New Age ideas on healing, but crystals and auras just don't fit with me. I haven't changed my diet and I've no intention on living off carrot juice because I hate it. It really pisses me off when people try to impose their ideas at a period when you are confused, and trying to deal with organising your life without letting cancer dominate everything.

Lynne was also put off by people who were insensitive to her situation.

> There was one person who decided that this illness would be my chance to demonstrate that I could heal myself. She and I had become friends when I'd been a massage therapist and naturopath, so she figured that this was my chance to prove I could do it right for myself. It was a really very mixed message. For some other friends there was the sense that they wanted to remind me that I had brought the cancer on myself so I was the only person who should and could cure myself. I think that

this is the influence of all this alternative self-help stuff. It's stuff that is seldom properly thought through but people are frightened and they react in extreme ways.

Beth 'didn't have that much of a problem with people's good intentions', but found there was a tendency to 'blame the victim'.

A couple of people gave me recipes for diets and treatments with the implication that if I want to get better I'll do this and if I don't I'll die and then it's my fault. And I've had a reasonable number of people tell me it's all in the mind, or that this helped Mary so it'll help you. The worst incident was the day I was going into hospital for my operation. Someone who I hadn't seen for ages phoned to say he was going to visit. He arrived with this fellow that I'd never met before. This man sits there telling me about his aunt and other people he knew who had cancer and he had advised them all against having surgery. They had radiotherapy and this and that, and they were all surviving. I'm sitting here, bags packed, itching to get to hospital because all I could think of was getting this cancer cut out. I knew that it was so big that I wasn't interested in any other means. I really got upset. My friend arrived to pick me up and she said, 'We've got to go.' This man said, 'Are you telling us to go?' I said, 'Yes, I guess I am.' He said, 'Well it's up to you, but if you want to live . . .' It was as though he was saying: 'if you don't listen to what I tell you, you will die.' That was upsetting.

The belief that a person is somehow responsible for getting cancer often goes hand in hand with the idea that if they do the right things they can 'beat it'. Annie found that a surprising number of people accept the 'notion that cancer can be beaten' and she became heartily sick of being 'bludgeoned with this idea'.

I think that is one of the stupidest slogans out because it's so simplistic. It doesn't allow for a discussion of what it actually means so people who don't really understand cancer think that you can use your mind to physically beat it. I don't believe that. Perhaps you can beat cancer spiritually and you can beat it intellectually and emotionally, but some cancers you can't beat physically. Nobody can. You can use the time during which you have cancer creatively by not focusing everything on the cancer and by being productive: that to me is beating cancer. Cancer is just a part of your life. You can't make cancer a career. You learn to live with it. You go off to work or you do anything that you normally do to the best of your physical capabilities.

In much the same way as these women had to learn to parry the good intentions of people who understood little of their experience of cancer, many also had to devise strategies for the stereotypes which accompanied the notion that 'cancer can be beaten'.

MYTHS AND STEREOTYPES

For most people, the word cancer conjures up images of pain and death, even though it covers a wide range of symptoms. A dictionary gives an answer to the question: why are there so many myths about cancer? Synonyms include words like tumour, swelling, outgrowth and excrescence, while the definitions themselves include: 1) any malignant growth caused by abnormal and uncontrolled division of body cells; 2) the disease resulting from this; and 3) an evil influence or corruption that spreads dangerously and uncontrollably. It is the superimposed images of contagion and decay, of being consumed from within, which people have to confront as soon as they are told they have cancer. Many of these ideas about cancer are inherited. For example, Annie found that she had to contend with her own background in nursing.

When I was nursing, I can't remember dealing with chemotherapy. It just wasn't around much. If someone with cancer came in, you went to the shroud cupboard, made sure you had enough shrouds and that you had the rellies' telephone number. It's a completely different, changed attitude now. There's not the assumption that because you've got cancer that's the end of it.

The task of dispelling the myths which surround cancer are made harder because it is not just one's own understanding of cancer that has to be reconsidered: other people's fears intrude into the process. Kaye recalled the pessimism she confronted, both in herself and in some people around her.

You find out that you're not going to drop dead exactly on that day, but it's still an iffy thing because you don't know when it's going to come back. It's like a hammer over your head. You don't know where it's going to strike next, or when. And, of course, you get everybody coming out of the woodwork with stories about someone that they knew who had something like that. I'd say to them, 'How are they now?' 'Oh. They died.' It gave me a horrible feeling. Very rarely did I actually hear of anybody that had survived these cancers. You needed someone to come up and say, 'Don't worry about that. I know someone and twenty years down the track she's still alive.' Then you might feel that there was a chance. It was so negative but I don't know whether these people even realised what they were saying. Instead of giving you encouragement or trying to keep your spirits up, they were actually dragging you down the whole time. You never seemed to hear about the people out there who had survived so when I got the second recurrence I didn't talk about it to many people: if they weren't real close family or friends, there was no need for them to know.

MAINTAINING INDIVIDUALITY 99

Anne K had been in Australia only a short time and was just beginning to make a few close friends when she was diagnosed with leukaemia. She also found that one of the major problems was other people's responses.

I only told close friends and once they found out they started avoiding me because they couldn't cope with the fact that I might be ill when they were around. I found that I had to take the responsibility for their being unable to cope. It meant I had to work very hard to be normal at times and periods when I was feeling very sick. With leukaemia you get a lot of bone pain and muscle wastage and I had to pretend I was OK. That made life a bit uncomfortable.

Annie also remembers how some of her friends 'ran a mile' when they heard she had lymphoma. Fortunately she had enough friends 'who didn't accept that nonsense and just carried on' but some people couldn't resist the ' "Oh dear, she's dying" stuff'. Similarly, Ann T discovered that 'some people found it very hard to talk to me or to look me in the eye: a lot of them had me dead and buried'. Marinomoana also recalled the difficulty of dealing with other people's sympathy.

I used to hate the sad eye looks when people found out. Cancer is such a horrible word, but it's become horrible because it's generalised to so many different kinds of cancers and they all get dumped into one idea of death. Cancer equals death. That also happens because of the names they give cancers. What does that mean? You can't even understand what you got. At first I didn't know what was going on and I didn't know anyone with cancer so I had no-one to talk to either. So one myth that I had to dispel in myself was that cancer is not a death sentence. Other people make it one though, usually people who don't have it: you have cancer therefore you are

> *going to die, end of conversation. A lot of older people, like my mother-in-law's friends, wouldn't come to the house if I was there. I don't know why and that was sad.*

On top of dealing with other people's reactions, there are specific beliefs about cancer to be contended with, particularly those which claim that psychological factors play an important role in the origins of cancer. Annie found 'some of the worst myths about cancer in books written by "alternatives"'.

> *I find them repulsive. They assume that the mind has total control over cancer! It's an assumption then that somehow you yourself have caused this cancer, therefore you yourself can fix it. My cancer was caused by a genetic fault and I don't see how as a foetus my mind could cause a genetic mishap! That's ridiculous to me. Before I was diagnosed I was probably overworking and under a bit of stress so my immune system wasn't able to cope with lymphoma which had probably been there since the day I was born. Previously my immune system had been able to deal with it but it was at this stage that the defences were down and it just slipped in and took over. But I enjoy working hard, like I enjoy doing a whole heap of things, and I can't see it's my fault for doing that. So be it if we take twenty or thirty years off my life: I'm doing things now rather than sitting about being a lump.*

Beth had similar reactions to some of the 'alternative literature' she read.

> *I can't stand people saying that if you are putting on weight, you can't have cancer, or people saying it's all in your mind. I read a number of books which made me very cross. They give advice like eat beans and meditate twenty-seven hours a day or*

you'll die, and if you do it's your fault. One book was about the typical person who gets cancer. They were all people who had dreadful childhoods, who really wanted to die, who were depressed. The people I know who have got cancer don't seem to be like that.*

Lynne, on the other hand, found useful strategies in some of this literature because it helped her combat some of the myths about cancer, leaving her free to find a healthy way to deal with her own disease process.

I used lots of Louise Hayes tapes and, although I think it's far too simplistic in the sense that she talks about the emotional roots of cancer, visualising your body in a positive way and dispelling negative ideas, it worked for me. All that stuff that says you get cancer if you're negative or if you're confused or if you're an unhappy person or if something's happened to you that you haven't accepted, I think that's bullshit. I really don't accept that because it blames the person for getting sick and there's no way that you can ever be well if you have that kind of strategy going on in your life. But I did a lot of thinking around what I really thought about cancer. I discovered the usual stuff about cancer being a killer disease; about it being something that you don't have any control over; about it being silent and insidious and something which can pop up at any moment; and about it not necessarily having any connections to other diseases in your family. They are all quite scary things really. I worked a lot on the mythological aspects of cancer because if you don't work on getting through the misrepresentations, the mythologies of cancer, then you do end up killing yourself, intellectually as well as physically.

Myths about the causes of cancer are added to by other people's ideas of how a person diagnosed with cancer should behave. Kaye

> *... got the impression from someone in hospital that there are ways people expect you to act if you have cancer. This patient was acting very cheerful and the staff kept on saying, 'You do know that you've got cancer? You know that you could die from this?' She knew, but they could not understand why she was cheerful.*

There are also myths about how standard medical treatments, such as chemotherapy and radiotherapy, will affect people. Although weight loss, nausea and ulceration are common side-effects, the greatest mythology surrounding treatment seems to focus around hair loss. Like Julie, many other women found that the only thing they 'knew about chemotherapy was that you lose your hair'. The prospect of this understandably appals many people, so considerable energy can go into psyching oneself up for a new bald identity. Carmen had been warned about hair loss and, still halfway through chemotherapy, wondered why she hadn't lost it all.

> *I really resigned myself to the fact that I would lose all my hair because I was told that would happen. I had long, thick, beautiful, spiral permed hair. They tell you how to look after your hair, so because they said you can't braid your hair back, I went and chopped it off. Sometimes I don't care but I liked my long hair. I hate short hair, although I have lost half of it so I'm lucky that I've even got it. Maybe it's my vanity that's been hurt but I am still losing the hair. Even at this stage when I'm halfway through the treatment, I don't know whether I'm going to lose it all. It hasn't worried me that much because I went and bought hats. I refuse to wear a wig.*

As every individual responds differently to treatment, there is no way of predicting the occurrence or severity of any particular side-effects, and many people experience side-effects that they had not

MAINTAINING INDIVIDUALITY

prepared for. Marinomoana remembers friends asking her when her hair was going to drop out once she started chemotherapy, and she fully expected it to happen.

> *I'm thinking I'll have to wear a beanie because they tell you about that. I found out that was a myth—it doesn't happen to everyone. What did happen to me though is that my tongue swelled. It was like a big blob and I used to bite it continuously. I still have scarring from it. I would choke and I was quiet because I couldn't talk. It was very hard for me to chew so I had to have lots of fluids. I lost something like thirty kilos in six weeks. I had three chemo doses in a very concentrated period, every two weeks and in that time I dropped weight because I couldn't eat. I was still playing netball. My nails were great and my hair was growing beautifully, but it was back to front! They were concerned about that. It was strange and I had not met anyone else who had that kind of reaction and they don't know why that happened either.*

Ann T coped with her initial fear of chemotherapy by acquiring as much information about the treatment as she could find. For her, knowledge was an effective way of combating the myths about breast cancer and she was grateful that there was a growing media focus on breast cancer around the time she was diagnosed.

> *I often said I didn't lose my hair because I didn't have any fear. I had an aunt who had a mastectomy and was still alive. They were writing to me from home in Ireland saying you'll have up days and down days. The fact that my aunt had it and was still alive helped me. I read everything I could on it so it really didn't scare me. At the time that I had the mastectomy, Nancy Reagan had hers, June Bronhill had hers, Simon O'Donnell had his lump removed and it was all in the*

papers. There was so much feedback on it and I realised then that people do want to hear the positive side. They don't need the negative side.

But even though breast cancer is so media focused, I still come across people who have lumps and they won't go and see about it just in case. They're frightened. They know what it can be and a lot of women can't handle losing a breast. I remember one friend coming up to me and saying, 'Oh, Ann, you're so brave. I've had a lump for months but I'm afraid to get it checked out.' 'Oh Jesus,' I said, 'you're a bloody idiot. Go and see about it. What's wrong with you? If it is cancerous, you'll die if you don't have it checked out. What are you doing?' 'Oh, I'm too frightened.' They've still that attitude. I suppose they're frightened of the unknown—of what it could be.

Although there is no doubt that a diagnosis of cancer can change priorities, Anne K is adamant that there is a substantial mythology surrounding the way cancer can mean sudden, radical, 'quality of life enhancing decisions'.

One of the myths about cancer is that it changes your life and that you learn to value things. I was so damned tired a lot of the time trying to keep everything going that I didn't have time to take that into consideration. I just got up every morning and thought, 'Okay. This is today. I've got to get through today.' I didn't think of tomorrow, or the day after. It was a day at a time for me. That's all I could cope with. Friends of mine used to make a date for down the track and I found that I lost interest because I couldn't think like that any more. It made life with my partner very difficult because he was a forward planner in everything. I don't think it ever occurred to him how I was thinking because I could never discuss my problems with him, never. I was simply a closed book.

As a sociologist, Lynne has written and published academic articles on the representation of AIDS and the way in which oppositions are constructed between diseased people and the general public. She believes a similar process operates in the representation of cancer and that a lot more work needs to be done on it: wading through the mythology of cancer takes energy, and that energy can be used more effectively finding 'healthy ways' to come to grips with a diagnosis of cancer.

> *I've worked with people who have AIDS or HIV, so the notion of having cancer never struck me as something that would necessarily kill me at this point. I thought, and I still do, that the chances are that I might die of cancer, but then again the chances are I might get run over by a bus or killed in my car, especially given the way I drive! I didn't have that horror of cancer that my mother had, for instance, and that I'd seen her as not being able to dispel. I'm sure that it contributed to her emotionally giving up at different points of her having cancer. One particular day, before I'd had radiation, I saw a sticker from the Cancer Foundation on someone's car that said: 'Cancer is a word not a sentence.' It's a brilliant slogan and I subsequently used it as a title for my journal. When my mother found out she had cancer, she treated it like a sentence. But you can even turn around the idea of a life sentence: it's something you're going to live with not die from.*

Noelle came across a few people who had to 'step back' from her because of the belief that

> *... cancer means death and not a nice death. That makes other people look at their own mortality and people aren't comfortable with that. We are mortal and we are all going to die and we are all dying. I think that's probably what is hardest for people when someone is diagnosed with something*

like this, whether it is cancer or something else. It is not so much, 'Oh! My God! This person is going to die.' It's, 'Oh! My God! I'm going to die one day.' I think that is why some people step back. They can't handle it.

The stereotyping has mainly come from myself, which I'm quite horrified about actually. I don't feel like a cancer patient because I don't fit the so-called norm. I'm physically fit and I don't look sick. My experience with other people with cancer is that they look like they have cancer. My partner's aunt has lymphoma. She's been battling with it for about six years now and I've seen her wasting away, being in considerable pain, becoming more bitter. Cancer is virtually written all over her. She's just a scarecrow of a woman. That's very much my image.

There's a man in my meditation class whose prognosis is that he could go any time. All he said for many weeks was he had health problems but when I first met him my reaction was: 'You are having chemotherapy. You have cancer.' These are the images I've got because I don't know that I've met anybody else with cancer who hasn't looked like they have cancer. I definitely took that on board. I have carried around this image of what a person with cancer should look like.

In contrast, Mara's major confrontation with the stereotypes which are inflicted on people with cancer came from friends in the form of subtle changes in their approach to her.

Once my friends helped me clean the house and did all the corners and everything after my daughter left. They really gave me good support but they treated me like an imbecile. They wanted me to sit in a chair and watch them do my house and I couldn't. I wanted to work along with them. They treated me like a total invalid. And also they treated me childishly. They'd say, 'How are you, my dear?' They would never do that if I had flu or if I had an appendix operation. They put a special tone in their voice when they talk to me and I don't like it one bit.

From then on I go visiting them and they come here for tea but I never call them to clean my house. They start treating you like a dying person straight away. You are now in a special league and there is a little barrier there between them and me. It took a while to forget that I had the operation. They don't mention it and I don't talk about it. Every now and then I meet somebody who I didn't see for a long time and they ask you how you are now. Straight away the tone of the voice changes and they treat you like you are on the way out.

Kaye had a similar experience, and found 'the things that people say to you can be quite surprising'.

The first time I went out socially after getting out of hospital, I was feeling very tired but I put on a good show of hiding it and tried to be bright and cheerful. A man I was talking to said to me, quite out of the blue, 'You know, I think you are very brave.' I said, 'What do you mean I'm brave?' He replied, 'You are so cheerful. I don't think I could be that cheerful if I'd been through what you have.' I laughed and shrugged it off, but every now and then I would catch him watching me. It was as if he was waiting for me to break down, as though he thought it was more appropriate for me to be sad and gloomy than happy. If only he had known that inside myself I was a mess. I did break down quite a lot, but only when I was by myself or with my husband.

When people said I was brave or coping well I was surprised. All I was doing was hanging on to hope—hope that I would get past the first three years, then the first five years into remission. All I wanted was to hear the doctors say, 'It's looking good. We think we've got it all.' How I would have coped with the news that it was terminal I do not know. If anyone should be described as brave, it is people who have been told they are terminally ill. One person comes to mind. This was before my problems. A friend of my sister-in-law was diagnosed with cancer and given six months to live. She had a husband and two young children. She was devastated and at first she went to pieces. Then she realised she wasn't helping her children so she sat them down and told them she was dying. She organised everything she could and carried on. I asked my sister-in-law how she could be so calm. My sister-in-law said, 'What choice has she got?' I only came to understand that after I had been diagnosed.

Several other people found that the worst attitudes came from their work colleagues. This was particularly distressing because all of them had gone back to work to regain a sense of normality. Carmen realised that her work-mates were

> ... probably as ignorant about cancer as I was but they looked at me like I was going to die and kept saying, 'Oh! Poor Carmen!' You don't want people to be saying that.

Julie was disappointed that her work-mates didn't have more faith in her and recalls how she dealt with the uncomfortable situation she confronted.

> I'd lost so much weight and I could feel their vibes as soon as I turned my back. I could feel the nudge, nudge, wink, wink— 'My God! Isn't she thin!' Thin means you've got cancer. Thin means you're not going to get better. I could hear the whispers. 'Did she lose her hair?' 'Is that still her hair?' 'Is that a wig?' A lot of work-mates said things like: 'Julie! You're back! Are you going to die?' It hurt a bit, and I had to keep my sense of humour but I ended up speaking to the administration officer

and being very firm about what I wanted. He kept saying things like, 'But, because you're sick, Julie . . .' I got quite cross and I said, 'Let me put it to you this way. I am not sick. I have not got cancer. I am on treatment that is making me sick and you must understand and expect that I am going to be sick one week in every month. That is through having the treatment that I need. I don't want anyone to say that I'm sick because I'm not.'

I tried to make them understand. I think that did get through. I went back to work thinking I'd start on half days because after so long on chemotherapy my white blood cells were right down and naturally I was very tired. I didn't do half days. I did full days right from square one. It didn't matter that I'd come home at six o'clock and go straight to bed. I'd done my day's work and I'd proven something to myself and that was very important. But I think their attitude spurred me on. I felt good by actually achieving what I'd set out to do.

Ann T was nervous about how people would react to her when she returned to the north west after her mastectomy and first round of chemotherapy. She considered that

. . . the hardest thing was the very first morning after I'd returned home from Perth, going down to the shops. I was shaking in anticipation of what people were going to say or not say. Once that was over, I was fine. I don't think I had problems with stereotypes because I put it more or less behind me. It's as if I never had it. I used to joke with friends. Going out at night, sometimes we went to the pubs, and sometimes there were skimpy barmaids. I'd just say, 'Jesus! I'd look good like that now, wouldn't I?' I used to make light of it really but because I had switched off. It didn't stop me. I still went to the pool. I still walked. I didn't run that much, mind you, but I

never let it stop me doing anything. I think people were quite surprised that I got back into life.

However, she found that going back to work while still on chemotherapy was another story.

Because I had cancer some of them had me already dead and buried, including the manager where I worked. The girl who relieved for me while I was in Perth having surgery was there when I got back, and the next thing I know is that she starts to say, 'Do this. Do that.' I said, 'Excuse me! Who's in charge here?' She started to redden so I asked, 'What's going on? Do you think you've got this job now instead of me?' She said, 'Yes. The boss said it's my job.' I said, 'Like hell it is! If that's the way you want it I'm going to fight you for it. It's not right that you move in and take my job. I need it now more than anything, as therapy if nothing else. If you want it that way I'll tell everybody that you've taken my job.' It was bad enough trying to battle the chemo, let alone to find that, lo and behold, I didn't have a job. I knew what the town would do because we'd been there quite a long time. They just don't like that sort of thing. I wasn't nasty about it and I'm not vindictive but to do something like take my job because I was sick—that was just not on. Anyway, she said, 'No, Ann, it's your job. You can have it back.' I said, 'I didn't think I lost it in the first place!'

It is not just lay-people who develop stereotypes of people with cancer. Medical professionals can also make assumptions about the people they are treating. Margaret's first specialist focused on her weight.

He was always going on about my weight and it was clear he thought that if you are fat you are brainless. Everybody knows that, because if you've got any brains you wouldn't be fat in the first place! There are a lot of people who stereotype like that but it's worse with a doctor because they have such power over you.

Marinomoana confronted some blatant prejudices when she first entered the hospital system.

At the hospital there was a presumption that I couldn't understand the medical terminology because of my ethnicity, being a black woman. There was a presumption that I was not educated, and therefore unable to understand. Not only that, I had people say, 'Would you like me to read this to you?' 'I can read, I can read very well!' 'Oh yes, I'm sorry'. Gee whizz! Or they'd sit down and start explaining forms. 'Excuse me but I can read the information and if I don't know, I will ask you for your help.' 'Are you sure?' 'Yes.' Every time you go there are forms about the last chemo treatment and I had nurses hovering around to check that I knew how to fill them in. I can read. And I can tick. The assumption from a lot of nurses was that I was strange. They had all been told I was very sick and I wasn't behaving like a very sick person.

Stereotyping on the basis of ethnic background and appearance did not always happen. After Mara's initial, unsatisfactory consultation with a specialist who appeared to assume her ignorance because of her accent,[6] she found that her second specialist and the hospital staff did not treat her 'in any way different' because she came from a non-English speaking background. Like Anne K, Mara learnt quickly that maintaining eye contact, being as articulate as possible and being assertive were effective ways of avoiding being stereotyped by medical professionals.[7] However, as Marinomoana discovered, what some people see as assertiveness others may interpret as aggression or bossiness. She considered that

6. See chapter 1.
7. See chapter 3.

> ... they didn't know quite what to do with an assertive woman. One day when I was feeling well I picked up the chart at the end of my bed. At the top it read: 'Very aggressive nature'. When the nurse came in she told me that I wasn't supposed to read it. I just said, 'It's got my name on it! Aren't I aggressive!' I think their problem was that they couldn't control me. I used to hate the way male surgeons would pat me on the back and say, 'There, there'. I would say, 'Don't touch me. I don't like that. If I'm sick fix me but if I'm not, it's goodbye.' But they kept trying to convince me that I was not well. I figured I was well as long as I could walk! I was left for hours waiting for an oncology appointment once and after that I'd never go on time again. When they rang to say I'd missed the appointment I said, 'After the last time, I figure that if I get down there about six o'clock it would be about the right time.'

Annie, who believed she needed to be polite but assertive in order to get the information she needed, found that on her hospital file she had been described as

> ... 'pleasant but pushy'. I was very tempted to write: 'Some people see it as pushy. Others see it as assertive'. I wish I had, and initialled it, because I don't think anybody would have known that 'the patient' was actually making comments in her own file! I did take it up with the hospital because writing descriptive, subjective comments in clients' files creates stereotypes which work like a chain reaction in hospitals. One staff member makes a judgement of your personality which all other staff read and then it is up to the client to do something about a personal assessment of their character which they know nothing about if they haven't seen their file.

Annie found that, for her, the best way to deal with the implications of other people's stereotypes of cancer was to tackle them head-on.

I got pissed off with stereotypes very quickly and, whether it's the medical profession, or friends, or people I don't know, I've learnt to say, 'I'm the one with cancer. You're not. I'm not going to accept what you think I'm about.' It's an important part of maintaining my independence and individuality and there are some strategies I've developed to do that. I refuse to be called a patient. I'm not a patient, I'm a client because I'm receiving services which people are being paid to give. I'm not there as somebody who's suffering! I hate the words 'suffering' and 'patient' because I'm neither of those and I refuse to accept a victim status. This seems to shock a few people.

Familiarity with their rights as clients of the health system also helped some of the women tackle another stereotype, one which Annie believes is all-too-common in the health system: the assumption that patients are stupid. This is particularly difficult because, obviously, doctors and other health professionals do have specialised knowledge: that is why they are there. Annie found that

... it can be a major battle when you meet a new doctor not to be arrogant back but it is more important to make them see that you're an intelligent human being with a grasp on what's going on. There's no reason why you shouldn't have a grasp on what's going on. I go and read my file every six months or so under the Freedom of Information Act. I request my file and I'm put in a little room and I sit there and read everything. I also get photocopies of test reports that I haven't had before and check that doctors aren't making subjective comments about me. If you want to be in control and in charge it's useful to keep a check on what's happening with your file and

there is no resistance to using the legislation, although I wouldn't do it more often than every six months because it is a hassle to get through the bureaucratic routine. Getting access to my file is really for my own personal interest because I can get a lot more information if I see it all out there in black and white. Although they'll tell you at the time what tests they are doing and why, it has helped me to understand better, and if I understand then it is not so easy to treat me as ignorant.

> **STRATEGIES FOR GETTING ACCESS TO YOUR FILE**
>
> *Write a letter to the Freedom of Information Officer in the Medical Records Department of your hospital requesting that you see your file for personal reasons. It will be much quicker if you provide your hospital unit number—or patient number—and your date of birth, or anything that can make you recognisable. Your letter will go through the system and in about a month you should get a telephone call or a letter saying that's fine and asking you to make an appointment to read your file. The time you need will depend on how big your file is. Annie allows a whole morning because her file builds up rather quickly. At some hospitals, photocopying is a free service and you are entitled to make a copy of your file for personal reasons.*

MAINTAINING INDEPENDENCE

Many of the stereotypes of cancer grow out of a heightened awareness of vulnerability, and thus, for many of these women, learning how to reassert their independence became of paramount inportance. This could require considerable readjustment because, while their bodies were under attack by cancer, the invasiveness of surgical, chemical or radiotherapy treatments frequently left them feeling sluggish and

MAINTAINING INDIVIDUALITY

uncertain. This combination could make it a real struggle to retain a clear notion of their own worth and value because their normality had been shattered.

Noelle avoided the problem by simply refusing to classify herself as ill. She found it was easy to retain her independence because, until secondaries took hold, she was not physically ill.

I have not had a day's illness for the last four years. I'm able to do my job, continue on with my life and be as physically active as I want to. I just try to retain my general good health.

Anne K developed a similar mind-set and emphasised the importance of not allowing cancer to dominate her personal identity.

It is really important not to lose sight of who you are. Don't let your cancer get bigger than you, ever. Maybe in your quiet moments let it all go but always keep your sense of self and find out what you can do to improve the God-awful situation you find yourself in. Get as much information as you can and don't ever let anybody not give it to you. Don't let them treat you like a sick person but ask for help when you need it. I didn't. Ask people to lighten the load a little and if they can't cope, then let them go. Somebody else will help.

While few would dispute the importance of keeping a 'sense of self', Margaret P found that it was difficult after experiencing long periods in hospital.

I was in hospital so much at one stage that it got very hard to maintain my individuality. Six hospitals stays in nine weeks is not funny. No matter how much you hate hospital and how glad you are to be home, if you are in hospital that much, you get used to it and you get at least some measure of being institutionalised. I was getting to the point where I expected to

> be in hospital, I had my bag packed with all the little things I
> needed and I was getting used to it. That made it harder to
> cope when I was at home because being in hospital is rather
> like being in a cocoon—it is safe.

Annie found that the best way to maintain her independence while in hospital was to emphasise her status as client rather than patient.

> One of the practical things I do to reinforce this is to never
> wear nighties during the day in hospital. I go in with a whole
> stack of tracksuits, soft trousers, shorts and tops and make it a
> rule that in the morning I get up, have a shower, change into
> street clothes, and then, if I'm feeling OK, I go outside for a
> meander around, and have a cigarette in the fresh air outside!
> At night I get into my nightie and go to bed, like I do at
> home. I generally treat the hospital like a hotel. Maintaining
> that normality is very important. My hospital stays are not
> going to decrease. In fact they are going to increase so it is
> important to be seen to be an individual who knows your
> rights.

Despite the difficulties, retaining a sense of being useful within the capabilities of new physical and emotional limits was vital to many of the women. For those who had been in the paid work force, continuing or returning to work was one way of maintaining their independence. Julie made getting back to work as soon as possible a priority.

> I thought a normal hysterectomy would be off work for about
> six weeks, so I aimed for a little longer. I was back at work in
> eight weeks. I told the people at work that I was going to be
> sick one week in every month because of the chemotherapy and
> I tried to explain to them that I wasn't sick, it was the

treatment that was making me sick. I'd get cranky because people would want to wrap me in cotton wool—'Julie's back and we have to create a job. There's really no job for her.' I said, 'I want to stand at the counter and serve the public.' It's a demanding public where I work and I wanted to prove something to myself. I didn't care whether I got the right level of pay for that particular job but that's what I wanted to do.

Work helped me deal with cancer because keeping busy stops me focusing on what I've got or what I've had. You can't afford to sit around and dwell on things and at work I deal with low income families: they've got a hell of a lot worse problems than I'll ever have and it gets my mind off myself because I have, and want to, focus in on their lives.

Despite the fact that 'lots of people assumed' she would stop work, Lynne insisted on working throughout radiotherapy.

I thought, if I don't work I'm going to go crazy because all I'll have to think about is this fucking cancer. Some people thought I was crazy but in the end I took a reduced teaching load, about half my usual students. I barely went into work, partly because I didn't have any energy. Instead, I read and marked at home. I tried to stick to my daily routine but really I slept most of the time. I offered some lectures from time to time although I don't know why. I did manage to get through them without anyone making any comments, despite there were a few moments when I'd get halfway through a lecture and think, 'What the fuck am I talking about?' The radiation left me weak and vague but it was the lack of a concentration span that got to me. Now, eighteen months later, my ability to concentrate is only just coming back. It was very frightening but maintaining a sense of who I was as an individual and sticking to my usual schedule gave me some backbone to get through it. I think it also helped my kids feel as though basically things were OK; I was sick, but I was coping.

Carmen also felt the need to go back to work while still undergoing radiotherapy after a lumpectomy. She found, however, that this confronted her with a confusing situation as she was given 'all the sympathy at work and the opposite at home'.

I went back to work because I wanted to feel like I was worth something and could produce something. Instead, I have found I'm having to create my own work to keep busy because they are not giving me work. I suppose I'm lucky that I'm not too busy because then I would be under pressure, but the basic line is that if they gave me work I'd forget that there is something wrong with me. They keep saying, 'Relax. You shouldn't be here. You should be at home.' I keep saying, 'I've had eight weeks off and I'm ready to work.' The worst part is when they try and chase me home. I hate that and I get so upset because I want to do the work. One man even said to me, 'How can your husband send you to work? Your life is more important.' I couldn't explain to him that I've got a loan and I want to work so that I can pay my loan off. The fact is that I've got a job and I want to do it.

At home it goes to the other extreme but at least they make me feel normal because they expect me to do the washing, the ironing, the cleaning and the cooking. Every now and then I can't cope and I need their help. If my husband gets upset when something is not done I say, 'Well! You do it!' I let loose and sparks fly but I've been able to handle them and I can cope at home.

Like Lynne, Annie is a university lecturer who found that continuing her work was central to maintaining her independence, both financially and intellectually. As a woman living alone she emphasised the importance of organisation and the role of her family and friends in helping her get through the various bouts of radiation and chemotherapy treatment.

> *I've been lucky at work because they've left it up to me to decide whether I feel capable of working full-time or part-time, and I've got the flexibility to do it. From the very beginning I decided that if this is going to be a long-term cancer, I've got to be nice to people or else they're going to drift away! I've got several rules. One is to be nice to people as long as I'm not in too much pain. Most of my friends have learnt about boundaries and understand that I am in pain and that there are times when I'm not nice to them. My second rule is that as long as I can do something, I do it, and when I can't then I call in somebody to help. I live alone so I do everything myself—except I can't do the cleaning any more so I've got a cleaning lady, and I can't do much gardening.*

As a retired, elderly woman who lived with her son, Margaret W had to contend with a range of issues which are particularly relevant to people isolated by age or infirmity. But she preferred to remain in her own home, where she could be with her son and do things for herself.

> *In hospital they told me they wanted me to go into residential care for a while but I didn't want to do that so they said they would get the Silver Chain to come three times a day. But they didn't. The Silver Chain[8] nurse came four times, once a day to see that I got a shower, as though a shower was the most important thing in life! When I first came out of hospital, I would rather have had somebody help with preparing my food and helping me eat. The house cleaning didn't matter because my son does his own flat and I have somebody come once a month.*
>
> *I have occasional visits from a support person at the*

---

8. A home nursing and care service.

Cancer Foundation and I can phone her any time I like. She says this cancer seems to have affected me more physically than mentally. A group called Do Care have been really good and they don't talk religion all the time. I'll get a newsletter every so often and they have a telephone group so instead of having people come to see you, you're contacted by telephone and you can ring them any time. That's good although I'd prefer a visitor.

My son would do everything for me if I asked him but I'd rather he only does things for me that I can't do, like all my errands or my clothes and dish washing if they get too much for me. He's there for me and he'll come if I yell for him. I find showering and dressing a terrible effort. I've got a chair in the shower and a chair next to it to place a towel and my clothes on. I manage but I wouldn't have a shower if my son wasn't in the house because I'm afraid of falling.

Eating is a bit of a problem. I can't stand for more than a couple of minutes at a time to prepare food so I keep it little and simple. I can make myself cups of tea and prepare a light meal. I like Chinese frozen vegetables and I buy thin pork or veal slices. I put the whole lot together in one baking dish. That's my tea. My son would do it all for me any time, but I think it's much better if you can keep doing things for yourself and be a bit independent. Otherwise, I could sit here, be miserable and groan and moan all the time. I do moan and groan a bit sometimes!

So does Margaret P. She has come to the conclusion that acknowledging the swings of mood that can accompany cancer and its treatment has given her the freedom to be herself while confronting the complex reality of cancer. She also learnt to transform other people's notions of 'positive thinking' about cancer into a way of asserting her right to deal with her cancer the best way she knew how.

People who pretend there is nothing wrong and who walk away from things all the time don't do as well as those who seek information. I think you need to be as curious and as positive as you can. By positive, I don't mean running around being frenetically cheerful all the time. You cry, you kick, you scream! I've had the bloody lot. Be depressed, so what? If people tell you to be positive while you are bawling your eyes out, just say, 'I'll feel better tomorrow, but I might feel worse the day after that!' By 'positive' I mean that you need to stick up for yourself. You have to be what you are. Having cancer does not turn you into an angel. You have the same negative personality traits that you had before. Why act? Why waste your time and energy? Be yourself.

3
Strategies for Getting Through the System

WHILE IN THEORY IT IS ALWAYS A GRAND IDEA TO 'BE YOURSELF', THIS is a problem once the medical system moves into gear. Maintaining your individuality can be difficult, particularly in the large teaching hospitals where many people with cancer eventually find themselves. Unfamiliarity with hospital administration and protocol can lead to a sense of being swamped, of being alienated and alone.

The potential for depersonalisation in the medical system is enhanced because it is a highly specialised world constructed around rigid hierarchies. There are also intricate networks between different branches of the health services, each responsible for different 'bits of the body' and these take time to get to know. In such a complex system, there is a whole range of situations or encounters which can trigger alienation. The women in this group developed strategies to help them deal with and manoeuvre around the system when it threatened to become overwhelmingly impersonal, or when it felt like there was a danger of their needs getting lost in the medical bureaucracy. Most found that, whether they were public or private patients/clients, the best way to deal with the system was to learn how it worked.

PUBLIC AND PRIVATE HEALTH CARE SYSTEMS

Many people have no choice whether they will seek medical treatment as a public or private patient. As Noelle put it, 'I have to go in as a public patient because there is no way I could afford private health cover.' For other people the issue is not so much one of the expense of private health cover as confidence in the public health system. Lynne comments:

> *Private health insurance is about the last thing that I would ever buy because I have this working class origin's blind faith in the public hospital system.*

All the women in this group who have sought treatment through the public system express confidence in it. Like Noelle, Margaret P has only dealt with the public system and she considers that she has 'nothing to complain about' because 'when you've got cancer, you've got priority. They don't stuff around.' Beth also expressed her confidence in the public system.

> *I know that they know me and if something goes wrong I can ring up the clinic or go down to the hospital and say I'm an oncology patient. I've got a big sign up on the fridge with all the phone numbers—who to ring any time, who to page. And the people in the public clinics are the best needle givers because they do it eight hours a day, five days a week.*

Although committed to the public system, Lynne found herself contemplating the possible differences between the private and public health systems when her diagnosis of cervical cancer led to 'a panicked flutter' amongst women in her workplace.

> *Some of the other women went and had smear tests and one of them found that she had abnormal cells. She had private health care insurance and went to a gynaecologist who gave her very good advice that dispelled her fears about the whole disease. But a couple of times it was said to me in the hospital that I was lucky that I was on Medicare and got rushed*

straight into the hospital because, a number of times, women had gone through gynaecologists who had not been able to give them the kind of instant support they needed at this stage of their cancer so the whole thing had been sufficiently delayed for it to become much more extreme.

The public system also has some drawbacks. Tiny felt that in the public system she sometimes had too many people 'batting' for her. While she was grateful for the care she received there were aspects of the staffing policy in the large public hospital where she was treated that she found increasingly frustrating.

Every six months you get a different registrar. They know nothing about you so there's not much point in telling how you've been, because they don't know your history anyway. Also, all our files get stuck on top of one another and the doctor that's finished with their patients takes the top one. It doesn't matter whether you've seen them before. You can specially ask for the one doctor but you might have to wait another hour. That's probably one of the downfalls of the public system. One doctor did a bone marrow biopsy but the nurses never knew I'd had it done because he didn't write it in the notes.

While Tiny was able to accommodate and adapt to the staffing policies of the big public hospital, other women wanted to retain more control over who they were treated by. For Ann T, who now works for a health insurance company, 'being able to pick and choose' her doctor is really important.

Some people won't go and have a second opinion because they think Medicare won't pay for it.[1] A second opinion might only be sixty dollars. What's sixty dollars out of your pocket? People think too much of what the bureaucracy has to do for them

---

1. As long as you have a referral from your GP Medicare will pay for a second opinion.

> *instead of taking things on themselves. If you feel you need something done and Medicare won't do it, go and do it for yourself!!*

In principle, the idea of paying whatever is necessary to ensure the most appropriate treatment is fine but many diagnostic tests and treatments are extremely costly, as Beth and her husband discovered. They had been insured with a private health company but Beth was advised to 'go public' when she was diagnosed, so both she and her husband dropped private cover. She has no regrets about the move or the quality of care she received in the public system. However, soon after her diagnosis, her husband developed health problems which could not be treated immediately as a public patient. On reflection she considers that

> *... we should have thought more seriously about how we did it: I should have gone public and my husband should have stayed with private cover so that he could get immediate treatment. Instead we are both public because we thought we couldn't afford the costs of private hospital benefits. Before I became a public patient, I had an afternoon of tests and they cost $600. Then, just after we went public, my husband had one little test that cost us $583. He was treated as a private patient in a public hospital because if he hadn't done that he would have waited three months for an appointment as an outpatient in a public hospital. In that time he might have been dead because he was really bad. He got charged everything because as a private patient without private health insurance he can't get all of it back under Medicare. All in all, finances have been difficult.*

Several women with acute cancers had been paying private health insurance for years and were content with both the level of care they received as private patients and the financial arrangements. Mara, for example, had been 'on the highest table of private health insurance since arriving in Australia thirty-five years ago' and was satisfied with the way it covered her costs. Rae had also been in a private health insurance scheme for 'a long while'. She was booked straight in for her operation, but is sure that if she had been in the public system she would have gone in straight away too because 'they get you in quick smart'. She went to a small private hospital.

> *They were absolutely marvellous: I couldn't have had better care if I'd given them a million dollars. There may have been more information available in the public system because they have greater resources. In a private hospital they don't have a cancer ward whereas the public hospitals do, so you don't get to meet other people with similar problems. It would be good if the private hospitals could put you in touch with people like that. One of the sisters gave me the address of the Cancer Foundation.*

Kaye had also always been in a private health scheme but because her surgeon was a consultant in one of the big teaching hospitals she found herself in the public system.

> *He had a clinic and operated out of there, so that's where I went. I think the health scheme helped with the cost but I'm going fourteen years back and it's all different now. I know it cost much less to see my surgeon at the clinic than at his private surgery. We still had a bit to pay but not as much as if I'd been seeing him privately because of all the anaesthesia and pathology tests. The financial burden wasn't that bad. We managed paying the balance. It may have been worse if I wasn't in a private health scheme but I'm not too sure. I wonder whether I would have got into the hospital so fast. I was pretty bad and he wanted to operate on me straight away. If I hadn't had private cover, I'm not sure how it would have*

worked. If I'd wanted a private room all the way through, I could have done, but I was in a private room just for the first days after the operation because I had to be looked after. As soon as I was on my feet they put me into the four-bed ward, which didn't matter to me because I like having people to talk to. I hated being in a ward by myself.

As a private patient, Julie found she also hated being in a single ward,[2] but other than that she

... didn't really see much difference between the two systems and, because I was fully covered expense-wise, there was no problem. We basically got all medical expenses back except for the ondansetron[3] tablets and a few pharmaceutical bills. I didn't find the gap between what Medicare paid back and what the doctors charged too horrendous and I think that being in private health care helped.

Anne K had been treated as a private patient for the first four years after her diagnosis. It was only when the time came to 'set her bone marrow transplant in motion' that she was transferred over to the public hospital system which had all the necessary resources. It was the public system which

... did all the following up of my siblings in my country of origin, getting their blood tests done to find a compatible donor. The people there were always very positive, probably because I was positive myself. I didn't really have any negative experiences. I had lots of delays when the waiting was dreadful—interminable some days, particularly in clinics, but you have to be realistic there because it's a question of economics. Public hospitals are run on public money and it's a very tight purse and there's only a certain number of staff and

---

2. See this chapter 'Being in the ward', p. 166.
3. Expensive anti-nausea drug used for some chemotherapy regimens.

there are so many patients. But I found that when you're really ill, they do try to put you first, make you as comfortable as possible, get you seen to, and get you out. There are glitches in it like everything else but, in all fairness, I think the public system does their best with what they are given.

Anne K also found that the public health sector had a very humane approach to a change in her financial circumstances. She had expected to pay for all costs associated with her brother's hospitalisation procedures as donor, however this never transpired.

I think because I was very unwell, and because my marriage broke down and I became a single person with two children, that the hospital decided to waive that fee. I never had to pay for it. I did bring it up twice with the haematologist and he said, 'Don't worry about it. You've got enough on your plate.' So I owe the government, and every tax payer, big time, I really do. This is why I feel I've been so lucky.

While Anne K had no choice about entering the public system for her bone marrow transplant, Marinomoana decided to change from the private to the public health care sector. She had come to the conclusion that the 'private system slugs you a lot' and that it 'was a big rip-off'.

When you are having the number of CT scans that I had in such a short period of time, even though the private scheme paid for most of it, if you've got to lay out thirty dollars each time, that's money out of our pocket. Plus medication. That was the big difference and that is why I went off private. I didn't believe that they were giving me what they had promised. After two years I became a public patient and I didn't find any noticeable differences between the two systems, except money and being stuck in a private room on my own. I didn't like that anyway because it left me too much time to think about myself. For me it was better being on a public ward. In terms of the care, there wasn't any difference except that as a private patient I was able to choose my own doctors—but I made some bad choices. A lot of doctors need to realise that they are providing a service not doing you a favour. It doesn't work like that, even in the public system. As far as I'm concerned I still pay for that because I pay big taxes. It may be public health but I am not getting this for free. Public or private—either way we pay for it.

Annie also chose to move from the private to the public system after initial treatment because she was not happy with the care she was receiving as a private client. It was not until a few years into her treatment that she realised how the cost of cancer accumulates: while she could cover her costs as a private patient comfortably enough at the start, over the years her medical expenses have escalated while her salary has decreased. In addition, she found that the private system wasn't as well 'geared up to chronic illnesses as the public health system' and considers that she has had better treatment since she 'went public'.

I've waited the same length of time in private and public clinics: both clinics have reasonable magazines but we get free coffee in the public clinic. And I don't have to pay GAP in the public system. Having had to go down to a part-time wage, I could never afford to go on any private system anyway. So I'm all for the public system. I think that it's brilliant and I really trust every aspect of the public system because I know I've got access to resources.

As a consequence, I have come to trust the place implicitly. I know that if any bit of me breaks up and falls to bits (which it has) then I'm immediately put into contact with a relevant consultant or treatment processes. What is more, it's all under the same roof. There's a whole range of departments I'm linked into: the ENT department, rheumatology, oncology and pathology. I've never had time constraints on any of my consultations in any of these departments although I am very conscious that there's rows of patients waiting and it's up to me to be efficient and not to waste unnecessary time. But I've never felt as though that's been imposed on me. I didn't feel that in the private system and my first oncologist was definitely clock watching. In the public system everything and everybody I need is there, available. I don't have the same trust in the private system because I don't think I'd have access to the sort of things I've got now.

DEALING WITH STAFF IN THE SYSTEM

Hospitals and clinics take on a new significance for people diagnosed with cancer. They offer hope of cure or remission, and yet the radical nature of many cancer treatments means that most people approach them with an understandable ambivalence: few want to be in hospital although none of the women in this group would reject the services they have to offer.

No matter how caring staff in a hospital are, there are times when the very structure of these institutions conspires against the patients' need for respect and individuality. In many ways hospitals appear to be worlds of their own. They function twenty-four hours a day, and seem to service all their own requirements without reference to the world outside. To their clients, this self-containment can at times feel like imprisonment, a safety net or a cocoon, or make them feel like an insignificant cog in a hustling, busy, important wheel. Unfortunately, highly bureaucratic and legally necessary admission procedures frequently set the scene for a 'cog in the wheel' experience. Kaye recalled feeling quite irritated by the admission procedures in one of the large teaching hospitals.

I had hardly ever been in hospital up until then but with having the biopsy and going back and having the stitch out, then going back and having the neck done I got sick of the administration always asking the same questions when it was all in the same file, in the same hospital, under the same doctor. They'd say: 'Have you been in hospital before?' I'd say: 'Of course! I was here a few weeks ago.' 'What was it for?' I'd think, 'Just look in the file.' They could improve the admission procedure for people who are in and out, even if they gave you your own file and said, 'Would you like to look through that and tell us if there is anything different?'

Even in the small district hospital where Noelle went to have her lumps removed, the paperwork and form filling sometimes seemed excessive, although she found ways to minimise her exasperation.

I go to the general surgical ward if I need a general anaesthetic or to the day surgery unit if the lumps are close to the surface and only require a local anaesthetic. For this type of surgery the paperwork takes longer than the actual surgery! The receptionist and I joke about this. We've decided we should have special forms printed up just with my name, or I could bring a rubber stamp so my surgeon can rubber stamp the forms. I have built up a lovely friendship with the ward clerk and so she is usually always prepared for me when I get there. I pick up the forms from the doctor and race them down to the hospital the day before so they pull the files that night. It is really nice because you go in and see a familiar face but it is maddening because you have to go through the whole rigmarole. I keep saying to the ward clerk, 'Nothing has changed since I saw you last apart from the fact that I have x more lumps.'

The form filling escalates with the number of specialists called in.

Particularly with some long-term or chronic cancers, years of treatment can bring a range of possible side-effects, each requiring a specialist. Occasionally it can feel as though your body is being split into separate components, as Margaret P discovered.

> *I did not have high blood pressure or diabetes before I got the lymphoma, but bit by bit, long term on all the treatment, these things started cropping up. So I asked the registrar if he could refer me to a physiotherapist and a dietitian and asked if they had a diabetes clinic at the hospital. This bloke spent ten minutes telling me what they couldn't do for me: I would have to go to my GP for blood pressure tablets, and somewhere else for this and somewhere else for that. They wanted to fracture all the different parts of me. That doesn't happen at the hospital I'm attending now. If you've got to be referred to anybody else, they will refer you to somebody at the hospital. Everything is intermeshed and that is really important for someone like me who is on drugs long term because you get a build-up effect and somebody needs a total overview.*

Getting to know how a hospital functions, where to go for particular services or what to do in an emergency is important for peace of mind, especially when you are first diagnosed and totally new to the workings of the hospital. Sometimes staff are so used to the system that they appear unsympathetic to simple enquiries about procedure. For example, Annie recalled how her concern about what to do in an emergency was brushed aside by one doctor.

> *The first oncologist I had seen simply told me there would be no emergency and then added, 'I don't give out my home phone number.' I said, 'I wasn't asking you for your home phone number. I was asking you what do I do in an emergency.' Now I know I could have gone to casualty at that hospital whenever I needed to but at the time I saw the*

oncologist as being a separate, private doctor and not linked to the hospital. For me it was important to have the security of knowing what to do in an emergency, even though there might not be one.

Lack of familiarity with the services available, combined with uncertainty about the changes taking place in your body because of cancer, can also lead to anxiety about how or when to contact the doctor, hospital or clinic. This uncertainty can be compounded by fear of being a nuisance or hypochondriac. Annie's current oncologist gave her a tip to help her make decisions about when to get to hospital or contact the clinic.

If you're feeling really bad, ring straight up. If you're feeling a bit funny, leave it for twenty-four hours, then if you're still feeling funny, ring up. Usually these things go but that's a good tip because sometimes it's really difficult to know when to ring the doctor. Now I generally leave things a week: usually they've passed in a week, and if they haven't then it is something to check up. But you have no idea until you get used to knowing what your body's doing at a particular time and whether there's a pattern to it. At first, everything new that happens could be a crisis, so you panic. Just to know that if you're really bad you go straight in, but if you're not wait twenty-four hours to see if it's still the same before you ring up. If it's not then you can wait until the next appointment.

In this way, she learnt to minimise her visits to the hospital—a strategy which allows her to get on with her life as 'normally' as possible. However, even similar kinds of cancers affect people very differently. Like Annie, Margaret P has a low-grade lymphoma but she is always in and out of hospital 'either having chemo, or in with an infection or getting the Infusa Port[4] done, or just for a check-up'. She has found that building friendly and cooperative relationships with staff at all levels has been a constructive strategy for ensuring she felt more than just another cog in the wheel.

The best way to deal with all staff is to treat them all like friends, whether they are or not. I'm manipulative. I have my ways of getting the things that I found I needed. I'm always amusing, I'm always nice, charming and friendly and I've never had to wait for anything.

In a similar vein, Margaret W believed in showing her appreciation to all staff. Her gratitude for the care she received was still evident months after her operations and, not surprisingly, she found that she had 'no problem dealing with staff' at her district hospital. They were all 'most helpful', as were

... the people at the Cancer Foundation, the Do Care people and the staff from Extended Care service at the hospital. The nurses were fantastic, and even the X-ray ladies sent me a beautiful bouquet of flowers and a card after my second operation. When I got home I phoned the Director of Nursing and told her how much I appreciated all that had been done. It is important to let them know.

Mara had a similarly positive experience with staff in the private hospital where she had two mastectomies in as many weeks.

I had my sixtieth birthday while I was in hospital waiting for my second operation. I didn't tell anyone but of course the hospital had my record and they took care to notice that. The kitchen knew that I was not allowed any sweets because I have

---

4. A small reservoir inserted under the skin, connected to a line ending up in a major vein, usually in the chest. It is used to administer fluids and drugs. Occasionally it is connected to an artery so treatment can be administered to an organ.

diabetes, so because they couldn't make me a cake they made an arrangement of cut fruit, like flowers in a vase. That was something to see—really magnificent. All the staff, the doctors, the cook and the nurses, all came in and sang me 'Happy Birthday'. I was embarrassed and then so thrilled because a sixtieth birthday is something really special and that time I needed cheering up. It was the best moment, one that I will remember all my life.

The cook was very good. He came every day and asked me what I would like. In hospital when you lie down your legs seem so thin and then I lost both my breasts after that second operation. The doctor come to visit me on the Tuesday after the second operation. I said, 'Thin legs and no breasts! My God, Doctor, I look like a fifteen-year-old boy!' The doctor said, 'You're cheerful enough! Don't worry, there are a lot of women who would give anything to have legs like yours.' One nurse was especially good. She used to watch my room, especially when I had visitors. If you have a lot of visitors, sometimes they really tire you, so this nurse told me, 'When you feel tired of your visitors you just say "I think I'll go to sleep now" and they will slowly walk out. If you enjoy your visitors, OK, but if you don't know how to send them off just ring for us. You don't have to say anything—you just press the button and we'll come in and say visiting hours are over.' If she saw me happy with visitors she would never barge in. If she saw me sitting and brooding or lying in bed staring at the ceiling, she would come in and talk to me. She would tell me about meditation, about positive thinking, she even gave me a book.

This sense of personalised care can be harder to achieve in the larger public hospitals where the bureaucracies are more obvious, and the pressures on staff evident. Even so, there are many small ways in which nurses in public hospitals extend their personal concern about their patients. Margaret P was hospitalised immediately she was diagnosed and was booked to have her first CT scan on the afternoon of her forty-second birthday.

> *You have to have a minimum of four hours with nothing but clear fluid and then you get this revolting mixture to drink. That was my birthday. Then, about ten o'clock in the morning, all of a sudden I hear whispers outside. Through the door came eight nurses pushing a trolley with an early lunch and a big ice-cream cake on it, complete with candles, singing 'Happy Birthday'. Course, I sat and bawled! A nurse had paid for that cake.*

Margaret P considers it 'rare that you get a nurse that's bad-tempered' and that the staff never ignore her because she is 'not the invisible type'. However, getting the attention of nurses can be a problem, even when the ward does not appear to be particularly busy. Marinomoana recalled an incident when nursing staff ignored her requests for assistance. Desperate and exasperated, she made sure that she did not get neglected again.

> *Usually I would get up and go to the toilet myself but this time I couldn't and I had been ringing that darn bell and asking repeatedly, 'Can I have a bed pan, please? I desperately need a bed pan.' There was a group of nurses standing where I could see and hear them chatting and none of them took any notice of me. So I wet the bed. Oh it felt good—ahh. It was just like—all right then—even to this day when I see them they mutter. It was so good! They had to get me out of bed, sit me on the commode, change me, wash me, fix the bed up, clean the bed down, and wash it because with the chemo and stuff you stink! It's a horrible smell and they had to clean it all up! I felt really good and after that when I rang the bell for a bed pan, or anything, they were there. They learned but it seems sad that you have to go to that extreme! But it served them right.*

Marinomoana considers that many of her more abrasive encounters with staff were largely a consequence of cultural differences.

Our cultural approach to being sick is different: if you are sick you talk about it. People seemed to find this embarrassing. There's none of this 'hold the pain in and grin and bear it'. Maoris aren't like that—well, this one isn't! We talk about what's wrong and where it hurts. If I was in pain, I'm in pain. I don't like pain, so I want something to dull it. I'd just keep on and they hated that . . . 'This woman never shuts up' etc. I got a name as a whinge but I got things done. If someone is sick I can't understand why they let you suffer. I saw lots of patients who suffered in silence, and most of them were women. Men don't tend to suffer in silence. I was told by one old dear, 'You know if you keep complaining, you'll give us women a bad name.' I said, 'Do you notice that we get ignored? Well, you do. I don't!' I thought, 'How can you be like that? They are here for us, to help us.' I saw a lot of women who lay there and suffered.

Ethnic and cultural background, class and occupational status can make a difference to the way some hospital staff approach their clients. Lynne recalls how

. . . there was a point at which they discovered I was a lecturer in sociology at a university and their attitudes changed. I felt bad about that because I knew that I was going to get better treatment than the woman across the ward from me. She was a Vietnamese woman in her late fifties with ten children and she didn't speak English, and she really didn't seem to understand what was happening to her. She was having a hysterectomy because she had cancer. She was totally dependent on an interpreter who could only spend half an hour with her and she was subjected to nurses and doctors who came in and

yelled at her in the most patronising, appallingly racist ways. They treated her like a moron but the reality was that she simply couldn't speak English.

In contrast, they treated me brilliantly the moment they found out that I was a professional, partly because I asked them detailed questions. I didn't always ask them questions that I really wanted to know the answers to. It was just that I wanted to keep them talking to me. The second time I was in hospital I took in a laptop computer and I sat there and I wrote about what was going on around me.

There are all sorts of subtle ways in which institutional norms of behaviour can operate to regulate behaviour in hospital, and many of these 'bring you down' in tiny but incremental steps unless they are combated. Marinomoana became aware of this possibility when she first went into hospital.

One older nurse said to me, 'You leave your dignity at the door and pick it up on the way out.' I said, 'No I don't. Where I go, my dignity is right beside me, inside me, behind me and in front.' I was really sick one time. I felt like shit and I just wanted to be clean. I really wanted a shower but the nurses wanted to wash me in bed. I was a bit shaky but I could still move about so I said, 'No' and got up off the bed and went for a shower. I felt so good! When you can't do jobs like that for yourself then it is good that the nurses can do them for you, but when you want to do it yourself, they ought to let you. Taking those little privileges away disempowers you. Like when you go to the toilet, they would say, 'Leave the door open.' No way! They can knock on it! You don't leave your dignity behind just because you are in hospital!

Kaye has no recollection of having to surrender her dignity in hospital, and recalls that the nursing staff were both technically efficient and generally helpful. However, a diagnosis of throat and neck cancer, together with radical surgery, left her feeling very vulnerable.

> *I'd been talking to a few of the nurses about the Tronado machine,[5] because I was interested in anything I thought might have helped me. One sister said, 'No, don't even contemplate that.' I asked why and she said, 'Half the time after you've had it, you are worse than before.' I think that if your position gets to the stage where you are willing to try anything you should be allowed to. I was hopeful about my future because the doctors had told me that they were pretty sure they had got all the cancerous cells and I told this to another sister one day. She said, 'You just don't know about these type of things, or which way they'll go. If I were you I'd go home and get my life in order just in case.' I thought, 'Thanks very much!' She was more or less telling me to go home and prepare to die. I went from being quite optimistic to practically digging a grave for myself. I was very upset and couldn't stand staying in the ward. I knew my husband was coming to see me so I went down to meet him. He was angry when I told him what happened. After that, every time that sister walked in the ward I walked out. I just couldn't stand being around her. She was so negative. You look to the nursing staff to keep your spirits up. You don't want them to lie to you, but a little bit of optimism goes a long way because you're needing to feel optimistic yourself.*

Despite the odd negative interaction with nursing staff, Kaye generally found that because nurses were in the front line of care provision, they were often more aware of changes in her condition than the doctors.

---

5. A form of microwave therapy first used in Perth in the 1980s.

Some of the doctors were all right, others I could have done without. Most of them only popped in and out of the wards. I often wondered if the nursing staff knew more than some of the doctors! For example, after the operation on my neck, I started to feel hot and sick and I didn't feel like eating. One lovely nurse checked my neck and commented that the wound was still looking very red. She said it seemed as though there was still a stitch inside. She called the doctor who said it was all right and that what I was feeling was part and parcel of getting over the operation. I could see the nurse was pulling a face, as if she didn't agree. The next day I was worse and I felt wet on my neck. When I put my hand up I could feel that the wound had opened. The sister said, 'I knew it!' The doctor had to remove an infected stitch and pack my wound. I was put on antibiotics because of the infection, but I never heard the doctor tell the sister that she was right. Even though she was sure of what was wrong she had to wait until the doctor gave the OK to treat it.

Sometimes, nurses are left in the difficult position of having to withhold important information from clients because it is the doctor's legal responsibility to fulfil this function. As Rae discovered, this can lead to intense periods of unnecessary anxiety if a doctor 'forgets' to visit.

I had the bowel operation on the Thursday and my surgeon went on a week's holiday after that. He thought probably late Friday night the results could come through and that his relieving doctor would come in and see how I was going first thing Monday morning. That was really important because at that stage I didn't know if it was malignant, whether they'd got it all, or whether it had started to spread. We waited the Friday night and the results hadn't arrived. We knew we wouldn't hear anything on the weekend. He didn't turn up on the Monday although the sisters kept ringing up. We waited right through till eight o'clock that night when the nurse came in and said he wasn't coming in. My husband was furious. The next morning the sisters got onto this doctor straight away and he said he would be in after lunch. My husband had been there for a while, and he was so tired. I told him to go and make himself a cup of tea and have a bit of lunch somewhere. He had only been gone ten minutes and the doctor walked in, before lunch. He said, 'You haven't been worried, have you? You are not waiting for any results, are you?' I looked at the sister, because she had known I was so upset, and I just said, 'You've got to be joking!' I was so uptight that I hardly answered him. Then he told me they'd got it all, it hadn't travelled and I was fine.

Afterward the sister told me that they had those results on Monday morning. They knew it was OK but they could not tell me. They knew all day Monday how we were feeling. I was upset because I didn't like that relieving doctor's attitude. My husband wanted to go and have words with him, but what's the point? If we had known straight away we would not have had that four days of getting uptight. It's the waiting for the results that is the worst because, whether it's good or bad, you've got to know the news.

In other circumstances, the problem is not one of the doctor forgetting to visit, but one of being inundated by visits from junior medicos. Being in a teaching hospital means that visits from trainee doctors and nurses become part of the daily routine. Kaye

... had a lot of young doctors and nurses coming in and saying, 'Could we have a look at your tongue? We haven't seen anything like that before.' They were very polite and always asked first. You could say no if you wanted to. I didn't mind as long as they didn't catch me at meal times. It was

usually the same kind of questions and they've got to learn somehow.

Public hospitals, in particular, are extremely hierarchical, and it can take some time before it is clear who fits in where, and even longer before familiarity with the system enables patients to become assertive about their needs. Medical students are the most junior in the pecking order, and usually the youngest. Next come the residents, then the registrars. If these young professionals have gone straight from school, then through six years of medical studies at university, many of them are barely twenty-five years old when they qualify. This can be quite disconcerting for more mature and worldly-wise clients. Right through the hierarchy of doctors, from medical students at the bottom to consultants at the apex, a great deal depends upon their personal communication skills and attitudes toward client involvement, as Annie discovered.

The only problems I've had with any staff in the hospital have been with residents, or interns, and a couple of consultants, who have come out of medical school with a degree of arrogance which has been nurtured. On the whole I have found registrars to be good and most of the consultants are good but I've developed strategies to deal with those that aren't and I don't stand nonsense. I don't have time to simper to a person because they're working in a job and getting paid for it. I can't understand why I should bow and scrape. In the long term, it's not in your interest to do that and I just keep remembering that. I also remind myself that these people have been trained on public money and they are earning money which is coming out of the public purse which I've worked and paid my taxes for. People are entitled to the best standard of treatment they can get, and you should make sure that you get it. That takes a bit of energy but if you can work up these stategies and get confident about using them, then even when you are feeling a bit down you automatically use them.

Margaret P summarises the range of doctors she has come in contact with, and the problems she faced in dealing with a specialist she felt intimidated by.

I've found most of the medical staff are pretty good. Some of the registrars are great because they're not only good with people but they know more. Some of them are dickheads—they look like young kids straight out of school but they don't really give you any trouble. My bad experiences come from the fact that I hated the specialist I had for the first three-and-a-half years. My first specialist was patronising, paternalistic, arrogant and just plain outright rotten. He gave me three-and-a-half years of misery. I fought with this doctor of mine, in my head. All the time, I was having conversations with him, reliving the rotten things he'd said to me, and thinking what I should have said to him and didn't. For me it's impossible to sort out a doctor who is examining you and dealing with such an important subject. I couldn't tell a guy off, or a woman, who's in charge of my life. I've got to trust them. I found it impossible to sling my weight around, or even to stick up for myself. You don't feel up to it in the first place, but you're not in any situation to do so because you don't want to upset them. The only thing I could do was walk away when I found out that even in the public health system you can change hospitals and therefore specialists. The bloke in charge of me now is a little darling and most of his registrars have been good.

It does not always take direct condescension or rudeness from a specialist to induce a sense of impotence, as Beth was perplexed to discover.

The way I respond to one of the doctors fascinates me because I act like I am powerless. I'm halfway through talking and he starts writing. He doesn't look at me and I feel like saying, 'Excuse me. I'm here. Listen to me. I'm important. Take notice of me.' I don't seem to be able to do that. I can with everyone else but he's my Achilles' heel. But there is a paradox because the staff absolutely adore him and have great faith in him as a skilled clinician. I think medical training teaches doctors to be distant. They are not taught to take feelings into consideration. It's that mechanical, biological model of health: if something breaks they try to fix it, but some can't see the difference between disease and illness. They can fix the disease but they can't all fix the illness. I think they are taught that death is a failure. They don't have to communicate with us, they can tell us. They don't have to explain or justify. They're the ones who have control over who we can see, what we can do, whether we have surgery, whether we don't, when we can go home. You can discharge yourself but in the normal turn of events they are the ones who dictate. They are a paternalistic power. It may be a benign paternalism but still it's paternalism.

It is usually assumed that because doctors have specialist knowledge they automatically know what is best. However, they need to talk to clients about preferred treatment options. Annie found her wishes being overlooked when a cyst in her ovary enlarged to uncomfortable proportions.

The first time that I saw the gynaecologist he just bowled up to the bed without introducing himself or anything. His first words were, 'We're going to take everything out.' Fortunately I was in fighting mode and I dragged myself up to my full height and said, 'Like hell you're ripping anything out!' Then a fight came about because he said he didn't 'rip' anything out, he 'removed' things. I said there was absolutely no difference. What really got to me was this assumption that because I'd had a tubal ligation and was beyond child bearing age, and because I was going to have chemo which was going to put me into menopause anyway, that it didn't matter if everything was taken out. I got really angry about this assumption that it doesn't matter. So I added several clauses on the anaesthetic form that if he was to remove anything that I was to see all pathology reports to make sure that there was a reason to remove it. It seemed to me that once I'd been diagnosed with cancer, every bit of healthy tissue assumed a greater importance than before the diagnosis.

Sticking up for herself made Annie feel as though she could retain some control over her situation. Lynne had a variation on this experience when she attended clinic for radiotherapy treatment.

Sometimes the doctors hear what I say if I ask a specific question but frequently they answer a question that I've never asked, and they do it in a very patronising way. For instance, the last time I was there, one of the doctors said, 'You will take Hormone Replacement Therapy.' I simply said to him, 'But why would I? I've read about Hormone Replacement Therapy and I don't see that it's necessary.' He looked at me and said, 'I'm writing a letter to your doctor. You will see him and he will put you on it. Don't worry about it, dear. It's only two pills a day.' I was prepared to talk on the level of bloody research into Hormone Replacement Therapy but they are clearly threatened by that.

There's something fundamentally wrong with the way that these men have power and act out their power over their clients and it seems like you have to act submissively in order to get the information you want. Subsequently, I've met up with women who've had cancer who've really given the guys hell and who have pushed and pushed to get the responses that they need. I think there are other ways of doing it but there's an awful lot more women who can't be articulate, who don't have laptops to take into hospital so they can write an account of what's happening to them, who don't read literature or sociology textbooks when they're waiting for their cancer results. And why the fuck should they? All women have got rights to the same information as more assertive women. It still makes me feel really angry.

It can take time and considerable strength of will to learn how to deal with a professional who may be technically competent but fails to inspire confidence. Annie found that

> Having a nursing background helped me in a strange way because when I was nursing I was this timid little meek and mild person. Thirty years ago nursing was very hierarchical in structure and you kowtowed to medical students and you weren't allowed to speak to doctors and it left me feeling very angry that I wasn't given due respect. I think that experience got me right into the conviction that no doctor was going to put me down. It gave me an energy to deal with doctors who I felt were incompetent. There are not many of them, but there are some.

Marinomoana didn't have any nursing background to bolster her confidence when dealing with consultants but she intuitively understood that it was crucial to her survival that she question everything the medicos told her.

> They gave people with anything on the brain such a minimal amount of time. After the first two years when I saw my neurosurgeon again he said, 'Oh you are still alive!' It was very empowering because it proved I was striving and living. I

had to show them that they were wrong. That was good for someone like me but maybe for other people, that negativity would have killed them. They really did consider themselves God. But I used to think, 'Sure, I'm going to believe you! You got it wrong the first time! I'm still here and I'm not a vegetable!' If anything, the certainty of the medical profession made me fight more. They could never keep me in the hospital any longer than I needed to be because, in my mind, hospitals are where people die! Sometimes I'd be dragging myself out feeling like shit!

This innate wariness of specialists and their language led Marinomoana to another strategy for dealing with the system. She enlisted the help of her GP and by keeping him fully informed she has been able to use him as her 'translator'.

He's the one that tells me what the consultants are talking about. There's been a few times when I've dragged him along when I've had to go for interviews to discuss more treatments. The specialists look at him like: 'You're not one of our club', because he is not down in the big hospitals. But if my GP doesn't know what they are saying, he checks up for me. It means that I don't always have to go screaming down the hospital if something goes wrong. I can go straight to my GP and he's got everything down. If he thinks it's more serious, then we contact the specialists. He has been with me the whole time, the same man. I don't know anyone else who's done that but my GP is my lifeline. He's a wonderful man.

When it came to understanding exactly what the doctors were talking about, Tiny had the additional problem of English being her second language. To get around this communication barrier, her daughter frequently accompanied her on visits to the doctor.

They must hate me by now because I am always asking the questions. I know Mum can't always express herself and I know the question that she wants to ask because we talk about it beforehand. I make sure that the doctor understands and explains it in terms that Mum understands. They have been good because they know Mum's English isn't that good. All of the doctors she has seen have explained everything properly, and if there's been choices to make, they let us have time to think. It's not like you're rushed through it. Most of the time you've got not much choice.

In any interaction with doctors, the issue of understanding what is being said is only one part of the story. The other challenge is making sure that they understand you and there are times when even speaking the same language seems inadequate. Carmen struggled along, not knowing what to ask, or who.

I really don't know enough and it's so embarrassing because people keep asking me, 'How's your cancer? Are the doctors saying you're doing well?' But the doctors don't say anything so I don't know how I'm supposed to be. They didn't say to me that I'm going to die, or that I've got a good chance. All the doctor said to me before I began chemo was that there were no guarantees. I didn't know what questions to ask. In the beginning the doctor told me to write my questions down and then ask them but when I go to the doctors I just tell them what I felt that week—like if I've had nausea or a headache or I'm missing my period. I don't even know why I'm missing my period. I feel too embarrassed to ask my doctor a question like that. I like him, he has got a terrific sense of humour and I've great respect for his knowledge but because he's a man I feel I can't talk to him about periods.

There is a female doctor that I sometimes see when I go to the hospital, so I tell her women things but I'm too nervous to ask questions. I know I should be assertive, but I'm just not! I don't like to complain a lot, I don't want to be too inquisitive and I don't want to waste their time. Those are the things that hold me back.

For different reasons Tiny also found it easy to communicate with a female doctor. This particular doctor had the skill to ensure her clients knew she thought of them as people, not just as illnesses to be treated. She conveyed this by the very simple device of

... saying things that a male doctor wouldn't say. My hair thinned and became brittle and very grey. I was not happy with it but she'd be really happy that I didn't lose my hair and would suggest little things, 'Maybe you should put a rinse through it. Try that.' She was very good at helping me to feel good about myself. If I saw her walking along the corridor she'd stop and talk, not about my illness but about how I'm coping. I think that was great. The doctor that I've got now is just straightforward. He tells you exactly and then you can go. He's not very sensitive towards your needs and I'm glad I didn't get this doctor straight away. I think I would have changed doctors if I'd started with this one. It's no good to stay with a doctor that you can't really be open with.

Lynne's experience left her doubtful that the gender of a doctor makes much difference to the way they exert authority. She found only

... two exceptions to the generally patronising attitude. One was a female doctor who worked under my specialist when I was having radiation. The moment she found I was a lecturer at a university, she stopped being patronising and she started giving me lots of information. Until then, I could have been an ant. There was absolutely no gender

bond or anything like that—it was really about being a professional. The other person was my specialist himself. He was brilliant. He anticipated my fear; he told me what he thought it would feel like; he anticipated questions that I might have, and he told me to write them down so I could take them in and then he could deal with them personally. But the reality was that I have seen him once since then and he didn't know who I was. He asked, 'Who's been treating you?' Then he looked at the notes and said, 'Oh, I'm sorry. It was me. I don't know all my patients.' I found him to be a totally gracious person but, in the course of my whole treatment, and all the clinics I've been to every three months since, I've seen him twice. So I know that there are important people in the treatment who are different but the chances are you're not going to meet them.

At the clinic, I have a different doctor every time I go and they give me different sorts of advice. Last time I went, the guy who tried to get me on Hormone Replacement Therapy said in a very patronising way, 'Make sure that you do keep coming back to clinic because there is a high recurrence rate for this cancer and there's no point in not coming back because we can't be responsible for you if you don't come.' What he was really saying was, 'It's not over yet.' However, when I saw my specialist he said, 'Your cervix area looks perfectly good. I think you've got a right to be optimistic now. It's looking normal. It looks as though it's healing well. You haven't had any problems? Are you taking care of yourself? How are you feeling about it?' So it seems the approaches of different doctors go across a huge spectrum, from scaring the hell out of you as a way of controlling your response through to doctors who say it looks great.

Given the diversity of doctors in the public and private health systems, less favourable encounters are inevitable. All too frequently, people assume that any problems they experience are their own fault. If they do not like the way they are being treated, they are being oversensitive or too demanding. One way to counteract this is to stop and consider what it is about 'good' doctors that sets them apart from their colleagues. As Annie points out

> ... one of the ways of knowing you've found a good doctor is whether you feel as though they recognise that your life is valuable to you. That might sound stupid but some people make you feel as though your life is of limited value. To me it's obvious that anyone's life is valuable but some doctors don't communicate that sense at all. You can sense it immediately and the only thing to do is to change doctors. There's no point sticking around a doctor who doesn't respect your life.

Doctors have a far greater impetus to 'respect your life' if they can 'see you' as an individual. Anne K found that the way she presented herself at each point in the system made an enormous difference to her relationships with all staff. By recognising some of the pressures operating on staff, she learnt that she could force them to see her as an individual.

> On some occasions in clinics they would bring around new staff, maybe a new haematologist or people from other areas wanting to look at your case. They were always interested and being a public hospital you have, to a degree, to act as a guinea pig for up-and-coming staff. Those staff learnt very quickly to treat a lot of patients as slabs of meat. That is something I was always very conscious of and I've never allowed it to happen to me. I grab eye contact straight away. I made a concerted effort to be really articulate and grab their attention. What I was really saying was, 'Don't dare dismiss me as a sick patient. Don't look at my disease, look at me.' I

found this was something I had to do a lot and I learnt that very quickly. I suppose there are lots of people who are unable to do that for whatever reason. Maybe they don't have the verbal skills. If they are from another country, they may have language problems. I can see that would be a real problem because they can be left sitting, unable to communicate.

It would be interesting for anyone with cancer, once they got over the shock, to take a walk through some of the clinics in a hospital and watch the body language of the people visiting those clinics. You see a room full of sixty people all sitting slumped, heads down, some looking visibly ill, others looking visibly depressed. If you think (and this is what I'd think to myself) that these people are going through the system every day, year in year out, and if medical staff see this all the time, they stop seeing you as a person. Doctors and nurses are only people and they have to switch off in order to be able to function. I think you have to turn that around.

I would love to be the sort of person who is able to go into clinics and say to people, 'Try not to shuffle up to the counter to present your card. Talk to the person who is there. I know you don't feel well. I know you hate life and hate how you are at the moment but try to grab hold of a little bit of power for yourself. Don't hand all your power away. Don't become powerless.' That is the key. Once you do that you really are sucked into the vortex of the system. You've gone—had it. You are just another sick patient. You don't have a name any more. Although in fairness to the clinics, they do try, they always call you by your first name. I think they do try but they only try for so long. If a positive approach is given to a patient and they don't respond over a period of time, then that disappears and you are just a person. Sometimes you're left sitting because they know you will sit.

THE FINANCIAL COST OF CANCER

Whether these women were treated under the public or private health system, many of them discovered that there were a range of additional costs which came with the status of being 'a cancer person'. For example, even as a public patient, some medications have to be paid for. Margaret P is a great advocate of the public health system because

> *... you never get a hospital bill and you get drugs to take home with you for up to five days. That's all free but I seem to be taking a lot of stuff for side-effects so I can pay a lot for prescriptions. My prescriptions are only two dollars seventy an item but even so, because I'm living on the invalid pension (which is $170 a week) sometimes it's impossible. For people who're missing work and not getting cheap prescriptions, it can be a real problem.*

Even for those women, such as Annie, who worked part-time, meeting the costs of additional but essential medications required considerable financial juggling.

> *The safety net for pharmacy is $600 whether you're on a half wage or a full wage. Without a health care card you are paying top dollar, but I'm not able to get a health care card because I work half-time; I get most of my pharmaceuticals through the hospital, but it's only a saving of $2 a script. I've got to spend $600 before I can get the safety net card. I get all my chemotherapy drugs free but when it comes to anything else, like simple analgesics, I pay.*

As a public patient whose only form of treatment was radiation, Lynne didn't face additional pharmaceutical costs because 'there was nothing to take'. However, she wanted 'alternative support' in the form of 'Chinese herbs, massages and counselling' and that was 'really expensive'. If she'd had to meet additional medical expenses from the health system, there was 'no way' she could have met the costs of the complementary therapies she sought.

While Lynne chose to spend money on those 'extras' because she considered them central to her healing process, many women discovered there were other unavoidable hidden costs. Marinomoana observed that

> ... it isn't only the cost of treatment, it's the other things that make your life bearable. There are pragmatic things that people don't consider. We had to move house because where we were living was on a hill and had steps which I couldn't get up and down during treatment. I still have trouble getting up steps, especially if my leg goes wonky on me. We have made this house very accessible. It has extra-wide doors and passages which we measured up to cope with a wheelchair because we had to think about the time when I will be in a wheelchair, a time when I won't be able to move about by myself. We had to make sure that we could fit ramps around the back so that everywhere is accessible. We thought about all of that at the time and it was a big cost and a big financial decision. I would hate to leave this area now because we've been here so long, but the cost was exorbitant and an added stress.

While Annie has been able to stay in her own home without making any major alterations, she has discovered other expenses which she didn't anticipate when she was diagnosed.

> There's expenses like taxi fares: after having treatment, I can't stand waiting for somebody to pick me up. I like to get straight home. If I'm on regular chemo that can be a taxi fare a week. Or I can't do the house cleaning any more, so I get a cleaner in once a fortnight. To do any handy work around the house costs money. I had to get another car, an automatic with

power steering and air-conditioning. Each of those has been essential equipment that I need to help me drive—they are not luxuries. That was a big cost. I've bought a lot of things, like my wig, when I was working full-time and I could afford it and I didn't mind paying for it. I could have got a wig much cheaper but there's so many people wanting wigs that if I could afford to buy it myself, I figured I should. When I was working full-time it didn't really matter, but now I'm half-time it's beginning to matter. Also you need a bit of cash for luxury items like a lunch out. Now, it really makes more of a difference to have lunch out than it did before but then I've got to save up for that. It really is a bit of a hole.

Annie touched upon several issues which have affected other women. The cost of transport became a major consideration for several, especially when on-going treatment necessitated regular trips to the hospital or clinic. Ann T was living in the north west in a mining town two hours' drive from Karratha when she was diagnosed so she qualified for the Isolated Patients Allowance. Even so she considered that 'it cost a bit of money travelling up and down to Perth'.

Even for those women who lived in the Perth metropolitan area, the cost of transport could become an issue. Marinomoana considered herself lucky because she had 'wonderful friends and parents-in-law who helped out with transport'. While she 'never had to worry about the cost of that' she knew people who did and they found it 'a big cost, even with the voucher system for taxis'. For women still in the paid workforce, assistance with taxi costs was not available. Carmen was one of those. As a public patient, she has been 'grateful' for the existence of Medicare because she has only had to cover the costs of additional medication which helps control the side-effects of her treatment. Carmen found

The major costs are from having to pay for transport to come in and out of town for the radiotherapy. I work so I can afford

it but it also wastes all my day in travelling. We live so far from the hospital that I won't use a taxi. I drive to the train station and catch the train the rest of the way—both ways. Travelling on public transport is tiring because you don't get the time to rest. There is a voluntary transport service but we live too far away to use it and we don't live far enough away to get the special discount. You have to live fifty kilometres from the hospital, and we live forty-nine kilometres away! I thank God we've got the train system. It costs me heaps in petrol and train fares, but I've managed. We can still cope because of Medicare.

As Carmen hinted, the cost of transport can be compounded because of lost income. It took time and energy to travel on public transport, and this could have quite dramatic effects because both ate into earning capacity. Tiny described the way this affected her small family business.

We have a vegetable stall at Midland Market on Sundays, selling the vegetables we grow, and my husband and I always went together. When I got sick, I had to stay home and my husband had to do all the work. And he had to look after me as well, and go with me to the hospital. The first year it was very hard to get everything together but we've got good children so we just made it. Now it is better and everything is settled. But it cost a lot of money because a lot of time was consumed getting from the hills to the hospital and then waiting around for the doctors. That can take a whole day when you are out and not able to do your work. That is lost production. So whenever I can, I go on the bus to Perth so my husband can work. My daughter works there so she comes with me in the morning. Then my husband will come and get me from the bus stop afterwards. But because we have our own business and work from home it is easier in many ways. When I was very ill my husband could look after me. If he worked in an office we would have to get somebody else to be around for me, and he can take me to hospital if I am not well enough to go on the bus. And because he was home he could cook for the family at night as well.

The loss of income and earning power was a fundamental financial issue for several women in the paid workforce. Cancer left them with little choice but to change their work status, either temporarily or permanently. Margaret P's health has deteriorated so much over the last few years that she has had to go on the invalid pension. Although she's 'extremely grateful' that she receives it, it has left her with 'a serious money problem'. She considers it farcical that this problem grows the longer she lives. While each new treatment managed to extend her life expectancy, she considered it

... disgusting that the fact that you get good news that you're going to live longer ends up being a problem: lack of money.

Fortunately she discovered that

... the Cancer Foundation does have provisions to help people financially, if you are on very limited funds. For instance, when my daughter was working away, they paid for the lawn mowing, and when the pump to the septic tank went last year, they gave me $300 towards the $470 it cost to fix it. I have been told that if I need money to keep the car going or physical work done around the house they can help. The social worker at hospital told me about this service, otherwise I wouldn't have been aware of it. The hospital social worker also got me home help at about quarter price for a few months. I paid three dollars instead of twelve dollars an hour and a lass would come for two hours cleaning one week and then three hours the next, when she would also do my shopping.

Financial and practical assistance for people on a low income or welfare benefit is available as long as they know where to find it. But for those who manage to keep working, there can be other pitfalls because of a reduced capacity to work. One woman described how her cancer had dramatically changed her family's financial status.

> *I now have to work less than I used to so my income dropped drastically. At the same time, my husband's employer increased their employees' hours and dropped their pay in order to keep jobs. Between health problems and changing work conditions, we've had to mortgage our house. That was hard. If I die the kids will get some superannuation and pay it off and if I live I'll pay it off somehow. I stupidly said we'd make the maximum repayments on our house and so we're actually living on the breadline to meet those payments. That was a silly move! All in all, finances have been difficult.*

For Annie the reduction in her earning capacity has been the central issue. She summed up the dilemma in terms which are undoubtedly applicable to other independent women with a progressing cancer.

> *I can't do a proper full-time job when I'm trying to live with pain. I just can't do it. It's not fair on the employer, it's not fair on those I'm working with and it's not fair to myself. So I've got to go part-time and that reduced my income by half. At the same time everything that I pay out for doesn't decrease and in actual fact I'm paying for more. Cancer really does change your whole financial outlook and the thing with this low-grade lymphoma is that it wrecked any earning potential I had. When I was first diagnosed but still working full-time I saved really hard and put away money which would act as a safety net for when I was on the pension. I didn't realise at all that there would be so much of a change in lifestyle because of the money I've had to*

spend on being a cancer person. Someone who goes in for surgery and can walk out the door again has got potential earning capacity. You might even be unemployed but at least there's a chance of employment and of doing a full-time job one day. There's no way that I can now do a full-time job and there's no way that I could get employment anywhere else at the moment except if it was very casual, very part-time and very poorly paid. Nobody would take me on. They'd be mad to do it! The most I'll ever earn is what I'm earning at the moment, and all I can look forward to is the disability pension.

ANNIE'S SUPERANNUATION SHOWDOWN

- One of the most difficult chores I had to do after I was diagnosed and had been given my prognosis was to cash in my superannuation. I had been advised to spend it while I was still fit and able and what I really wanted to do was take my children on a luxury holiday.

- The problem came with cashing in my private superannuation—to which I had been contributing $3 000 a year—whilst still wanting to work. It was possible to do this but taxes were going to make an enormous hole in the final pay-out. There was no way that I was going to see my contributions—which had already been taxed twice—taxed yet again, especially when I had a very legitimate reason for terminating superannuation.

- After three months of letter writing involving the Commissioner of Taxation, two federal politicians, my doctor, financial adviser and friends, I finally received my superannuation pay-out, taxed at the normal rate.

- It took a lot of tenacity and courage (especially in having to be honest with myself about my prognosis) but it was worth it. We had a wonderful holiday.

ATTENDING THE CLINIC

For many people with cancer, the clinic becomes an integral part of life. Considerable time is spent in the waiting room whiling away time between blood tests and results, waiting to see the doctor and receiving treatment. Annie associates clinics with

> *... waiting time. Sometimes you don't wait, sometimes it's five minutes, sometimes it's two hours. It's part of the game and it's pointless getting frustrated. The thing is that when you actually get into the consulting room you want as much time as you can with the doctor so in order for everyone to have their due time, you've just got to wait.*

Tiny was also relaxed about the time she had to spend at the clinic.

> *I'm not worried about the clinic. Sometimes you have to wait too long, that's for sure. One time I went, we had to wait for four hours. I don't like that. So the next time I went early and said I had an appointment at twelve o'clock and that I had to catch the bus at eleven o'clock. I was on that eleven o'clock bus! Most of the time I don't worry because I could not do much at home, so I read a book or magazine, or go for a cup of coffee. When I see people that I know, I talk and sometimes a friend will arrange to meet me there because where I live is too far for her to come. That is good.*

Even as a private patient, waiting seems to dominate the experience of the clinic. As Julie recounted.

> *I would go into the private hospital where my specialists have*

rooms for my blood tests and check-ups prior to having the chemo. Sitting in those waiting rooms is a real eye-opener because of the amount of people that come through: young, old, people with headscarves, people with bald heads, people with hats on and people with hair. When a couple comes in, it was like a game. I would wonder, 'You're here because you've got cancer but I wonder which one of you has?' You could see the great interest. If I walked in by myself, they'd think, 'She's got hair!' You could almost read people's minds. It was like, 'Gosh, you don't look as though you've got it!' and I'd often think, 'God, you don't look too bad either!' You are always summing people up, checking them out and thinking, 'I think you'll get over it. I really think that you've got a good grasp on it.'

Many people find clinics depressing. It is not just the association with cancer which creates this atmosphere. The physical environment adds to this joyless atmosphere: stark walls, a TV to fill in the silence of waiting and rows of plastic chairs which further discourage communication are hardly conducive to cheering people already feeling vulnerable. Beth maintains

The clinic I go to is the most depressing place I've ever seen. It's got brown carpets, brown chairs and these horrible baby-poop yellow and mustardy brown walls. The nurse has tried to cheer it up by putting nice bright quilts on the beds and postcards and pictures on the walls. That's the only nice bit. Behind the oncologist's chair is the most depressing painting of dead, burnt trees. Now how appropriate is that! The waiting room is like an 'L' shaped passage with seats in it but at least they have the trolley with coffee and sandwiches. People sit and stare or read their book. I decided I wasn't going to have that so I always say hello to every person there. If they don't want to talk to me, that's fine. Some chat and some don't. I find them very depressing places. They could have it brightened up with music and pictures. But the staff are actually terrific and they try to relax you and make you comfortable.

Anne K preferred to keep to herself on clinic day although, like Beth, she found the staff in the clinics were an important support mechanism throughout the duration of the treatment.

> I never looked at the clinic as a social gathering. In fact I didn't want to get involved with any patients at all because they were sick. On clinic day I would put on something really smart because I was damned if I was going in looking sick. I wouldn't talk much and would bury my nose in a book till it was my turn. A few people did approach me but I just said what I had to say and got back to my book. That was something I couldn't handle very well. I had built a huge thick thing around me. I had to, to keep going. If that showed any chinks then it might all come tumbling down.
> However, I did find that clinic was one area where I could talk about being ill to the staff. It was usually the nurse while I waited for the haematologist to arrive. They'd sit and ask, 'How have you been since your last visit? What's happening? What have you noticed?' I could let go and actually talk about being sick and they were always supportive. I got to know them very well because I was going over such a long period of time. I did set up a relationship with a couple of them, in particular when they found out my marriage had nose dived. They were concerned and invited me to their homes for meals, they asked if there was something they could do. Outside of that, I didn't encourage anything.

In contrast, Margaret P, who describes herself as a Yorkshire woman who 'likes to get her feet under the table and be at home', considers that the clinic can be an 'enormous support and source of information'. She did not always think this. Even though she is 'not the shrinking violet type', she attended one clinic for three and a half years 'and never spoke to another person'.

When she moved hospitals and started attending another clinic, the atmosphere was different. Now she finds that

> ... *attending the clinic can be good fun. That's the way I meet people, make friends, learn things. It's just a regular thing that I've got to do. You go for a blood test, then you go around to the oncology clinic, you wait until you see the doctor and then you go home, unless you're coming in and they send you off to a ward. There's no problems apart from the fact that the more ill you are, the more time you're at the clinic. I'm there just about every week, and I have been for a long while.*

In contrast, Carmen's experience of the same clinic has been far less sociable.

> *I read a book and drink coffee from the coffee machine because nobody talks to you and it helps to while away the time as I wait for my blood test to come through. All the time I've been there I haven't made one friend at the clinic. I go on Wednesday afternoon and it's usually the same old people and they sit there and complain about the voluntary service being late. I can't blame them but I thought I would have some sort of interaction attending the clinic. The only other communication I had there was on my first and second visit: a woman was complaining about how life sucks. I thought, 'Poor dear, if she can't see that life is wonderful.' About three months later I was feeling the same way! Now when I'm looking at people in the clinic I wonder if they're going through the same depressed feelings as I am. Are they wishing it was all over or do they really desire to live?*

After visiting clinics on and off for eleven years, Marinomoana still thinks they are 'really horrible'. She believes that they could be organised so that they are more sensitive to the needs of the people who have to use them.

> *They ought to have separate areas for people who are at different stages of their cancer and their treatment in the clinic. I think it'd be more comfortable for those patients who aren't too sick yet. At one of the major clinics in particular, it can be really hard when you are sitting looking at patients with beanies and things on their heads. I felt terrible about looking well, with all my hair. I sat there thinking, 'I really am sick! I really am supposed to be here!' The other clinic has got a little garden where all those deadbeats who smoke meet and you talk about what you've got and how your treatment's going. In fact you talk out in the garden but you don't when you're inside, you just wave at each other.*
>
> *It's really strange. I think it's the walls and the seats around the edge and the tellie on the wall. They always have those soaps on. I always sit down and wish they would change it to Oprah! I don't think the hospitals will do anything that'll be satisfying to everyone, but if they had a common area outside or in an atrium where people could go and wait with their families, I think that would be a lot better than the clinic waiting rooms.*

Just as some people's experience of the clinic is more sociable than others, so not everyone finds the clinic depressing. This may reflect the atmosphere in different clinics because, as Annie found, some clinics are more hospitable than others whether you strike up friendships or keep to yourself.

> *In a public clinic on a regular basis you get to know the people who go on that day so you form a very informal support group. People order coffee and sit around in the garden and*

you can make it a chatty, weekly social time. At the moment I don't go to the clinics on a regular basis so I don't know anybody well. Instead of talking I take marking, reading or sewing and I listen to a walkman radio. I say to myself, 'I'm here for the duration. Don't worry about it.' The clinic is in an old part of the building and has a very small waiting room. The walls are lined with postcards from people who've gone away all over the place. People know everybody's first name, or whatever they want to be called. We've got a TV and video, a coffee machine, and a little garden outside. It's not depressing.

When I was diagnosed, the first oncology clinic I went to had rows of seats, just like a train waiting room. It looked so inhospitable, and everybody looked as though they were on death's door. At the time I called them 'sticks with beanies on'. I'm sure if I went back now they would look completely different but at the time it looked like everybody was on their last legs. They looked absolutely awful with no hair, or they were yellow with liver involvement and I was the healthy person sitting there saying, 'What am I doing here?'

I didn't feel that when I changed to the public system and moved hospitals. When I first walked into the public clinic there was nobody there but the receptionist because they book you in for a first consultation and the whole afternoon is taken up with looking after you, as an individual. The receptionist came over and said, 'Would you like a cup of coffee?' Then she gave me a little pamphlet about the oncology clinic. It had the names of all the oncologists, of the current registrars, of the residents on the oncology ward. It had all the phone numbers you might need, told you who your social worker was, who your physiotherapist would be, and told you about the oncology dietitian. It even told you the best place to park your car when you come to the clinic and what to do in an emergency. It was all there in this lovely little pamphlet. I *felt as though somebody had bundled me up and said, 'We're going to take care of this nuisance, don't you worry.' It was just a joy.*

Annie was being treated as a client who needed certain information to help her find her way through the medical maze. A device as simple as an information card gave her greater control over her situation because it was empowering to know who the people in the system were, and where they fitted in the scheme of things. This sense of empowerment is important if and when treatment shifts from the clinic to the hospital ward.

BEING IN THE WARD

Although few people enjoy being in hospital, the sense that you are in the right place to receive the necessary care, combined with the fact that you are suddenly in a community of people who have had things go wrong with their health, can do much to ease the transition into the ward. When the women in this group were 'in the ward' they were all at different stages of different cancers, receiving treatments that were specific to their needs. Beyond that, their reactions to hospitalisation were influenced by their personalities and their status as public or private patients.

Some people on private insurance discovered that they did not like the privacy offered by the smaller private wards. Julie recalled her reactions to being in a two-bed ward.

I was in a private two-bed ward the first couple of times I went for chemotherapy and I was always in with a very sick person. I didn't want to be in with non-positive people who would say things like: 'What's wrong with you? Have they given you any treatment? Is there any time set on you?' At this stage I didn't want to talk about it and wasn't ready to talk about my illness.

168 Songs *of* Strength

Although in a public ward, Carmen found that

> *... the first time I was in I met three ladies who'd had mastectomies about twenty-five years ago—I was the youngest in the ward. So I knew there was a really good success rate and that gave me a hell of a boost. The second time round most of the other ladies were older and in need and it gave me a tremendous feeling to be able to help them to the shower and to eat. What I had felt like nothing compared to what they had, so I was able to overlook my troubles and help them. If you can help other people then that gives you the best therapy.*

When Anne K went into hospital to have a Hickman line[6] placed in her chest before her bone marrow transplant, she found therapy of a different nature through observing the way other people in her ward were coping with their health problems.

> *I noticed some people are unable, for whatever the reason, to handle their illness. They seem to fall apart. I watched one woman who was undoubtedly ill and feeling rotten complain continuously. She wasn't capable of making any effort, but it sort of feeds off itself and then the staff become negative. I always thought that the staff were going to do their best for me so it is up to me to do the best for myself. I would keep it light. A few times I went under. I had my moments when I absolutely plunged but I always tried to do that in my own time when there was nobody else around. In my own bed, quietly sinking into this black abyss.*

Tiny found that she particularly liked the weekday ward, even though the accommodation 'wasn't brilliant', because

> *... they put lots of people with cancer there. We all had the same sort of problems. Sometimes I would be sent to a different*

---

6. An intravenous tube used for giving chemotherapy drugs to avoid damage to veins.

ward and you don't meet other people on chemo. It was good to be able to share some of the way I was feeling with other cancer patients. I found that useful and I was very happy with the hospital.

Annie came to the conclusion that sharing with other people and the business of the ward was

... not a problem because I've got to know the system and I know how far I can take things. Like the last ward I was on had a balcony outside. It was summer and I wake up very early in the morning. So I said to the nursing staff, 'I'd give anything to sit out on that balcony in that beautiful early morning sun.' There aren't a lot of safety devices out there and a couple of people have hurled themselves over, but those nurses used to come every morning at six o'clock with a cup of coffee, unlock all the doors, wheel me out and leave me there till I was ready to come in again. I used to take the walkman, the fags, the coffee and the morning paper and they would bring me another cup of coffee an hour later. It was just brilliant.

Doctors and nurses in the hospital system have to tread a fine line between sympathy and empathy and some are able to do this with more grace than others. As a long-term, and at one stage regular, resident of an oncology ward Marinomoana developed an acute awareness of the sympathy/empathy issue.

I think that the rigidity of the hospital system encourages staff to become desensitised for their own mental health. I only saw one nurse stop and cry when a patient died and in fact that endeared her to me. It was like at least one person who works here will miss that patient. The others were cold. I understand why they have to do that. They're dealing with this every day and it's a survival technique for them. But when you are on top of the bed, it's like: 'Are you real?' You don't want to be treated by robots.

Staff turnover was another problem for Marinomoana. Even though she expected this when visits were months or even years apart, she recalls that it was always nice to recognise the few nurses who remained. And while understanding that nursing staff, like young doctors, have to learn different areas of medicine, and thus have to move, she still considers that they are not left in one area—

> ... long enough for you to get to know them and for them to know certain case histories. One time I had explained what was wrong with me to three different sets of nursing staff. THAT was HARROWING. It causes a lot of distress when you've got to repeat everything all over again. It drags a lot of stuff that you are starting to deal with back up to the surface again so when they ask again, 'What have you got?' I found myself saying, 'I don't know!' You don't mean to be angry but it's like, 'You're hurting me. I don't want to talk about it now. This is how I deal with it.' They don't seem to understand that either—the different ways people deal with their sickness. They could go and look at the case history and find out themselves. There NEEDS to be something done, though I don't know what.

In comparison, Tiny considered that

> ... the nursing staff was very good and they know what they're doing. Everyone was very supportive and had time to listen to you. The nurses were pretty good about letting my family visit after hours because my daughter worked at night and couldn't get in till ten o'clock sometimes. On New Years Eve my husband stayed till one o'clock. They seem to know that

you need any support that you can get. They know the people that have got lots of family and the people that don't and they'll sit on their bed and just talk about everything. People need that.

Not only do people receiving treatment require emotional and practical support; they require awareness that they may become more sensitive to a range of different stimuli, such as colour, texture, taste, or some unexpected combination of these, as Julie recalled.

I can remember laying there after one chemo session looking at this beautiful flower arrangement that somebody had delivered. It was a lovely arrangement with beautiful big yellow dahlias. Suddenly I felt very nauseated by looking at it. I couldn't stand the smell. I couldn't stand the sight of the yellow flowers. Another friend has told me that she couldn't stand yellow daffodils. Perhaps yellow is not the colour to give a person on chemotherapy? I also couldn't stand the stainless steel covers that they put over the food dishes, the stainless steel soup bowls and the thick, chunky crockery. I wanted fine glassware and china to drink out of. Maybe because you're having a metallic drug, the fact that you've got to touch stainless steel makes you feel nauseated.

Tiny got so sick with a lung infection during one stay in hospital that she couldn't eat. Although she blamed her condition rather than the food, the hospital staff chose to send her home when her family convinced them that they could feed her better on their fresh produce. Margaret W's unpleasant experience with hospital food suggests that there were some disadvantages in her choice of a smaller, local hospital where there were no specialist oncology nursing staff who could advise her on appropriate food after a stomach operation.

After the second operation I was finding eating very difficult and I was talking to one of the sisters and she said, 'How about scrambled eggs?' So I said, 'Oh yes, that sounds nice.' She scrambled some eggs for me herself and about half an hour after the scrambled eggs I was screaming in agony and the nurses were rushing about. They phoned the doctor and he said that was the worst thing they could have given me because the operation was on my stomach and egg protein is very difficult to digest.

Most larger hospitals, and certainly those with an oncology department, have specialist dietitians. Annie never has any problems with hospital food because she has got the oncology dietitian 'on-side'. Her observations, however, apply to hospital services and relationships with hospital staff in general.

I think it all boils down to knowing how the system works, knowing how far you can take it, and knowing that there is a boundary and that you can't go over that because that's getting into the realms of their work. They've got a role and you've got a role and you have to meet on a certain ground. I think that the trick is saying, 'I'm an expert of my body and what is going on with my body right now but I'm not an expert in how to diagnose it and how to treat it. They've been trained to do that.' I think if they recognise that, and you recognise that they've got the training and the skills in dealing with that then you get along fine. Beyond that is knowing how a hospital operates, and the various resources you can call on—like knowing that there's a dietitian and how to get hold of her. It didn't take me long because the first time I was in hospital was for three weeks. By the end of that time I had got it all worked out.

Knowing how the hospital works includes knowing what is permissible in terms of creating a more hospitable environment. All the women in this group who have had to go through regular periods of hospitalisation developed techniques to make their time there more pleasant and more comfortable. As Tiny observed

> *... I don't like the hospitals—not at all—but you have to go. You know that and then you make the best of it. I take everything I need for the whole week, including my sheepskin, so nobody had to worry and I tell my friends I go on holiday for one week!*

Annie sees time 'on the ward' as an intrusion which had to be borne for the sake of treatment. The only way to tackle it is head-on.

> *I'm an organised person so I have a bag which I have set up with a card in it. On that I write everything that I need to take into hospital with me to keep me sane. I take comfortable clothes. I always take my walkman because I find at night when I can't sleep I can plug into the radio so even if I don't sleep it doesn't matter because I'm sort of drifting in and out. That walkman's essential. I have a stock of novels that people give me for my birthday and Christmas which I leave for the ward. I have a card with all my mates' phone numbers on and I nearly always order a phone as soon as I step foot on the ward. I don't order a TV because I find I don't use it. I do other things. I take my own cup because I like fine china. I always take a rose and a little vase, so as soon as I get into bed I can look at one of my roses. Most of the time the bag is packed, but the card is there with everything I need in case there's any emergency so somebody else can see what I want brought in, pick up the bag and bring it.*
>
> *I take my own soft pillow, and I will be taking my own sheepskin next time because they can be quite rare in hospitals, as can wheelchairs. A couple of years ago I bought a wheelchair because I smoke and I don't like being in a ward*

all day. Even if I didn't smoke I'd find it confining and claustrophobic. I rarely use it, but it's nice to know that I've got a wheelchair that somebody can bring in if ever I'm in a situation where I can't walk and I want to get out of the ward. Another thing I've done is to take in some thin foam to go on top of the mattress because I find that the heavy plastic really digs into parts of me and I get sore. And I take my favourite pillowslips so I don't have to use the standard white hospital things. I guess what I try to do is make this part of my life as livable and as normal as I possibly can.

Margaret P has developed similar ways of making the ward as agreeable as possible.

I go into hospital regularly so I take four of my own pillows in and I use their two as well; and I have a sheepskin I take in. I set myself up really comfy. Sometimes the noise of the other people can annoy the shit out of me, so I take ear plugs. It's simply luck who you get to share a room with. I found it easier to mix with cancer patients, probably because we are all going through similar things anyway. You need to know what you can and can't do. You need to know what's reasonable, when it's just red tape that you're bucking or when it's something important.

For Margaret, the issue is one of patients' rights and advocacy, not just one of personal well-being. Like other women in this group who have had extended periods of contact with the medical system, she has learnt that getting to know the system has made her more confident. All of these women devised some strategies which helped to normalise the ward and clinic environments, thus making them less intimidating. This in turn made it easier to be assertive about their individual needs and right to have a say in the way their cancers were managed. As Anne K emphasised: 'Don't let yourself be dismissed as a sick patient. Don't look at my disease. Look at me.'

STRATEGIES FOR GETTING THROUGH THE SYSTEM

- Get to know the hospital system, public or private. Find out what facilities and services are available to oncology clients. As the bigger hospitals, much of the information you will need to familiarise yourself with 'the system' will already be compiled for you in a pamphlet.
- Make hospital as comfortable as possible. Taking in soft, comfortable day clothes (tracksuits etc) can help you feel less like a patient and more in command of the situation. Hospital beds can frequently feel hard after too long spent lying on them, and sheepskins can be a luxury item. If you take your own, then you can ensure your own comfort. Similarly, if you enjoy drinking out of fine china or glass, take your own in with you: hospital crockery is designed for durability, not culinary pleasure.
- Uncertain about when to contact a doctor, the clinic or hospital about a change in your condition? If you are feeling really bad, then ring straight up. If you are feeling a bit funny, leave it twenty-four hours and if you are still feeling funny, ring up. If you are feeling better, then you can wait until your next appointment.
- Getting along with staff in the system—recognise the pressures operating on staff, try to be cooperative and friendly but assertive. Be aware of your body language, grab eye contact right away, in every interaction with

staff, try to ask questions or at least talk with the staff so that they see you as a person not a disease. Try to take control of your illness.
- Your appointments at the clinic will normally take time: you have to wait for results of blood tests, wait to see a doctor, wait for treatment and during treatment. Make life easier by accepting the fact that you are unlikely to get out in a hurry. Patience may be a virtue but it is also a simple stress management technique.

BLOOD TESTS, BIOPSIES AND SCANS

As the women in the group discovered, blood tests, biopsies and various imaging techniques are an integral part of the cancer process. Like all aspects of cancer, there are no 'right' or 'wrong' ways of experiencing these tests.

For some women blood tests became part of the cancer routine. These are used to monitor the side-effects of treatment and to check the function of liver, kidneys and other organs. As Anne K found, blood tests were so routine after her diagnosis of leukaemia that they simply became

> *... a way of life. I had to have blood tests all the time and some other procedures, like blood pictures and screening, because there are certain intravenous things that you need for quite a while with leukaemia.*

On the other hand Lynne found that every time she went to the clinic she had to have

> *... blood and urine tests and pelvic examinations. It was distressing, especially having to repeat my story each time to*

whoever was taking notes or consulting—it was never the same person.

Blood tests can be a problem for people on chemotherapy because surface veins can collapse. Carmen faced that problem soon after she started treatment for breast cancer.

I had trouble when I had blood tests. They were quite painful because they never could find my veins and, because they were students doing the tests, they don't know how to do it properly. I know students have to learn, but can't they learn on non-cancer patients? Cancer patients have to go through enough needles without the added trauma of someone who is learning how to do it properly. The ladies that give you the chemo are experts and they find my blood straight away, no hassle. I don't even feel the needle. They are so good in finding the veins that they should do the tests. Maybe they can't? Maybe they haven't got the time?

Biopsies are also common. These involve the removal of tissue to determine the presence, extent or cause of disease. The procedure may consist of a simple needle biopsy or a small operation, but where the cancer is in a less accessible organ, such as the bowel, a larger operation is required. If there was adequate forewarning about the likelihood of pain or discomfort, and if appropriate pain relief was given, the women found it easier to accept the procedure as a kind of diagnostic 'gain-pain'. This did not always happen. Beth recalled her experience of the biopsies which confirmed that primaries in her bowel and ovaries had already spread to her abdomen.

I was lying there in absolute agony and the doctor said, 'This will be a bit uncomfortable.' Then he stuck this needle deep into my abdomen! He did three biopsies, one after another.

> *Wham! No warning; no pain-killer; nothing. It was excruciating. I would like every doctor or nurse to have things like biopsies and babies so they can understand exactly what we are experiencing.*

Lynne experienced the opposite end of the pain relief options. In the first few weeks after her diagnosis of cervical cancer, she had a laparoscopy to 'explore the scene', then another just less than a week later during which three extensive cone biopsies were taken.

> *When a cone biopsy is done a cone-shaped piece of the cervix is taken from an area suspected to be cancerous. It's then spread open into a fan shape and examined. If the cancerous cells extend beyond the borders of the specimen, it is assumed to have spread widely into the surrounding cervix. In my case three biopsies were taken and they all revealed that the tumour was much larger. Sometimes if the tumour is small, a cone biopsy may remove the cells entirely. At that point I was told conclusively that I had advanced cervical cancer. Fortunately the scan (dye injected) taken to ascertain how far it had spread showed that it had not gone beyond the parameters of the cervix although I was told my cervix had enlarged to the size of an orange!*

For all these procedures, Lynne was given a choice between an epidural and a general anaesthetic. Even though she 'didn't take very well to the general anaesthetic', she rejected an option to have an epidural because

> *... my experience of it when I was pregnant with my first delivery was fairly horrendous. I didn't want to be paralysed and have people talking about my cancer while I couldn't bloody do anything. I'd rather hear about it later.*

Exercising the right to choose the most suitable form of available anaesthesia could require considerable powers of assertion. When Margaret P was first hospitalised to have a lump in her neck removed, the doctors decided a bone marrow biopsy was needed to gauge the precise nature and spread of her lymphoma. She had

> ... *heard of people who'd had lumbar punctures, and they went through hell. I thought there's no way they are getting near me with a big metal drill on a local anaesthetic, so I refused unless they gave me a systemic drug to knock me out. Actually, it's a very narrow drill, like a corkscrew, which they use to go into the bone, but is not a pleasant experience under local anaesthetic. They gave me pethidine and valium that first time, and I ask for it every time I have a bone marrow biopsy. I've had trouble with doctors because of this over the years, but I stick to it and I've never had a bone marrow biopsy under a local. I think when you've got cancer you have got enough problems without having unnecessary pain.*

Annie has also had

> ... *several bone marrow aspirations which I'd never have without this magic little intravenous mix of pethidine and intra-venous valium. It knocks you out for the duration so you don't remember anything. I'd wake up with a sore tummy but that must be from the tension of having it. For me, bone marrow aspirations are painless but I couldn't imagine having it without the needle.*

Anne K remembers that the 'dreaded bone marrow aspiration was a very unpleasant procedure' which she coped with by going onto 'automatic pilot'. She found that if she 'just bore with it' she could 'get a little bit above it', a reaction very similar to Tiny's. Tiny was quite emphatic that to be forewarned was to be forearmed.

> *The doctors told me beforehand that it was going to hurt. If they tell you that it's not as bad when it gets uncomfortable because you think it will be a lot worse than it actually is. If you lie very still it doesn't hurt that much.*

While pain relief is available for biopsies, there is nothing to help people get through the various imaging techniques that are used to produce pictures of the body's internal structure. These procedures include conventional X-rays, computerised scans (CT scans), nuclear scanning, ultrasound examinations and, in the larger hospitals, a new method called magnetic resonance imaging. Pain relief is not considered necessary because these techniques involve lying still while the equipment scans the appropriate part of the body. Many of these techniques involve injection or ingestion of a dye or radioactive material.

However, it can be an intimidating experience, as well as an extremely uncomfortable one. Several women recalled the panic that accompanied their first appointment with the CT scan, and the physical environment in which these scans were conducted did little to help. Marinomoana had to have 'ten or eleven' CT scans in a two-year period because her doctors wanted to 'keep a check on what was happening' to her brain tumours. She hated the CT scans, finding them 'worse than chemo'.

> *They gave me the dye through my arm. It's uncomfortable but it has to be done. Then they make you lie on the bed and strap you in so that you keep perfectly still. It's important to be still. The machine's at the back of you 'cos they put me in head first so you're looking at the people in front of you behind the screens. That used to amaze me: how come they are behind a screen and I'm not? It made me very fearful. Every time I was in tears.*

Claustrophobia seemed to be a common reaction to a CT scan. Marinomoana, a 'bouncy, talkative, fidgety person', found being strapped down and having to keep still was very claustrophobic. However, she discovered that if she didn't keep still—

> ... we'd have to do it all over again. There was one time someone had strapped my ankle so I asked them why. They said, 'Try not to talk. Your ears are moving.' I burst out into fits of laughter because I didn't realise your ears move when you talk! These are the things that go through your brain. They had to bring me out, sit me up, and get the giggles out. Later I found a strategy: all-up the scans would take a couple of hours by the time the dye has worked so I used to go to sleep. That made it easier for them. The only thing was the strappings were bruising my legs badly. I was very anaemic because of the chemo they were pumping into me so I'd end up with bruising on my legs from the straps. The bruising was so bad that I couldn't shave my legs for a long time.

Tiny recalled how daunting she found her first CT scan.

> I was very sick, with pain in my back and I had to lie still in a position that hurt. I had tears rolling all over my face and they were saying to me, 'You have to try.' I was trying but to be in the machine for one and a half hours was really hard. After twenty minutes they took me out for a bit and asked: 'Is it all right?' I say, 'Yes, it's all right.'

The length of time spent having scans varied, depending upon the age of the machines used and the extent of the images being sought. After years of having CT scans, Margaret P decided that they were just 'an uncomfortable nuisance'.

> If you're having your chest and abdomen scanned, you've got to have nothing but clear fluids for at least four hours beforehand and sometimes they inject iodine into you, and it

all takes time. I find an abdo/thoracic scan takes about forty-five minutes.

Annie's first full scan took about an hour.

I was terrified out of my brain because I didn't know what a CT scan was. I'd read about these huge machines. Now I look back on it I think 'stupid'.

Since then she has become an old hand, having now had a range of different scans at regular intervals since diagnosis. She has devised some strategies to cope with the experience.

What pisses me off is that they can see what's happening inside my tum and I can't. How dare other people have secrets! Now I've got them to wheel the screen and monitor so that when I'm going through I can see what they see. I get the monitor right by my head so I can see my guts going past! I can't read it and I would hate to be able to read it, but I find it very interesting to see my liver and lungs and heart and bits and pieces. I find it all fascinating.

It's the same with the bone scan. The first bone scan I had was at the first hospital I went to as a private patient and it's a different bone scanner to the later ones I had as a public patient at a different hospital. With the first one I had to go into different positions for the scanner and that really did something to my back. I was in agony for months and months. For the scanner at the second hospital you just lie straight on the table. Some of the staff don't like to but some of them will leave the screen so I can look at it and see where the hot spots are. The arthritis that I've got comes up as hot spots of bone activity. These show up on the screen as a concentration of dots in my head, feet, ribs or whatever. It turns the staff into a panic because it's also a signifier of bone cancer but we've worked out that with me it's not bone cancer.

I've also had a Gallium scan.[7] *Like the bone scan, they use radioactive dye for a Gallium scan. Low-grade lymphoma can turn into medium or high-grade lymphoma and the Gallium scan will pick up intermediate and high-grade lymphoma, although it doesn't pick up low-grade lymphoma. I watched the Gallium scan too: it's all by computer and can home in on various bits of the body. That's fascinating.*

For people with chronic incurable cancers, like Annie, fascination with the changes taking place in her body has been one way of managing her situation. Repeated visits to the radiology and nuclear medicine departments have meant that it has been possible for her to get to know the staff there well enough to ask to see the screen. Lynne had little time to get to know staff. The alienation this caused was made even worse by the straps which immobilised her limbs.

I was having tests where they pump all the gunk through your kidneys and it goes through and then they take pictures of all of your organs to see how far the cancer's gone. There I am strapped to the bed and the oncologist who'd been assigned to my case came in and said, 'By the way, Mrs A,' (because they never called me anything other than Mrs A, even though I told them repeatedly that I did not want to be called Mrs anything! It's appalling. It's not even my married name!) 'your tests have come back and you do have a cancer malignancy.' Even though I knew this was the case, I thought this really was an inopportune time to tell me. Maybe he thought it was safer to tell me when I was strapped down! Then he disappeared. I burst into tears and was really miserable. The radiologist who was doing the tests coped by telling me about his mother who'd had both breasts removed and cervical cancer and she'd still

---

7. Gallium—a radioactive isotope used in some nuclear scans to indicate some tumours and inflammatory activity.

survived to live to a reasonable age. Then the nurse who was helping him related a story about her mother having cancer. There I was, strapped to this bed, having dye pumped around my body with these people telling me their favourite cancer stories. I couldn't believe it. There was an awful lot of that and you have to be able to laugh. It's just too absurd.

Beth's early encounters with radiology were made more traumatic by the manner of some staff.

I don't sleep well before a CT scan because they're absolutely vital to me: they tell me if I am going to be all right or not. So I worried and fasted and arrived at the hospital to be told that the machine wasn't working and I would have to wait for another appointment some weeks later. I was very upset and said: 'Doesn't this hospital have a telephone? Couldn't you have rung me yesterday when you knew the machine wasn't working? Don't you realise that people fast, that they worry and lose sleep over the test and the results?' I was really upset by the delay and felt I was not being considered as a person with feelings and rights, that it was a case of the power of technology and the mystification of illness versus the lack of concern and thought for the individual's feelings and rights.

This sense of subservience to the priorities of medical technology left a profound impression on Beth after a particularly unpleasant experience when she suffered an allergic reaction to the dye.

Another time I was on the table for a scan, dressed in a trilby [hospital gown], with IV running, lying still, following the lights on the machine. The technician told me what to do and left the room, telling me to yell out if I had any problems. My trilby caught in the machine and was riding up and down leaving me partly naked and exposed, but I couldn't call out because my tongue had swollen up and gone all numb and I couldn't talk. I felt terrible. The pre-test drink made me feel sick and gave me diarrhoea and I had a dreadful headache. When the technician came in she growled at me and said, 'Why didn't you call me?' With my swollen tongue I couldn't answer her so, still in the hospital gown, they put me on a trolley in the corridor. They left me there for about an hour and came to check me out periodically before letting me go home. There was little thought to dignity. Put into a gown, given a number and left in a corridor, I felt stripped of my roles, my identity, and my personality. I felt de-humanised. I didn't feel like a person who happens to have cancer: I felt like the cancer on the trolley.

As Beth's swollen tongue indicates, no-one can predict how any individual will respond to a particular test or treatment. Not knowing that reactions are possible can lead to women putting up with extreme discomfort. Marinomoana found the radio-active dye she was given prior to her scans 'burned' her vaginal area.

I don't know if it happens to anyone else but for me it was like sitting on a hotplate. Afterwards you've got to sit and wait because of the drugs they give. I'd take off my panties and sit with my legs open, fanning myself with my skirt, wishing that the breeze would cool me off! But hospitals are always body temperature, so it's hot in there and you are burning. It took me a while, but after about the fifth time I mentioned it to one of the nurses and she said, 'We do have bidets. Maybe that would cool it down?' It did. It was lovely. I never ever thought to ask anyone else if they felt this sensation but for me, that was the worst part. I really used to hate that.

No matter how intimidating scans are at first, and no matter how uncomfortable they remain, all the women learnt to cope with the physical processes involved. But, as with blood tests and biopsies, having the scans is only step one. For many women, the time between the completion of a test and receiving news of the outcome is the most difficult part of the process, particularly if there is some delay. Kaye had 'quite a few needle biopsies' and found that

> ... *waiting for test results was always stressful for me. I remember clearly a lump I had tested just before Christmas one year. I was told to phone for the results a week later. Exactly a week later I rang up, only to be told that the lab had closed for the holidays. The receptionist who answered the phone couldn't give me the results and told me to phone back after the holidays when the lab re-opened. That was the worst Christmas.*

Kaye learnt to cope with the anxiety of waiting for results by thinking back to her first needle biopsy—the one that showed she had cancer. On that occasion she was 'told the bad news about twenty minutes later', so she 'began to think that if test results took a week or longer to come back' then she must be clear. 'It was,' she reflected, simply her 'way of coping with the waiting'.

Annie also found that there were times when waiting for results 'got to her'. At one stage she was experiencing a lot of pain which no-one could explain and she got so anxious that she knew she had to do something to deal with the situation.

> *I didn't know if I was going mad and the results of a CT scan really worried me. I didn't think I could wait two days to get the results so I rang up the oncologist and told him I was freaking out. He rang the radiologist and got the doctor to come out and tell me the results as soon as they had done it. That was magic and I'm getting better at them each time. Now I'm all right as long as I know that the scans haven't been read, or the results are in the mail—as long as no-one is*

sitting on them without contacting me. That has been a strategy for reducing the anxiety of waiting. But if I know they will have the results, I phone if they haven't contacted me. Sometimes the system is so busy that it doesn't recognise that the client has got a problem with not knowing, so it's up to the client to ask. It all gets back to good communication and knowing the system.

Precisely because imaging procedures are concerned with plotting the presence or progress of cancer, it is easy to forget that there may be a therapeutic value in seeing how the body has responded to treatment. Ann T realised this, but even her experience illustrates the tumble of emotions which can accompany the scanning procedure.

The thing that really helps you get through is peace of mind or knowing the positive things of it. If you don't do anything about it you could go around for years thinking, 'What if those cells are in my bones?' Instead of doing that I said, 'I'm worried about this. What do you think?' My doctor said, 'What about a CT scan? Would that ease your mind? We know there's probably nothing there but have it just the same.' I had a CT scan of my middle area from my abdomen down to my pelvis within six months of my operation. I felt good about having it because there was one more thing eliminated.

Then, because I was reading and getting information for myself I'd heard that secondaries can pop up in the spine. I decided I wanted a bone scan exactly a year after I had my mastectomy so I went down to Perth for one. Coming up to those sort of tests I was so on edge but afterwards it was like I used to feel as a kid going to confession: you would go into confession worried about what the priest was going to give you today. When you say your three Hail Marys, and you go out, you feel like a weight has gone. This is the way I felt after the CT and bone scan: absolutely on a high. Those scans really helped me a lot. I did have a positive attitude about my breast cancer before, but the scans really clinched it because they showed there was nothing there. After that I relaxed. I could forget it and get on with my life.

4
LUCY'S DIARY

THIS IS A DIARY KEPT DURING OCTOBER AND NOVEMBER 1989 WHEN I was being treated for a tumour in my left breast. Having discovered the lump, I saw a GP then a specialist. Both initially believed the lump to be a cyst.

MONDAY 2 OCTOBER
   The doctor tries needle aspiration. Finds solid lump. Takes needle biopsy and sends sample to pathologist.

THURSDAY 5 OCTOBER
   Results through. Atypical cells. Mammogram lined up.

MONDAY 9 OCTOBER
   Mammogram. Cysts show up, also unidentifiable large lump.

THURSDAY 12 OCTOBER
   Appointment with the doctor. Decides to take out lump next week. Feeling fine. It appears lump not typical cancer. No emotional problems.

MONDAY 16 OCTOBER
   Night into hospital. Edgy, not particularly nervous but not sleeping. Woman in same room having same operation. Great source of comfort from being with someone in same boat.

TUESDAY 17 OCTOBER

Morning ... apprehensive ... fear as wheeled down corridor into lift and down to theatre. Feel very vulnerable on a trolley and watching ceiling flash by then theatre lights. Doctor explains that he will simply take out the lump ... nothing more in this operation. Operation over soon ... back in grim recovery room. Nurse has bright red lipstick ... a source of cheer. Back to ward and feeling good. Little pain, no drop in morale. Doctor says lump was most unusual, will tell me when he gets results. Heart sinks a little ... this man gives nothing away. Still have fellow patient to talk to.

WEDNESDAY 18 OCTOBER

Home.

THURSDAY 19 OCTOBER

Back at work feeling fine and waiting for appointment on Friday to hear that all is OK. Phone call mid-afternoon. Lump malignant, treatment removal of breast. Find it hard to understand what he is saying. I'd been interested in the process so far but this wasn't in my imagined scenario. Like a game I didn't want to play any more. Felt like saying, 'Look, stop here. This isn't what I want.' Arranged to see him Friday afternoon after work. Hard not to cry at work and on way home. Dreadful night ... tears and fear uncontrollable ... shaking, sweating etc. Very little sleep.

FRIDAY 20 OCTOBER

To work, functioning reasonably well. To doctor at four or so. Tears begin. Doctor tells me this type of cancer is rare, doesn't tend to spread and is treated by mastectomy. I cannot understand logic but believe him. I bring up idea of partial mastectomy. He doesn't agree. I end up pleading for something, a vestige of femininity like a nipple, but no go. It seems there is to be a boney expanse with a large scar. I've seen pictures of these in books, they look so unattractive. I find it incomprehensible it should be happening to me.

Doctor tells me this sarcoma is, if you have to have cancer, the least dangerous ... something to be grateful for, I guess. Finding it hard to be grateful for anything. Finding it hard to think of anything. I go to sleep, using valium, with cancer the last thought on my mind. Before I open my eyes at 2 am, which seems to be the time that those with cancer all seem to be awake, I am consciously thinking about it.

SATURDAY 21 OCTOBER

The children are told ... Mum will cope ... Daughter (11) asks, 'Will you have some stuffing put in?' I don't know, maybe. Small son tells me he loves me about fifty times a day and sits and holds my hand. I know he'd love to be cuddled on my knee but that's impossible. Older boy says little, thinks much, comes out with blunt questions, 'Will you die?' Unable to look me in the face. I explain to them separately that this operation is not pleasant and that I'll look a bit odd after it, but that if I don't have it then I could die. They say they don't care what I look like because I will always be the most beautiful person in the world. But they are still children and as the deadline for the operation has been set for Tuesday week and the Royal Show is on, the show is uppermost in their thoughts, with talk of showbags, fairy floss etc. Not callous, just children. Crying in shower, toilet, anywhere private ... not in public. Went to dinner in pub at night. Become idiotically obsessed by women's breasts. Envy of what looked like perfectly healthy pairs of breasts. No appetite to eat ... unlike me. More valium and some sleep.

SUNDAY 22 OCTOBER

Still functioning as normal. Emotionally thoughts dominated by this wretched cancer.

MONDAY 23 OCTOBER

First thing woman from Cancer Foundation rang offering support. Rang back at night. In spite of her being busy we spent a long time sorting out a few fears and reassuring me that life goes on after. She says crying is good but I don't do much of it.

Week at work passes fairly normally. Find myself commiserating with people who have colds. Then feeling angry that anyone would complain about a runny nose.

THURSDAY 26 OCTOBER

Went to get second opinion. Same as first. Difficulty in getting more than one opinion is that if one doctor offers a more attractive, ie less drastic, treatment, you would well be tempted to take it and die regretting it. Fortunately both doctors agree. Two interesting pieces of information from visit to second doctor: 1) Surgeons working on breasts have regular meetings to discuss cases and progress . . . good to hear that they are not acting in isolation 2) Talking of reconstruction, second doctor describes silicone bag as having 'quite a sensual feel'.

FRIDAY 27 OCTOBER

Ring doctor to make arrangements for Tuesday. Getting attacks of the weeps now.

WEEKEND 28-29 OCTOBER

Spend time rubbing down brass bed to paint ready for return from hospital. Determined to pamper myself a bit. Weekend drags on. Getting very tired. Wish it was over. Cannot bring myself to look at sacrificial boob. If I have a mastectomy, does that mean that fourteen women will be spared on the basis of 1 in 15? I feel like a sacrifice to the god of quotas.

MONDAY 30 OCTOBER

Wet and miserable. Public holiday. Everyone in cheerful mood at work but me. Everyone eager to get off home but me. Home early, phone a couple of friends, great morale boosters which give me a high for half an hour or so. This is the best thing, to talk to friends and family, some people who have some knowledge and insight into it all. Packing and off. Tension as soon as I am in hospital. Up to room and unpack. Send off family. Can't get into bed ... beginning of end. Pace up and down corridor. Try to read. Read a complete D. H. Lawrence, which, even though no heavyweight, was skimmed rather than absorbed. Notice darkening sky. Tears well up then subside. Anaesthetist comes. Tears again ... feel a fool and a coward ... this is not a major operation such as heart surgery etc ... angry at my weakness. Ask for double dose of sleeping pills for tonight to avoid the two o'clock horror stretch. Ask for as much oblivion in the morning as possible. Explain fear of trolley ride, operating lights etc. Anaesthetist and nurse look slightly perplexed ... am I overreacting? Anaesthetist promises oblivion. Cowardly way out as I have always had an interest in experiencing whatever was on offer. But after corridor trip last time two weeks ago that's enough. Anaesthetist leaves. Phone call from friend made in hospital last time. Again a source of courage.

Talked at great length to woman in same room ... family history of breast cancer and is having fourth lump out. Sister had a mastectomy so I found out a bit more. Knowledge is all in this case. Doctor comes in. Puts mind at ease and tells me he is not taking lymph glands as I thought he was. This news fills me with quite out-of-proportion joy. I have been so wrapped up in this breast cancer business, particularly at an accelerating rate lately, to the point that it is all I think about, and things like lymph glands become enormous issues. I had barely heard of them until the last few weeks. They regulate the fluid in the arm and if removed can cause swelling, stiffness and reduce use of the arm ... nothing to look forward to. This news sent my mood pendulum swinging high and it fortunately lasted until I had talked, watched TV and taken enough sleeping tablets to cope with the night.

TUESDAY 31 OCTOBER

Morning ... awake without a watch and not knowing the time. Two pills to put me semi conscious. Shower and hospital gown. Feeling pretty calm though eyes fill with tears occasionally. Cannot remember much of trolley ride to the theatre, certainly doped up enough not to feel fear like when the lumpectomy was done with theatre doors closing ... like gas chamber of Treblinka. Not much recollection of returning to ward. Drip in, drain out, nuisance impeding movement more than anything else. Left ex-breast padded but little pain, only a pulling feeling where drain is attached.

Feeling surprisingly calm and relaxed, mainly because of dope, I imagine. Nurses very good, backward and forward with solicitous attention ... a universally kind lot, nurses. Blood pressure, temperature all taken often. The feeling of being cared for is good. Feeling tired and groggy. Mother comes, also kids. No appetite but then not much pain either. Day passes in haze. Night comes. No sleeping tablets, drip one side, drain the other. Back pain starts, cannot get comfortable, cannot roll from side to side. Dreadful backache. More pethidine. A nightmare of a night ... fortunately no-one else in the room with me.

WEDNESDAY 1 NOVEMBER

Nausea and vomiting in morning. Cannot stand up properly, feeling dreadful. Feel a little better after breakfast. Have wash, walk about a bit. Head clearing, fear gone. Chest certainly flat ... not the courage to look at it. This is the part I've been dreading most ... that hideous gash. Still difficult to move about in bed, like in advanced stage of pregnancy, every move must be plotted to pivot and heave out of bed with least discomfort ... in this case with least pulling on tubes and stitches. Lots of visitors ... good to see. Feel very cheerful about everything, genuinely so. No really low moments yet ... is this the pattern? Will ask Cancer Foundation people when they come. Phone calls, talking to friends, nurses, other patients etc give a great boost. I sometimes stop and tell myself to do a bit of serious thinking about this operation and its consequences, but it doesn't worry me still. Maybe the anaesthetic is still protecting me a bit. Try to walk up and down the corridor, very slow of course and doubled up. Any pulling on wound is not painful but extremely unpleasant. The whole area feels vulnerable, but I guess men have had to cope with nothing much protecting their rib cages and heart. We are so used to that comforting padding. I'm glad my children are not so young they need constant cuddles ... a boney rib cage is hardly a comfort.

Wound feels so fresh and open somehow. I wonder if the sutures have come undone leaving the thing gaping. Always have hated scars ... cannot touch them even years later. I have a scar on my ankle that is 40 years old and I still cannot touch it. This new scar will be the hardest thing for me ... it may never get washed. Drip is out, which is one less burden to carry about. Drain is still in though, diminishing in amount. Night still difficult even without drip. Turning over a problem still. But discomfort is all I can complain about, the pain is nothing.

THURSDAY 2 NOVEMBER

Wake up feeling tired and headachy but determined to be a good patient. Get up and wash myself as much as possible, clean teeth. Feel better. Doctor in, asks how I am and laughs. Comments that everyone always says they feel fine when they don't. Was amused at one of his patients last week who told him she felt awful. He assures me that the wound is healing, seems bemused that I query it. Takes off dressing. I watch the nurse's face. She's very young but whatever she sees does not worry her at all. I ask what it looks like ... 20cm long and a nice cut ... some comfort. Still I cannot look. A lighter dressing is put on. I go for a walk, a bit straighter, and come back feeling a bit better. Surprising lack of pain, headache only problem apart from awful pulling sensation of scar/wound. Makes me want to curl up and walk like I have curvature of the spine.

Still feeling emotionally good. Lots of flowers and visitors help. Wonder if I am to be spared physical pain and tearful outbursts. Expected to go through boxes of tissues but have not shed a tear. Ask nurse who has had a lump removed and is generally a cheerful person to talk to about 1) Lack of emotional outbursts and 2) Lack of pain. Apparently both normal although she says the scar sighting will be a test of emotional strength. She's a one-day-at-a-time person. Also practical . . . reminds me that there are still the results of the pathology tests on the tissue etc to be seen and that check-ups are needed for some years before I can be pronounced clear. This is a worry. It seems that the hurdles are never quite cleared.

Tomorrow come the mastectomy ladies from Cancer Foundation. As nurse says, they are good to talk to—having been there, done that. I look forward to seeing people who have got back to a normal life after this enormous upheaval. It shows courage too that they remain in the cancer circle when they could break out and put it behind them, ie not make any unnecessary contact with reminders of what is an extremely unpleasant experience for anyone. Read of death of one of Monty Python people from cancer. He was I think on the TV a few weeks ago looking great and talking about his recovery from cancer and his new, healthy lifestyle which was going to promise him longevity.

FRIDAY 3 NOVEMBER

Wake up with headache and nausea. Feeling down considering previous couple of days' good progress (I consider anyway). Expecting doctor first thing, must ask about pathology reports on tissue. He does not arrive. Woman from Cancer Foundation arrives. Same person I spoke to last week. Pleasant woman but I still feel I don't want to be drawn into this exclusive club of mastectomy ladies ... give me mainstream normality please. She obviously finds me depressed, especially a flippant reference to suicide seems to upset her. She speaks of me getting some more help if I still feel bad later ... I didn't realise I felt bad now. Am not cheerful, but headache and nausea not conducive to conviviality. She is patient and explains the processes of leaving hospital, temporary prosthesis ... a sort of cotton wool sac, permanent prosthesis ... an alarming looking (picture only) orange plastic mould with a nipple, intricacies of bra renovating etc. I find it difficult to maintain an interest, was more interested in this aspect last week. Maybe too close for comfort now.

Uppermost though, I don't want to be in with this particular group of maimed humanity. Much as I admire these women who can not only get through the trauma, but can subject themselves to it again by visiting and counselling others. If I could shut the door on it I would, but then this is not a very productive way of looking at things. Poor woman sticks it out in spite of my lack of enthusiasm. We end on a better level though, talking about neutral matters. Nausea worse, eventually get an injection from nurse which seems to settle nausea and headache. Feeling depressed still. Nurse tells me third day after operation is often a downer.

Doctor comes ... pathology report shows no spreading of cancer, so that is clear, good news. Now I can get some energy sorted out—feeling very tired all day—and think about getting back to work and getting my mind on something other than my tiredness, stitches, pathology reports, sleep, nausea, temperatures, drain bottles etc. Drain bottle to remain. It is a nuisance, every move must be planned to accommodate it ... unclipping it from side of bed, not catching it on a corner and tripping over, or even worse ripping it out ... it's stitched into the wound. If wound doesn't drain properly there is possibility of haematoma[1] or some other problem which adds time and trauma to the whole business. Feeling a bit better this afternoon, wash my hair, which always has a remarkable recuperative effect. Everything is such a business though, with drains and bandages and an arm that's not working properly. I envy the nurses and visitors their freedom of movement, but who knows, they may end up in my position themselves.

Go for a walk in afternoon, an ambitious effort, not just around the floor but downstairs, out the front door and next door to the chemist's to look over the magazines and get some fresh air. Conscious of being so slow, bent and ill-looking ... everyone moves briskly past me, doing things, going places and apparently whole. I catch a reflection of myself in a window ... what the hell am I doing, in a dressing gown in the middle of the day, shuffling along, bent over and clutching a bag of blood? In chemist's I pick up a magazine. Unbelievably, 'How I beat breast cancer' is one of the articles ... put it back ... shuffle back out into the fresh air. A cool, damp day—feels delicious after the cloistered hospital wards with windows that can't be opened for fear of upsetting the air-conditioning.

Shuffle back upstairs, feeling very much an object of curiosity and probably pity by the 'unmaimed' public. Back to bed. Put on television and find breast cancer being discussed in a forum. Getting heartily sick of this emphasis on illness. Watch a bit of basketball and read some Fay Weldon—really is a treat, the sort of wit that hits the right spot. Still haven't looked at the wound. Take first downward look at the dressing, a neat oblong gauze bandage covering a flat, or probably concave, spot on left chest. It looks curious more than anything else.

SATURDAY 4 NOVEMBER

Restless start to night. Drain still in ... perforated plastic tubing sticking up under wound to drain off any fluids that might collect. If feels like it's starting to stick through my skin. Also plastic tape

---

1. Accumulation of blood.

holding bandage has got all rucked under armpit causing a burning. Call a nurse after a couple of hours . . . she takes a look. An earnest Irish girl. 'It's a lovely suture line,' she says, 'really lovely', and gives me some panadol. Sleep till morning. Day looks good. Sun for the first time in days. Birds, butterflies etc around. Auspicious start to the day that I have expected to be one of the worst. I really dislike scars. How will I cope with a twenty centimetre effort? Doctor in, takes a look, all OK. He's off on a couple of days' holiday. How I'd like to be doing that instead, or anything normal. One of the nurses is going to spend today topdressing her lawn . . . most times this sounds pretty dull but now it sounds fine.

Dressing comes off . . . scar looks surprisingly like those I have seen pictures of . . . a thin red line, not the hot-iron-on-a-piece-of-terylene effect I had thought it might be. This is not to say it's pleasant, it's not, especially when it's you. But I'm pathetically pleased to still have the pectoral muscles which lend a tiny bit of contour to the flatness. Also count the lymph glands among my blessings. Doctor says drain to come out. Good news as drain is very restrictive, not that I'm going far, and depressing. Having your bodily fluids draining into a jar is not pleasant for the patient or anyone who visits I imagine.

Drain comes out. This involves stitches being taken out . . . not a problem, a couple of deep breaths and whoosh, the tube is pulled out. Not so bad, and better out than in. Arms feels freer and so do I.

Next step, shower. Do it solo, though manage to avoid looking too closely at scar. Get a good steam-up in shower so that mirror fogs up and there are no nasty surprise glimpses of it all. Feel increasingly better after shower . . . (Is it only Australians who see showers as a cure-all? Do the Finns or Brits say, 'You'll feel better after your shower?'). Anyhow, *do* feel better until a particularly solicitous nurse asks me how I feel. I'm not sure how I'm supposed to feel. Lack of tears seems to cause more concern than tears ... the 'have a good cry and you'll feel better' idea has not completely gone. I bought a box of one hundred tissues some weeks ago and it has survived a trip to the hospital for the lumpectomy and another for the mastectomy and I reckon there are still about seventy left in the box. This is not intended as a show of personal strength, I had expected gales of tears but there have been few ... Maybe they come later (the delayed reaction!!), maybe not at all.

Making more of an effort to walk more ... mindful of home and work ahead. A short walk is one lap of the floor ... a long one is two, not at a fast pace and most of the time clutching my chest so it doesn't feel like it's falling apart. The terrible tearing feeling is not so pronounced ... Seem to be more agile. Will have to get a spurt on to be fit enough to tackle things later.

SUNDAY 5 NOVEMBER
Home day. Farewell to nurses who have shown care above and beyond their call of duty. Pack, shower and into mufti. Clothes hang ... some weight loss. Feeling fine. Still not over-anxious to look at wound/scar. Outside hospital cocoon where self-absorption is all. All attention directed at oneself ... doctors, nurses, visitors etc. Nice to feel that invalid status has been discarded. Air fresh too. Hospitals have their own slightly stale atmosphere, perhaps hothouse is a better description. Nurse has taken off final dressing from wound. Feeling very vulnerable. She laughs, knowing me and saying that I probably wish the dressing could remain, as I do. It seems like a child's bandaid to comfort. Very conscious of bumping myself. Hand goes up to protect side from anything coming. Guess this will continue for some time. Temporary fluffy prosthesis at least gives some semblance of protection, also makes me look a little more normal. Never be misled into thinking your breasts are small ... the remaining breast looks quite voluptuous next to the dead area. Feeling physically pretty strong, go for long walk in afternoon without much trouble.

TUESDAY 7 NOVEMBER

Still dread mornings. Lie in bed putting off moment of getting up and having shower. Force myself to look in mirror. To be honest, I look very like I expected to look. It's very simple ... one normal side, one like a boy with a slash across from near the breastbone to up under the arm ... no nipple, just a thin red line. I try to think of this as a lifeline, this operation has after all given me my life back, but the cost seems somehow such a cruel one. I try to think of others in worse circumstances, there are many, but this does not do much to cheer me.

I think of the possibilities of reconstruction. These involve the use of existing muscles, either from the back or the spare roll from the stomach, which are flipped somehow into the chest area and attached with the blood supply kept intact. Even the diagrams of these look horrific. The second (soft option) is an implant, which involves an operation during which a bag is inserted under the skin, filled gradually with water to stretch the skin, then filled with gel, which apparently gives a 'good feel'. Nipples are added extras.

Before the mastectomy this seemed like a good idea, some regaining of normality, though everyone is quick to point out they are not perfect. However, the people who have had them seem unanimously pleased. Now the thought of a trip back into hospital and a revival of that fear does not seem worth it. Will give it some thought later. Ring up and make appointment to get prosthesis[2] fitted. This will be a trying day, I think. Have trouble sleeping ... aches and pains around area of wound, like bruising after an accident.

WEDNESDAY 8 NOVEMBER

Shopping ... first venture into real world. How normally people seem to go about their business! Find myself again very conscious of other women's breasts and of clothes in shops ... swimsuits and low-cut dresses catch my eye constantly. Have become very

---

2. Artificial replacement for a body part.

aware of people with disabilities, limping especially. Seems a lot of people have something wrong with them. Maybe my hidden disfigurement is not so bad.

THURSDAY 9 NOVEMBER

Dual visits today—to doctor and to prosthesis fitter. Also the day which should see the end of the 'in-patient' phase of this whole business. Doctor to be visited to get general all-clear and idea of what if any further treatment. Visit passes without trauma. Doctor declares himself pleased with suture line, adds as an afterthought ... 'from a surgical point of view'. He seems more approachable today, to the point of admitting that mastectomies are operations he hates doing. He also, under pressure and somewhat amused, agrees with me that this terrible phase will finish and that in a few months I will feel completely different, ie more like a functioning human being rather than a self-pitying emotional mess.

I also manage to feel guilty that I feel bad ... double punishment ... the patient surgeon tells me, as he has before, that the type of cancer I had is the best sort to have (given that there are grades of it) in that it does not spread like the more common form of carcinoma and is very unlikely to recur or flare up again. I should feel more grateful but it's hard to forget the hideously scarred body and feel relief that I did not face death or the likehihood of it. So, in a slightly less miserable state, with self-pity still intact but eyes relatively dry, no further treatment and a follow-up visit in three months ... the intensive all-action four weeks or so have finally finished. It's been a terrible time, without doubt the worst period in my life, but even now I am hopeful that my life will take on a more positive look from now.

Second phase of the day and one I had been dreading as a tear-producer ... the visit to the prosthesis fitter. I am still loath to look at my scarred body, although the doctor looking at it and the prosthesis fitter seeing it doesn't worry me. I just don't enjoy carrying this deformity about with me. The visit was actually quite entertaining. Feeling a little like a youth entering a chemist's shop to ask for condoms, I enter the very frilly and frothy lingerie shop and ask for the fitter. She is blonde, attractive, brisk and cheerful ... and is also a mastectomy victim. Very businesslike, probably an approach she has found best when dealing with the maimed creatures who have lost so much of their self-confidence when they visit her. She whisks me into a fitting room. I strip. She, like the nurses, shows no sign of the horror I feel at the scar, just assesses the damage and works out what to do about it. We try on bras ... not the lacy type. Something more substantial and practical. Then comes the prosthesis, a neat silicone form packed according to size like a bra. It's fitted and a critical appraisal made. 'It's terrible when it's too big,' says the fitter. A few sizes are tried before she pronounces things satisfactory.

All this is going at such a pace ... the fitter has half hour appointments ... how many mastectomies are there in Perth? There really is no time for self-pity. There are even a few laughs. The next booth is occupied by a cheery soul of sixty-five or so who loudly proclaims she had a mastectomy in the early 1960s. She hears of a new recruit to the lopsided ladies league and bustles in to say hello. 'Look dear,' she says. 'I had my operation twenty-five years ago and look at me ... I'm perfectly fit.'

And so the visit passes. The day I'm pronounced fit and fitted out. This is now the end of the two-week post-operation phase and I've allowed myself to lick my wounds and sort out a few feelings. It has been a bad time but already I feel that the worst is over.

5
ENCOUNTERS WITH TREATMENT

SPECIFIC TESTS AND TREATMENTS VARY, NOT ONLY BETWEEN DIFFERENT kinds of cancer, but between individuals with the same general diagnosis. Physiological and psychological responses are highly individual, influenced by factors such as life circumstances and the respect and compassion shown by medical professionals encountered along the way. Blood tests, biopsies and scans are all part of cancer diagnosis and management. Apart from varying degrees of physical pain which many of the women described, tests were associated with the anxiety of waiting for results. Surgery, chemotherapy, radiotherapy and biotherapy—the standard medical treatments for cancer—were found to be unanimously unpleasant. While many of the women in this group offered candid, and sometimes disturbing, descriptions of their experience of tests and treatment, hope, in its various guises, helped to carry them through.

When it comes to treatments, neat categorisations which dealt with specific experiences of surgery, chemotherapy, or radiotherapy proved artificial because many women had a combination of these regimes. To break up each woman's experience of treatment into kind or phase meant that the full force of their impact on each individual was lost. Hence, treatments have been dealt with by dividing cancers into broad types and then presenting each woman's recollection of her personal encounter with treatment.

The major forms of treatment for cancer fall into three categories: surgery, chemotherapy and radiotherapy, with a fourth category, biotherapy,[1] increasingly moving from experimental research to an increasing range of therapeutic applications. Although the actual procedures involved with each of these techniques are pretty standard, each person has different reactions to, and perceptions of, even similar forms of treatment. What is more, the medical management of similar forms of cancer varies from case to case. What may be straight-forward for one, may have a significant impact on another. A treatment which causes few side-effects and works wonders in one instance may have little therapeutic effect on another, or lead to periods of sickness. Treatment is a highly individual experience which there is no 'right' or 'wrong' way to accommodate.

The women in this group approached discussion of their treatment in a way which reflects their uniqueness. In an attempt to capture the intensity of their experiences, and the ways in which they strove to come to grips with each development, each woman's story is presented as a discrete, though abbreviated, 'whole'. Some talked at length about certain aspects of their treatment and skated over other issues. Others commented only briefly on their treatment, or touched upon it in relation to themes which have been covered in other chapters.

CANCER OF THE STOMACH AND BOWEL AND MELANOMA—MARGARET W, RAE AND NOELLE

There is no routine chemotherapy for cancer of the stomach so Margaret W had two operations in the effort to arrest the spread of her stomach cancer. The first removed a large portion of her stomach. Eighteen months later she had a second operation when it was discovered she had secondaries in her liver. A pragmatic woman, she did not discuss her feelings about either operation although she did discuss the most immediate consequences of them.[2]

---

1. Biotherapy or biological treatment includes the interferons, blood cell growth factors, tumour necrosis factor, interleukins and erythropoietin. See Lowenthal (1994) pp. 60–65 for some basic information.

2. See chapter 6.

Surgery has also been the only form of treatment for Rae. She had two melanomas removed and an operation to remove a cancer of her bowel. She did not need follow-up chemotherapy because her specialist was sure he had caught the cancer at an early stage.

Post op was fine. I was up straight away, and everything was functioning very well. I had to eat ice for four days after the operation. The funny thing was that I wasn't even hungry and it didn't worry me that the other ladies in the ward were eating meals. Isn't it amazing? To me that is nature's way of saying you can't have it anyway, so why think about it. I lost some weight, but I've put it all on again now.

Rae continues to have regular examinations to check for a recurrence of melanoma.

For Noelle, recurrent operations became par for the course eighteen months after she was diagnosed, when a lump in her groin indicated that her original melanoma had spread. Most of these operations were conducted under local anaesthetic in the day ward of her local hospital, although larger or deeper lumps required removal under general anaesthetic.

The lump in my groin had pigmentations which showed that it had definitely come from my toe. They presumed that my melanoma was still contained within that lymph gland but there was always the possibility that it had got into the surrounding tissue and into the blood system. So, a week later I was back in hospital to have a good section of my groin removed because the treatment for melanoma is a block dissection to remove all the surrounding tissue and glands. By doing this they hoped to cut down the chances of the cancer cells travelling through the rest of the system. It was a two-week wait for results from that tissue. They came back negative which was a great relief at the time. Later I found out that of the huge amount of tissue that they took from my groin, only a small portion was sent away for testing. It would take years to test all the tissue so they only take small sections which meant that they did miss other cancer cells.

Since then I've been having recurring outbreaks of the melanoma. About six months after the lump from my groin was removed I had a lump come up next to my parotid gland, on the ride side of my jaw. That was removed by general anaesthetic and proved to be malignant. By that time I realised it had left the lymph system and had travelled through the blood. Three months after having the lump from my jaw removed, I had two removed from the top left hand thigh and left hand side of my stomach. A month later I had one removed from my right armpit and the left hand side of my jaw. Today I will be going to show the surgeon some more that have come up on my right hand and between my fingers. They're coming very quickly now and it's not giving me much of a chance to get myself onto an even keel. I'm quite angry about that.

With so few treatment options, Noelle sought further possibilities in complementary therapies.[3]

BREAST CANCER—MARA, ANN T AND CARMEN

Surgery was also the first stage of treatment for these women. Mara had a double mastectomy, conducted in two operations over the course of a week.[4] She recovered from both operations quickly. Her treatment did not involve any chemotherapy or radiotherapy but she was placed on the anti-hormone medication tamoxifen, which she continues to take. In contrast, Ann T and Carmen, who were younger, pre-menopausal women, underwent different surgical procedures and forms of follow-up therapy.

3. See chapter 6.
4. This decision is discussed in more detail in chapter 2.

Ann T was admitted to a private hospital in Perth to have a modified radical mastectomy of her right breast.

I remember going into the waiting room before you go into the theatre. There were trolleys everywhere and I thought, 'Jesus! I hope I'm going into the right theatre and they do the right thing here!' Anyway, I fell off to sleep and that was that. I woke up and all I could hear was my husband saying, 'It's fine, Ann. Everything's fine. They got it all.' From that moment, when I heard him say that, it was fine. I had no hassle with it. I had my operation at eight o'clock in the morning and I was actually sitting up in bed having my tea at five o'clock that afternoon. I was all right. There was nothing wrong with me! Then my specialist came in and said, 'We're ninety-nine per cent sure we've got it all. But of course, when you're ninety-nine per cent sure, you have to do something about the other one per cent, so we're going to put you on chemotherapy.' Of course I went, 'Urrgh!' But then I thought, 'God! What if I'd left it till January to get a second opinion!'

When the doctor said I had to have chemotherapy I panicked a bit. I thought that because I was having chemotherapy I still had cancer, or that the cancer was definitely there, or it would definitely come back. The nurses couldn't tell me anything about it because it wasn't a cancer ward but one of them got as many leaflets for me as she could. I sat there and studied them and I wasn't scared any more. I found out they were only giving me a six-month dose of chemotherapy which meant it was really a preventative rather than a cure for cancer that was already there. That relaxed me.

I had my first lot of chemotherapy in hospital on the Monday following the operation. I remember one of the doctors saying, 'God, this is powerful stuff! If it gets on our skin, it's going to burn us.' I thought, 'What the hell is it doing around my body?' But then I'd think, 'No. It's killing all those little cancer cells. I'll do this, get over it and everything will be fine.' The chemo didn't react for about six hours and I was walking along chatting away. I don't know what I did but I felt very tired and everybody looked at me and said, 'You're going back to bed!'

After that I was to go as an outpatient once every month, two weeks on, two weeks off providing my blood count was all right. Some ladies I'd get talking to in outpatients had been having chemo for two or three years so I thought, 'Jeez! I am lucky.' I stayed in Perth for the first lot of chemotherapy and then I went back home.

We lived so far up north that I got the isolated patients allowance so I flew down for the second round of chemotherapy. But I hate flying so the third time, I exchanged one air ticket for three bus tickets so my husband and son came down with me. After that they arranged for me to have my treatment at the medical centre in our town. They didn't like doing it but it was too far for me to travel all the time. They had to do a blood test before any chemotherapy was given so I used to get up at five o'clock in the morning, go down to the medical centre in town and ring the bell for one of the sisters to take my blood. Then my blood had to go by plane out to the mine site, get flown over to Karratha and then down to Perth to be tested. They would phone back within four or five hours to say if my blood count was all right and I could have the chemotherapy. I got knocked back twice and I'd have to wait another week because my red blood count was down. I was looked after so well up there.

Through the chemotherapy there were days when I reacted badly to it. I went back to work part time until the chemo was over. I was on my second lot of chemo and I felt so sick that I felt I had to lie down. Afterwards my doctor said that was the worst thing I could do. He said, 'Don't lie around on your *tummy. Move. Get going.' So I thought, 'That's it, I'm going back to work full-time.'*

One particular day was dreadful. I was at work and there was nobody else to take over. There was nothing I could do so I just had to keep going. Once my doctor had told me not to lie down while I was having chemo, just to get up and go, I did. I actually had a sixteen kilometre run in the middle of treatment because I felt running would get it out of me sooner. By the end of the chemo I couldn't face Mylanta or any of that white, gluggy gunk that you had to take. The thing I found most beneficial were the little Quick-eze tablets.

Carmen had a different experience. Her breast cancer developed secondaries.

I had a lumpectomy and I had a bad experience with the anaesthetic. I was nauseous for about thirty hours and I couldn't stop vomiting. That was terrible. It was the worst nausea I had experienced in my life and I was going to give up there and then. Three days after my operation my husband noticed that the battery that was used to drain the lymph fluid from the operation site was flat, but they didn't replace that battery until the next day so my wound leaked all over the bed linen. Even after they had dressed the wound again and changed the battery, nobody noticed that the lymph fluid still wasn't draining properly: although my bandages were soaked, the container into which the fluid was supposed to drain was empty, so the doctors discharged me. Three days later I noticed swelling up under my arm so the next day I contacted the hospital and was told to come in immediately to have it drained.

So twelve days after my first operation, I was back at the hospital having fluid drained, my stitches removed and being told the results of the pathology tests. The doctor said that I would have to go on chemo because the cancer had gone into the lymph nodes. I had my first chemo injection on the Wednesday and I had tablets to take on the Thursday and Friday. The nausea was terrible but I was so proud because I'm usually really forgetful, and I had taken them all at the right time. On the Friday morning after I first started chemo I went for the radiotherapy planning session. I was numb and I wasn't really aware that my arm was all red and swollen because I thought that it was supposed to be sore as I'd had an operation. I was too scared to complain so I put up with it. When the doctor saw it he exclaimed, 'She can't have radiotherapy. Look at that infection!' They sent me down to oncology and they put me straight into hospital for five days. I didn't have time to get pyjamas or anything. The next thing I know they'd taken my chemo tablets away from me and put me on antibiotics.

For the antibiotics, they stuck needles all the way up both arms, and all the fluid went into the tissues because my veins collapsed. Oh, the pain. I'm trying to be a saint—not complaining—but in the end I had to say that I couldn't face another needle so they sent me home on tablets. Before I could start chemo again I had to have a port put in. They put it exactly where you adjust your bra, and they bruised me so badly that they couldn't use it. So, altogether, I had a break of four weeks from the chemo because of that infection and my veins. By then I was terrified to go back on it because of the nausea that I had experienced the first time. I don't like to think of the bad side so I've been telling myself: 'I'm okay. There's nothing wrong. Three more months I'll be back to normal.' To be honest, I'm totally confused!

I stayed at home for about eight weeks when I was having the radiotherapy and I lost interest in life. I just wanted to stay in bed and sleep. I didn't want to get dressed. Sometimes I could have got up but you lose interest because there isn't anything to get up for. I really didn't have the energy to go to the kitchen to wash the dishes and when I did wash them I was panting. I really did need somebody side by side with me to take me for a little walk or something. I was alone most of the sick period. It hasn't been very nice in that respect. Then the phone calls were too many! It was a very mixed up period for me.

Now I'm halfway through chemo. I've had three months and I've got three months left. I'm counting these three months to get them over with so that I can start living again. I'm just getting up, coming to work, dragging my feet. I go in as a day patient—two weeks on, two weeks off. They don't tell you that in the beginning, so you don't know what your procedure is and when I asked the doctor she said: 'You'll soon find out as you go along.' I was totally confused about when I was going to have it or when I wasn't, and how much I was having.

My first reaction to chemo was a terrible sore stomach right in the middle, and I wanted to go to the toilet badly. I just managed to get to the toilet. The nurse had to carry the chemo bag right through all these people at the reception. When I got to the toilet it was just like water but so painful. It hasn't happened again but in the beginning I was absolutely terrified that I was going to have bad accidents. They didn't warn you about that reaction.

I was at the peak of fitness when I was diagnosed and I think that's why I'm handling the chemo so well. I didn't have a lot of nausea but when I did, it was terrible and it came on me so suddenly that I didn't have time to combat it. They did give me tablets for nausea but in the beginning I didn't recognise when it was coming. I was confused about my feelings. I didn't know how I felt because I was in shock. You want to get better but you're tired and everyone's throwing thousands of questions at you, trying to help. In the beginning I found there were too many interruptions. You needed to have *peace and quiet because everybody is so anxious to be so sympathetic. I found that very disturbing.*

CANCER OF THE TONGUE AND NECK—KAYE

Kaye didn't have to have chemotherapy, although she had two rounds of major surgery to excise growths in her tongue and neck. Both operations involved lengthy periods of hospitalisation, with follow-up radiotherapy after the second operation.

I had to have skin taken from under my arm and grafted on my tongue because, along with the cancer, the doctor had to remove a major part of my tongue. When I woke up after the operation, the first thing I said was, 'Did you get it all?' They were ninety-nine per cent sure that they had but I could never get them to say they were a hundred per cent sure. My doctor told me it had been a big operation, but that he'd left me some taste buds. I hadn't even thought about that side of it—that because the taste buds are on the top of your tongue I could have lost them all. I was glad that I didn't because it would have been terrible not being able to taste anything. I was in hospital for quite a few weeks because they had to make sure the skin graft would take and that there wouldn't be any infection. It was a very boring time but the staff were very nice. They gave me work to do to keep me busy.

Funnily enough there wasn't much pain from the operation. In fact my tongue was numb for a long time. I was fed through a tube down my throat because no food was allowed to touch the graft while it was healing. The tube was irritating at first—I think it scratched my throat as it went down. I was given some painkillers for this. The liquid they put down the tube came straight out of the fridge and was cold. I couldn't taste anything but they told me the liquid was nutritional and would give me a feeling of fullness. The smell of the other patients' food, and watching them eat, was hard, so I was fed early and then I would go for a walk while they ate.

When the tube was finally removed I was able to eat soft foods. It sounds awful but with all the stitches and the numbness it took all my time to make the food go down because it would catch on my tongue. The doctor watched the skin graft closely because, as the new skin grew underneath, the old skin would slough off. Finally I was allowed to go home, and was told to come back for check-ups.

It was during one of these check-ups that a biopsy on a new lump confirmed that some 'rogue cells' had escaped so Kaye was booked in by her ear, nose and throat specialist for a second major operation.

He more or less explained that it was going to be quite a radical operation. It didn't worry me. All I could think of was, 'I don't care what type of operation you do as long as you get all the cancer out.' The worst part was having to tell my husband that I had to have another operation and then get through the time waiting. What upset me was that when I first went in they put me in a private room. To me, the real sick people went into a private room. They told me that when you come back from the operation they like to keep an eye on you so the private room is better. The registrar came in and explained to me what was going to happen and how much was going to be cut out. I just said, 'Oh yes.' He was surprised that I wasn't more upset.

They took me down and then I remember them calling me to wake me up. I vaguely remember them putting me in the bed and the doctor saying, 'Kaye? Smile for me.' I was wondering what I was meant to smile for, but I obliged as best I could. He said, 'That's not too bad. You've got a bit of an Elvis Presley smile.' The incision had gone from under my chin up to behind my ear and down to my collarbone and they were worried that they had cut a nerve that could have affected the side of my mouth. At the time, of course, I was so dopey that I couldn't figure out what he was talking about.

That first night after the operation I was propped up in bed with drains in my neck wondering what my wound looked like. The nurses were reluctant to give me a mirror and I couldn't get up by myself. I was still very sleepy so I didn't press the issue. When my husband came in he had our son and daughter with him, as well as his mother. I asked why he had brought them in so soon and he said that he had intended to leave the kids with his mother but that they had all wanted to come and see me. I was upset that the kids were seeing me looking the way I did: as soon as they walked in the door their faces dropped in shock and my mother-in-law said: 'Ooh! You poor thing.' I had no bandages on so what they were seeing was a long wound with stitches up and down my neck covered in mercurochrome, and drains coming out.

Seeing the look on their faces I asked: 'What do I look like?' My husband answered, 'It's all right. It looks worse than it is because of all the red paint on it.' My kids acted as if they were too scared to talk or touch me in case they hurt me. It took a while to get them to relax. When I next saw the nurses they told me that my specialist always tried to make the least possible scar so he used minimal stitches. When I was able to see myself in a mirror I realised what they meant. I was too scared to move my head in case the stitches would break and my wound open up. My doctor took my stitches out as soon as possible so they wouldn't leave marks. He said that even though it was a tiny lump he had gone that far because he was trying to get ahead of the cancer to make sure there wasn't any left. I was glad I had him.

Once I had physically recovered from that operation, I had radiotherapy for my neck at a private clinic. They were very good. I went, I think, every day for two weeks. It was something like that. Of course I was worried I was going to lose my hair but they said that only happened with chemotherapy. They did the therapy on my neck and had to block off my shoulder and jaw with a lead pad. They left an open square that they would target with this plastic piece with dots on it. Then they'd push a few buttons and walk out of the room and leave me there. It didn't hurt or really burn but it made the skin go dry. They told me to use only baby soap, if I had to use any soap at all, and to put lanolin on it to keep the skin moist.

Of course the radiotherapy had side effects. I lost my taste again. I think it took about a week after I stopped treatment to regain it. I was very tired and would sleep all the afternoon when I went home. I had a little bit of nausea, but I've been told it was not as bad as chemo. Thank goodness I never had to go through that. I think radiotherapy did affect me because I had to have all my teeth out when they went all chalky and crumbled. Still, all that treatment was in 1980 and apart from a few scar tissue lumps there hasn't been any recurrence. I'm still very self-conscious about my scar although people say they can hardly notice it. I know it's there.

BRAIN TUMOURS—MARINOMOANA

Marinomoana has no scars to mark the site of her treatment.

I won't allow any surgery because they just want to have a look. In my BRAIN! The tumour is not like a large solid mass. Apparently it's more like spaghetti. So what are they going to look at if they open me up? It's bad enough that they stick needles all over you and stick that hat thing on your head for the electroencephalograms.[5] That also hurts.

---

5. The trace obtained when the electrical activity of the brain is recorded by means of electrodes placed upon the intact scalp.

Nearly two years after she had first been to a neurologist because of her deteriorating reflexes, a CT scan indicated that Marinomoana had developed two new 'dark areas' at the back of her brain. This made a total of four pin-sized growths, enough for her specialists to give her a very bleak prognosis.[6]

All of a sudden they wanted me in for chemo. One of the things that they kept worrying about were the migraines that I didn't have. That they kept insisting I should have. It was really strange! After a couple of bouts I started thinking, What are you going to give me and why are you giving me these doses of toxic waste? It seemed like they don't even know what they're doing. That's the impression I got when I was asking them why I had to have all this. I only had three actual treatments of chemo. I don't know what sort of chemo they gave me. I don't think I ever asked and even if they had told me I don't think I would have remembered. During that time I went through a really big blockout period when I tried to push people away from me. I know now that was wrong, but I was doing it because I was going through a terrible time and I just didn't believe that this was happening to me. Chemo was one of the things I really wanted to block out.

I had three rounds of radiotherapy because my tumour multiplied to eight areas and I was very, very sick. They hit panic stations and thought maybe we could stop it with radiation therapy. I wanted them to try anything. They had to be very careful about the concentration they used because of where the tumour was in the brain. I was so anxious that they gave me tranquillisers or sedatives so I was asleep through the whole procedure. But, you know, they fry you! It feels like you've been toasted. For me the saddest thing is that the radiotherapy treatment took away all chance of having more children. That's no longer an option. Radiotherapy stopped in 1992 and I have been declared in remission because I've had

---

6. See chapter 1.

nothing go wrong with me for the two-year period. The tumours are still there and that worries them but there's been no new growths and I still don't suffer headaches.

MULTIPLE MYELOMA—TINY

Tiny had a combination of radiotherapy and chemotherapy in the treatment of multiple myeloma, commonly called cancer of the bone marrow.

At first, although they had taken CT scans and X-rays, they weren't sure how spread the myeloma was through my body. They thought it was quite a light dose but afterwards they found out that I have one of the heaviest cases they'd seen. The first five weeks in hospital I had to have radiotherapy once a day, five days a week for two and a half weeks. They had to do it quickly because otherwise I might lose the feeling in my legs completely. I never feel anything with the radiotherapy. I was so surprised. My skin went brown, like it was burnt on the back. You can still see a dark spot after two years. I couldn't keep my food down so I lost a lot of weight. They are not sure if the radio worked because there is still a little dark spot showing on the X-ray which might have been from that tissue, left after radiotherapy. Or it might be the start of MS. That is the reason that I ask for the CT scan again: I'd like to know what it is because when you leave it too long maybe it is worse then. They're very supportive except when you talk about herbs or carrot juice or something like that!

After the radiotherapy, I went onto oral chemotherapy. I had just over a year of tablets when they decided that it would be better to give me the highest dose of chemo through IV. Every month for one day I went to the hospital for blood tests because if my white blood cells weren't high enough I couldn't have treatment. I have had chemo nine times, three times through the Hickman line and then they had to take that out and start again for another six times. I had tablets that were supposed to settle my stomach down, but they didn't seem to work because I would bring everything up. I couldn't keep any food down at all. I was on so many tablets at that time that I can't remember what they were.

Everything the doctors said would happen didn't happen. They said I was going to lose my hair: I didn't. One time they said that my white blood count was so low after a blood transfusion that I had to be sick but I wasn't: I felt quite well. Another time when I was not so good they said I'd feel better after a blood transfusion, but I never noticed any difference. After the heavy chemo you're supposed to feel really sick. The main problems I had with that intravenous chemo was that my bones got sore two days afterwards. I got out of hospital on Fridays and on Sunday my bones would be sore. And I got infections every time about a week after treatment. The first time I got an infection in the IV site, where they put the IV line. The second month it was infection in the eye. It was very bad and I had to stay ten days in the hospital with it. The third time, they had trouble with the Hickman line so they put in a port. But then I got blood clots down my neck and they had to thin my blood so much that I couldn't have chemo for over six months. I've had so many infections. I think my white blood cell count was so low that I was susceptible to bugs, although I didn't get the flu.

I did not like being hooked up to the IVAC[7] machine for chemotherapy. That was not nice. I was happy when I got off. You have to take the machine every step you go on your own, and when you have to go to the showers, the nurse has to go with you to take your nightie off. I didn't like it. It is like being on a leash. And if I wasn't on that machine it would be a drip to flush the chemo through every two hours during the night,

---

7. Equipment which regulates the amount of intravenous fluid entering the body.

and every three weeks for a year and a half I had to have a blood transfusion. Even when I wasn't hooked up there would be something else to make me sore, like a bone marrow biopsy, so that I couldn't sleep properly even then. I just had to laugh.

LOW-GRADE LYMPHOMA—ANNIE AND MARGARET P
As with multiple myeloma, surgery is not an option for cancers of the lymphatic system, except for the removal of specific tumours which are causing discomfort. For Annie, whose lymphoma has been complicated by the development of an associated arthritic condition, spondyloarthropothy, treatment has involved radiotherapy and ongoing regimes of chemotherapy.

I've had two lots of radiotherapy. The first one was really scary. All I could see when I was having the actual blast was the Hiroshima Peace Memorial and Museum. That's all I could picture for this whole minute of having to lie very still, knowing that you're being blasted with the stuff that killed millions of people. But you get used to it and it doesn't become scary any more. With the first dose I got radiation burns that required some burns dressings. It was a huge patch under my arm, up to my ear and halfway down my neck. It's weakened my bottom jaw so that my teeth are not as firm as they used to be and I've had both sides done so that the whole bottom jaw is now weaker.

Getting radiation isn't painful. You don't feel anything. I had two days of radiation sickness during which I slept. Then it was over and I was absolutely normal. If I had a choice, I'd go for radiotherapy any time because I can handle it much better than chemo. It's quick and clean and it's all done in a month or six weeks and then you're on your way. It's not like chemo that drags on for months. At least, that's the way it's been for me.

I've been on seven different regimes of chemo so far. I remember being absolutely terrified when I started even though the first chemo was just a pill which you took at home. I remember sitting here and forcing myself to put this pill in my mouth. I didn't have a clue what would happen to me. I imagined that I had a headache, although it really had nothing to do with the chemo. That chemo only lasted one session because the cancer seemed to thrive on it. I had three different regimes of intravenous chemotherapy which didn't really work then an oral lot of chemotherapy called Etoposide which I took for eighteen months. I took one tablet every day for three weeks and then had a one week break and it worked brilliantly. I could work full-time and take chemo and have no side-effects. But it's got to the stage where the lymphoma has become resistant to it so from now on chemotherapy is going to be really heavy hospital stuff for several days.

On chemo, my hair thinned but I'd always had to have it thinned at the hairdresser so it saves all the hassles! I did have severe vomiting after one regime of heavy chemo—enough to go into casualty. I had the most incredible, violent vomiting I've ever experienced and nausea, like, you can't describe it. It consumes your entire body. You've got no control over anything. It was dreadful, and I was straight into casualty on both occasions. Even with direct medical intervention, with all the Maxilon and Stemetil injections, there was still nothing that would stop it! I just had to ride through about eight hours of these vomiting fits, every fifteen minutes on the dot. I learnt how to ride through that by not fighting it. But I was getting too many side effects so they stopped that particular chemo regime. Over six months of having different regimes, each one getting heavier and heavier I developed a routine: for the first week after I'd had chemo I'd be in bed for three days and then gradually get up. The second week was building up my strength. The third week I was back to normal, and then I had chemo again.

The last lot of chemo was in-house stuff every three weeks, for three days in hospital hooked up to chemo for five hours a day. There were two big side-effects—extreme boredom and I completely lost my hair. I handled the boredom by going for endless walks around the hospital when I wasn't attached to the drip. When I was attached, I would try to sleep. I listened to my radio endlessly and became a full bottle on current affairs. Losing my hair was traumatic. It came out over a two-day period. Most of it came out under the shower when I tried to wash it after it became sore. Sore hair? It felt like it was going to break. There was masses of hair and I was scared that it was going to clog up the bathroom drains. I rescued most of it, put it out on a tray to dry in the sun and then put it in a plastic bag. I cried solidly for two hours and then tried to get on with it. But there is a good ending to the sorry story—it grew back darker than before and it's curly. I've never had curls—always straight hair—and I love it. But it was not easy to have a bald head, no eyelashes or hair anywhere else. It was such a relief when it started to grow back.

TIPS FOR DEALING WITH HAIR LOSS

- Not everyone loses their hair, even with heavy chemo. Only two women in the Women's Cancer Group completely lost their hair. Others found that their hair thinned or changed in texture. But it is better to be prepared.
- Either buy, hire or borrow a wig which matches your hair colour and style before you go on chemo—even if you don't have to use it. It is the sense of security that

you have something in the top of your wardrobe. Although a purple wig with long bouncy curls might seem like a good idea to cheer you up, you might have to actually wear the wig every day for months and it is better to have something that you and others are used to.
- Make a couple of beanies from T-shirt material. They are soft and warm and good for wearing around the house.
- If it is summer and too hot to wear a wig, beanie or scarf, or if, like Noelle, you believe in turning any crisis into an opportunity, you can always 'paint your pate'! Noelle had a beautiful, colourful dragon painted on her head by a talented loved one.
- After the initial shock, friends easily adapt to seeing you bald. Don't be afraid to go bare-headed if it suits—and it is the latest fashion—half your luck!
- Hair normally grows back, sometimes better than it was before. You might get lucky, like Annie, and find you've had a permanent perm!

Margaret P's lymphoma has a relationship to leukaemia. Her story illustrates how different kinds of treatment can be used at different stages of a lymphoma and indicates the varieties of chemotherapy used. It also shows that no-one can predict precisely how a person will react to a particular combination of chemotherapy drugs, nor how long any given individual may be able to tolerate them.

The only surgery I've had is two biopsies from the side of my neck. The second one they actually took a big lump out while they were doing it. That's fairly minor surgery, just a couple of stitches and a drain in your neck. They did that under a general. I had one session of radiotherapy on the back of my head where I had three small tumours pressing on a nerve causing bad headaches. I lost my hair across the back of my head and I got bad ulcers so that I couldn't put my teeth in for weeks. I used to slap gel in so that I could eat but I had to leave them out the rest of the time, which is not flattering.

When I was first diagnosed in 1988 I was put on prednisolone, which is a steroid, and Chlorambucil, which is an anti-cancer drug, three times in a row because each time my lumps went down. In that time, I had a three-month remission and then, after another dose, a whole year without any treatment. After about three years, that combination stopped working so in 1992 I was put on Etoposide. That was brilliant, just tablets with hardly any side-effects. I took it for six months which enabled me to get over the steroids.

Then, in April 1993, my lymphoma got a lot more aggressive. They'd tried everything they'd got right throughout 1993, and none of it worked. In August I started on a slow infusion of a mixture called MIME.[8] The slow infusion meant that I had to be in hospital several days for treatment, having an infusion of each drug every day. One of those drugs looks like Indian Ink and you pee electric blue for a couple of hours. Obviously it is pretty tough on your kidneys. That treatment stopped me from getting any worse but it didn't knock any of the tumours back and my white cell count got very low, which meant I had a lot of infections. I was in and out of hospital, six times in nine weeks, and the registrar came to the conclusion that I was in more danger from the treatment than the illness so we stopped the treatment. I felt so much better for not having that treatment but two months later I realised that everything was on the grow so in January 1994 my oncologist decided we're going to do ESHAP.[9]

I felt really depressed because nothing so far had worked

---

8. MIME—based on initials for Mitazantrone, iphosphomide, mesna (which is a recovery agent to help minimise some of the negative effects) and ETOPOSIDE.

9. ESHAP—Etoposide, Solu-Medrol, H only stands for high dose, ARA-C and Platinum.

and my oncologist said this was the last treatment they had: there was nothing else. ESHAP takes about four-and-a-half days to administer and by the end of that first week I couldn't even drink water without feeling sick. I decided I was going to tell my oncologist to stuff it. I thought, 'If I've got to die, I might as well do it without all this chemo. This isn't living.' When I went home I had given up totally but then two or three days later, out of curiosity, I started having a feel around and I thought, 'Where have these lumps under my arm gone?' I didn't believe it, but when I went back to the doctor the next week they were still going down and I'd lost about six kilos. My oncologist looked at my neck and said, 'Your neck is a lot thinner.' He had a feel and said, 'You have made my day!' I said, 'I'll tell you what—it's made mine!' He showed me the CT scans from the previous week, and you couldn't count those lumps. They were all around my throat and neck. So it was a good job that the ESHAP worked because I was worse inside than we thought.

The ESHAP was working brilliantly on me. But it was interesting because, although they did slightly change the medication for my second dose of ESHAP, I felt nowhere near as bad in hospital the second treatment, and I have to wonder if that was my mental state. My lumps had gone down so fast it was ridiculous and, although I was desperately tired, I was floating on air. I could feel the lumps going down day by day, and I could stop taking Panadeine Forte for the pain, except at bedtime. I had been taking it three or four times a day. So it looks as though I can have six lots of ESHAP if my body can stand it, although platinum is tough stuff.

It sounds silly, but there's one thing I dislike about the ESHAP: They give you a three-litre plastic jug and for twenty-four hours before you go in you have to pee in it. Sometimes they put something like acid in it and the smell is *absolutely nauseous. The jug has a narrow neck, which would be fine if you were a fella but isn't so easy for a woman to aim at. So you have to take a bowl out of your supplies, pee in the bowl and then pour it into this jug. It's one of those silly little things which don't sound as if it matters much but you can imagine what it's like when you get up in the middle of the night. You're wide awake by the time you've finished farting around, and I am usually up at least three times during the night. They give you a blue plastic bag to carry the jug around in so nobody knows what you are carrying when you go to the hospital the next day. They have to do it to measure your output and check that your kidneys are doing all right.*

Margaret P went on to have eight regimes of ESHAP and then no treatment for six months. The price of this was some nerve and bone damage and hearing loss, but as she said: 'I'm still alive so it was worth it.' In March 1996 she was placed on another less effective but less damaging chemo regime which has kept her lymphoma just under control for a few months. By June she was back in hospital and facing the prospect of whole body radiotherapy to inhibit the growth of tumours which have 'cropped up all over the place'.

CHRONIC MYELOID LEUKAEMIA—ANNE K

Anne K was diagnosed in 1986. She had four years of oral chemotherapy whenever her 'white blood count would start climbing very high'. This treatment would give her periods of remission, sometimes for eight months, sometimes for as long as fourteen months, before her leukaemia would start to reactivate.

I was living from one remission to the next but I found ways to manage. The bad days I absolutely refused to lie down. On my worst days I went to aerobics. It sounds rather crazy but I was like a lunatic. I didn't just go to aerobics—I had to be in the front row kicking and stretching. I can see it now. This stick woman saying 'no way, Rae!' I kept very busy with the kids and running around. I pushed as much into every day as I could and I just wouldn't let it get to me. There were days when I was very bad and I had to say 'OK. Fine.' But they were few and far between, and I would hold out as long as I could to give the boys time to grow up a bit because they were very young. Also I wanted my husband to be more established in his work. But then you reach a point when you can't do this any more. You've two choices: you either have the bone marrow transplant or you die. Eventually the day came when I couldn't put it off any longer and I had to bite the bullet and go for the transplant.

The transplant was quite dramatic. I think there would probably have been twelve to fourteen people present during the transplant. I was in a little private ward and I was conscious, sitting in bed. You get a mega dose of chemotherapy which kills off cancerous bone marrow. You reach what they call the critical point after all the chemo has gone through and your own bone marrow is dead, then you get your transplant. They feed the medium via the IV to the Hickman line in your chest. That goes directly into the main valves in your heart and pumps it around your system.

They predetermine a nurse who is going to look after you for that period. She is allocated solely to get you through that procedure and through the next few days. She was there all the time, helping me through like a guardian angel. I grabbed hold of her hands and wouldn't let them go. She was wonderful, a skilled nurse who talked to me all the way through. She kept the conversation very light. Nobody talked over my head; that might have been a team effort or it might have been her refusing to let them—it's hard for me to decide. Everybody spoke to me during the procedure so it wasn't a cold or inhumane experience for me. I felt as if I was part of the group. I didn't feel alone. There wasn't any member of my family present because my husband didn't make it in time. He had intended to be there but they moved the procedure up by about twenty minutes and it was all over when he came. I think he was quite shocked to find it was over.

When the transplant is over, they whip you off to the life island[10]—my little glass room. From that moment on you're pretty much on your own. You don't have too many visitors because your system is going to crash. Then, a few days later you start the follow-up chemo. The staff are very much aware you're on your own and I found them very supportive. If I had to ring for anything they would be there instantly. They popped in all the time to keep an eye on me and to talk to me. I had very specialist nursing from a few nurses. They obviously take it seriously and did anything that they possibly could to make an uncomfortable situation more comfortable.

I was in the life island for three-and-a-half weeks. It was terribly spooky. There are times when you think: 'Is this transplant going to take? Will I reject or will I hold it?' It's a difficult period of waiting to see what is going to happen. I can't remember how often I had to have chemo but I used to dread it. It was all injected from the other side of the glass box through tubes tied up with the Hickman line. That was really unpleasant. I hated it. Sleeping was the biggest problem I found in the life island but there were other problems from the chemo. Your oesophagus gets burnt all the way down and you get mouth and gum ulcers. You have a regimented mouth care regime which starts two weeks

---

10. The life island was a 10 by 6 foot glass cubicle designed as a sterile environment to minimise risk of infection. Advances in marrow transplantation mean that life islands are no longer required. Now bone marrow transplants are managed in specialised single rooms.

before your transplant, to make sure you are not carrying around any bugs, and goes on indefinitely afterwards. If you are carrying around any bugs they take off as soon as your system crashes. That ulcerated throat was very painful. Life in general is very uncomfortable, very unpleasant.

I'd get through by thinking, 'Tomorrow will be a better day. Never say die!' I used to lie on the bed, this stick woman with a bald head and a swollen face from all the drugs, saying to my nurses, 'I'm not going out of here in a wheelchair.' They would say, 'Most people do, Anne.' I would lie on that bed and, if I had a good hour between procedures, I'd lie there doing my leg exercises. I had no muscle so I would do leg lifts and lift books to build up my arm muscles. Then I'd walk up and down for maybe three or four minutes before I'd have to sit down because I was too sick. When I felt a little better I'd get up and walk up and down again. When I think of it now, I must have looked like a lunatic but it worked for me. You do what you have to do and that was making me feel good.

I remember one of the nurses passed by one day and shouted, 'How are you going, Anne?' She couldn't see me because of the curtains on the inside of the room. She didn't hear any reply so she came in. Now, it's freezing cold in the life island, although the cold is also a condition of the patient—your body temperature drops and it is very hard to keep warm. There I was with two pairs of socks, two big thick sweaters, lying on my back doing my leg lifts. She shook her head and said, 'What are you doing?' I said, 'I am doing my leg exercises. I want to walk out of here!' When they finally broke the barrier and somebody could actually walk into the life island they said, 'As you're so keen on aerobics, we've decided we're going to bring you up an exercise bicycle.' They brought up this little exercise bike for me and I used to sit there pedalling, trying to get my legs back. It was difficult but it was good. I didn't just walk out of there, I skipped out!

CANCER OF THE BOWEL AND OVARIES—BETH

Beth was admitted for exploratory surgery after blood tests, an ultrasound, CT scan and a biopsy indicated that she had primary cancerous growths in her bowel and ovaries.[11]

The nurses were great. They spent a lot of time trying to allay my fears when the enormity of the whole thing hit me and I fell into a bit of a heap. And the anaesthetist was great. He told me what he would be doing, asked if I had any problems, warned me that I would have a lot of pain and told me how they would deal with that. I told him that I get bilious after surgery and so he gave me tablets instead of an injection pre-med. The tablets made me very light headed and chatty and, even though I am told I didn't make much sense, I talked to everyone who would listen and chatted away to the staff, introducing myself to the orderlies and people in the lift on the way up to theatre. I was also wary of having an epidural for pain but after the surgery I appreciated the help with pain control until, one day, I looked up and 'saw' thousands of black ants crawling up and down the walls. That was scary and the apparent movement of all these ants made my eyes hurt. I think I must have been getting too much pethidine because the ants disappeared when we turned the drip down. Now I think I know what a bad trip must be like. It was an awful feeling.

I had a lot of pain after surgery. I had been fit, walking most days and going to aerobics three times a week. The surgeon said this level of fitness had helped to get me through. As I recovered from the operation I started gentle exercise again but I started to get a sharp burning pain

11. See chapter 1.

> near my suture line which stopped me. I told my surgeon about it and he said, 'It looks like a pinched nerve which will probably go away in a few months. You're actually very lucky. We didn't think you'd be here so you should be grateful. A pinched nerve is nothing.' I hesitated to make any further comment. He said they could open up the scar and try to find the nerve, but as long as I know what it is and that it is not something to do with the cancer, it doesn't matter. I can live with it as long as I know. It is while you don't know that you worry.

After her operation, Beth started chemotherapy.

> I've lost all my veins through chemo treatment, so it hurts when they're putting in the chemo line. After a few months I've got black vein burns up my arm and the nurse—who is the best needle giver I've met—can't always get the whole dose into one vessel because they collapse. This means that some weeks I have to have two or three needles, and that hurts. I have a shorter chemo weekly for two weeks and then a long one for the third week and then I have the fourth week off—which is great. I'm not as sick as some people although I get bad nausea, some vomiting, and mouth ulcers if I eat spicy or acid foods. I haven't lost all of my hair but it has gone grey, thin and lifeless. I don't like having chemo. I know I have to have it but I dread Tuesdays. I do visualisation and relaxation to get me through, and the nurse is great—she rarely leaves us alone.

CANCER OF THE FALLOPIAN TUBES—JULIE

Julie had more problems with the chemotherapy regime she was placed on to treat cancer of the fallopian tubes. Before that she had a hysterectomy during which a tumour was removed. Uncertainty whether she had cancer of the ovaries or fallopian tubes, and the need to find out if the cancer had spread, meant she had to have a second operation.

I had three weeks before my next operation and I was determined to make the most of the time I had before the second operation. I couldn't do much but I sat near the pool to take in the sunshine. I was not looking forward to the second operation and I had lost about three stone in weight and was very weak. In fact I said to the oncologist who was to do the next operation, 'I don't think I'm strong enough to get through this.' If he'd not been positive I don't think I could've coped. He cut me vertically from the pubic hair line up past the navel to remove the omentum which could harbour cancerous cells, and to check some of the lymph glands. I recall waking up from the anaesthetic and hearing the doctor say, 'It's all over and we haven't found any cancerous cells this time. Can you hear me?' Do I hear you! That was very important because I was hearing something positive for the first time. For almost a month I'd sat in fear waiting for this second operation but I seemed to recover incredibly well and I only stayed in hospital for about twelve days.

Hearing the positives was a plus for me but I didn't like the word chemotherapy and I didn't want to hear of radiotherapy. The doctors would come in and say, 'We're still not quite sure which way to treat this. We're working on it.' That frightened me. I guess you're frightened of the unknown so I decided to adopt the attitude of one day at a time. Whilst I'm in this hospital I'm going to rest, sleep, eat and get all the strength that I can. I'm going to get well and then I'm going to take the next step. This is how I mentally handled it. During this time Mum's lymphoma was getting worse and my husband's blood pressure shot up and he was sent to hospital, which left my daughter at home to cope. It certainly didn't help things.

The first chemotherapy session was about three weeks after the second operation. I had a mop of hair and I was pretty proud of it. Vanity was really taking over and I don't think I remembered to ask anything else except, 'Oh, God! Am I going to lose my hair?' My oncologist said, 'I don't know. I don't think so.' That's the first time I realised that not all chemotherapy patients lose their hair. I didn't realise that there were different types of chemotherapy. At this stage they thought I was going to have eight to ten months on intravenous chemotherapy and a further six to eight months on tablet form. But they said they'd work it out as we went along and saw how I was going on it. So, I was admitted to yet another hospital with yet another bunch of nurses to get used to. On the outside I was so brave but I really was frightened. I'd had two shocks and I really didn't know what was going to happen with the chemo.

I was admitted into hospital because this was my first treatment and I had to stay overnight to see how I'd cope with it. A very abrupt nurse on the cancer ward came along and introduced herself. She said she would have to wait for the doctor to put the bung[12] *in. (I can't stand that word bung because I can remember this tube in my hand . . .) Then she said that they would connect me to a bag of saline which would wash through my system, then they would put a bag of chemotherapy up and that would run through and then they would put another bag of saline to wash me through again. The whole procedure would take seven hours, or something like this. Then I was left. I was really frightened. I didn't know whether it was going to make me sick straight away, whether I was supposed to be sleeping or whether I could have the TV on. They just told me to relax!*

---

12. A stopper used to block off an intravenous tube.

They put this intravenous injection into the tube in my arm. Whilst they were administering the drug, they warned me, 'Brace yourself. Your vagina could suddenly contract or be quite painful. This drug could make you itchy down below.' It never did, but I'd always be frightened at that stage. I used to get bad indigestion which was an indication that my stomach was beginning to get upset. Then the hiccups would start. They'd become more frequent, and then it would be the dry retching stage, and that would be it. Within half an hour of the drug going through me, I would be so sick that they couldn't keep up with the bowls. I can't remember anything except ringing the bell, changing the bowl, being sick and ringing the bell. It was so violent and I was absolutely exhausted. There was nothing left in my stomach and I could smell the drug coming up out of me. I couldn't stand the smell of the drug. People say they can't smell it but I can. I can remember my hair hanging in the bowl. I thought: 'Oh God! Let me die! If this is chemotherapy, I've really had it.' I asked if they could give me something, but they said they couldn't and that it just had to wear off.

I wanted someone to tell me again what was going to happen, how long it was going to last. I didn't know whether to ring the bell or just leave all this sick in the bowl. I didn't know what to do. The wards were so busy that they couldn't be with me all the time. I really needed attention full-time and I could hear them in the distance saying, 'She's sick in there again. We'll just have to leave her for a minute.' I didn't want to be left with this full bowl. Then they said, 'Most patients sleep while this is going through.' When they finally disconnected it, I thought that was the end of it but I was sick right through the night.

My husband couldn't come and pick me up the next morning, so a couple of friends took me home. They just about died when they looked at me. I was still feeling terribly *nauseous and wondered how the hell I was going to get home without throwing up in the car. They packed me up with plastic bags and I was sitting up trying to be normal, thinking, people are watching me through the windows. The more I looked at the plastic bags the more I thought I was going to be sick. When we got home I did the polite thing and asked if they'd like a cup of tea. Thank God they said they'd get going! I put myself on the bed and I slept and threw up, and slept and threw up. It took about a week before I felt better. Gradually, it became less and less. By the time three weeks went by and I had picked up and was starting to feel fine again, it was time for the next dose!*

The second and third treatments were exactly the same, and then I had to visit my oncologist and he asked me how I was coping with the chemotherapy. When I told him he said, 'You're a candidate for the new wonder drug, Ondansetron, which has just come out from the UK. Don't wait for the doctor to ask you. You ask for it.' So the next visit I said: 'I am so sick. Can I have this Ondansetron drug?' He said, 'Sure!' Apparently it was twenty-five dollars for each tablet and not many people got it so I was fortunate. After that, I'd go in on the Monday morning and I'd be allowed to come home at night. I thought, 'This is marvellous!' But it was like a delayed action. By Wednesday afternoon at precisely twelve o'clock the nausea would start again and that would go through to the Saturday.

There was nothing else they could do so I just had to put up with it. That meant I was going to be in bed, not able to do anything. I couldn't look at TV, I couldn't turn my head, I couldn't even move my mouth. All I could do was move my eyes. It's ridiculous when I think back. Then the phone would ring. They'd say, 'Are you having chemo this week?' I'd say, 'Yeah! See you later,' and plonk the phone down. No-one would ring that week. I love company, but if somebody had called, I've have wished them to hell.

Every month I'd pack my little bag with my 'jamas, hop in the car and put on this brave front. The whole time I could picture this bloody chemo machine and the saline, and I knew I was going to feel absolutely awful. I could imagine how dry my lips and my mouth were going to be. I used to be really good at drinking water, but even to this day I feel drinking water is some kind of punishment because I used to have to force myself to take even a little sip just to wet my lips. I was so bloated with the water we had to drink and the bags of saline through my body that I could not stomach anything. From the Monday after a chemo session, probably till about Thursday night, I might have two grapes, picked out of a fruit salad. That's basically all I ate. Then by Friday I'd suddenly want Chinese food. It was always curried prawns and rice! The funny thing was, I'd recover as quick as I got sick.

As time went by I got more confident because I knew what was going to happen. I asked a few more questions and I became more positive. I always liked going to the oncologist because he would say I was doing fine and that would keep me going for the next three months. But just before my next three months I wouldn't feel as cocky, particularly if I was tired or if my blood tests weren't right and showed that my white blood cells were down. That would mean I couldn't have chemo for that month. The first time that happened was a big blow because it set me back another month before finishing chemo. In time I got more philosophical and thought, 'Well ... next time the white blood cells are going to be all right.'

CANCER OF THE CERVIX—LYNNE

Lynne had to wait four weeks from the time she was told she had advanced cervical cancer before radiotherapy started.

It was incomprehensible and terrifying to me that I should have to wait for an appointment to have radiation when I'd been told that my cancer was advanced. I argued without success about getting an earlier appointment. I didn't have private health cover, so there wasn't any option but to wait. The hospital was quite unsympathetic. After two weeks I had an assessment about how much radiation and where it was to be beamed. Then I waited another two weeks until I could start the treatment. It was a bleak and anxious time, especially as my vaginal discharge became heavier and my body started to ache and feel very bloated and miserable.

Each weekday for five weeks, Lynne had external radiotherapy. Then came the final and most invasive aspect of her treatment.

The internal insertion of radiation rods into my cervix was the worst experience of my life. Until that point I can truly say I had never been afraid of anything, or anybody. Now, nearly four years later I still feel vulnerable about the experience. Basically it goes like this. I was readmitted to surgery with yet another full anaesthetic (this made three in two months) and had several rods of radiation inserted into my cervical area. The pelvic and vaginal spaces were then packed with padding designed to protect the surrounding tissues from radiation damage. It felt as though a fencepost had been shoved inside my vagina. It felt like rape. I felt hysterical and totally silenced at the same time. I was heavily drugged and can vaguely remember being trolleyed through the hospital for X-rays to check that everything was in the correct position. At some point someone said something negative about my appearance and one of the two nurses flanking the trolley bent over me and apologised for what was said. I can remember the horror of realising I didn't know what was happening to me and I tried not to focus on the dull indescribable pain between my legs.

I was taken to the ward to be installed in the radiation proof rooms I had been shown earlier. For a claustrophobe the smallness of the room, its huge radiation warnings, notices of protocol and flashing lights was a torture. I was placed on my back and told not to move. There was a telephone and a television set. I took a book with me, that I've never picked up since—Marge Piercy's Body of Glass, *a wonderful tale about cyborgs, a posthuman technological world and battles over science and ethics. My dose of pethedine blunted but didn't remove the pain or my fear. In front of me red and green lights continually flashed. I was told that if the green light went out it indicated a radiation malfunction and found myself transfixed by that light for hours on end. From time to time nurses came to check. I vomited a lot. I phoned my family and had what I thought was a reasonable conversation that freaked them out because of how little sense I made. I was given egg sandwiches to eat and lukewarm tea, which I had neither ordered nor was really capable of enjoying. The cabinet on which they were placed was on an almost impossible angle and I was terrified of moving my body to try to reach it. Later someone apologised and I can remember thinking, or perhaps saying, it was lucky I wasn't hungry during the twenty-one hours I was there.*

Shortly before I arrived, another woman had been admitted to the room next door. She was there for only twelve hours during which she constantly moaned, screamed and sobbed. It was so distressing that I began to imagine she was inside my body and it was me panicking. After a while the horror of the experience began to seep deeply into my consciousness, my whole body felt as though it was pulsating and I felt very angry. I was angry at the anaesthetist who gently asked me if anyone had told me how painful it would be. I was angry at the constant surveillance by the ward nurses through the video camera in the corner of the room. I was angry that women were experimented on with this kind of treatment, which seemed a fitting part of the apocalyptic future world tale I was reading. I was angry that this was apparently my only option for treatment and its after-effects were still being discovered.

At the end of the time the machine which had squatted dull grey and sinister at the foot of my bed was turned off. Nurses came and took about half an hour to remove the rods and then the padding. I was given more pethidine for the pain but by then felt almost delirious with relief that I was getting out of the room. I can remember thinking that I did not want to remember the details of what had happened there and that if I became healthy I would let the experience go and not dwell on it again. It's because of this that I've resisted learning the medical language to describe the treatment, but of course my own account of it is ultimately more important to me—the treatment happened inside me in more ways than one, and that's where I've learnt to deal with it because, whatever else it's done, it helped keep me alive.

No matter how gruelling aspects of many cancer treatments can be, each of these women agree with Lynne: the hope that treatment would at least arrest, if not cure, their cancer gave them the determination to continue. Although medical professionals could provide certain kinds of information about the likely effects of treatment, noone could predict exactly how each woman responded, either physically or psychologically. In this sense, although there are common threads, all treatments take place and are integrated at a deeply personal level.

6
TRAUMAS OF TREATMENT AND OTHER PAIN

NO EXPLORATION OF THE EXPERIENCE OF CANCER SHOULD UNDERESTI-mate the very real traumas associated with it. Physical and emotional pain is a reality with most forms of cancer so how each person combats or learns to live with pain is important. Although 'pain' may well have been a precursor of cancer, this is not always the case. However, the tough nature of many treatments means that even where pain was not explicit beforehand, treatment may well provoke it. It is useful to look specifically at the kinds of emotional and physical pain these women experienced as a result of treatment as well as the strategies they developed in order to survive it. For some women that meant contending with the effects of surgery, radiotherapy and/or chemotherapy; for others it entailed learning how to live on drugs for extended periods of time. Although all the women went through, and stuck with, the conventional medical systems of treatment, some turned to a range of complementary therapies to assist them.

THE TRAUMA OF PHYSICAL AND EMOTIONAL PAIN
The whole experience of cancer—from diagnosis through treatment to its uncertain outcomes—is accompanied by a kaleidoscope of different forms and intensities of physical and emotional pain. Individuals feel and confront pain in their own way and each woman in this group had a different interpretation of the pain they associated with

cancer. While physical pain can normally be managed, there is a loneliness about the experience of cancer which means that many more personal strategies have to be developed to deal with emotional pain, no matter how much support is received from other sources.

Kaye, who had two rounds of surgery, anticipated more intense pain than she felt. She discovered how drugs could dull outright pain, although she felt fragile and vulnerable, especially after her second operation.

> *The physical pain was very unusual after the first operation on my tongue. I don't know what they used but maybe it was some sort of anaesthetic on my tongue so I couldn't feel anything. Someone told me that with the shock of the operation, the body tends to numb everything a bit. There was no taste and there was no feeling. My tongue felt swollen so I could hardly speak. It was a funny feeling but because I had expected to come out in absolute agony it wasn't too bad. When I finally got some feeling back in there, it had practically healed. With the neck operation, there was more an ache than a pain. It was a very weak feeling and I couldn't support my head. I had to sleep sitting up because if I laid flat I couldn't get up. I still can't. The muscle has gone in my neck. I have to either put my hands on the back of my head and lift myself up, or roll. The first night, they laid me flat and I panicked. I had to ring the bell for a nurse. After that I said I'm not sleeping flat any more. I didn't have an extreme lot of pain but I was in a lot of emotional pain trying to figure out what's going on and what the future's going to hold. Clearly I have been lucky so far.*

Margaret W viewed her physical and emotional condition as largely symptomatic of her age. As her disease progressed, she was philosophical about the physical pain.

> When I wake up in the morning I feel as though I could jump through the roof. Then I get up and start walking about and by tea-time I'm confined to this bloody armchair. It takes me all my time to walk into the kitchen. I'm blaming the heat! I think that part of dealing with my illness and recovery is my mental attitude. With cancer you can perhaps give up more easily than with anything else because one's grown up with the fear of cancer. But I'm eighty-three and if it's not cancer, it could be arthritis or something else. I could suffer much more with arthritis than I'm suffering now. My main trouble is weakness and a horrible taste in my mouth all the time. I would like to be more interested in the things that I used to do but it doesn't worry me that I can't. I used to be very active in a women's association and I wrote plays and poetry. Now the days just slip by: it's bedtime and then it's morning—nothing seems to worry me too much.

Julie found humour helped her cope with emotional and physical pain during and immediately after treatment.

> The physical pain was covered up by my sense of humour. I didn't like to feel that I was putting the staff to any trouble. I could feel how busy they were and I thought I'm just one little pebble on the beach here. I could see what was going on and I'd think, 'Gosh, those poor girls! They're really run off their feet.' When they'd come and say, 'How're you going, Julie? I know I've been neglecting you,' I'd say, 'I'm fine,' while I might actually be thinking, 'God, if I don't have an aspirin soon I'm going to scream or something.' If it got really bad I might complain but I tried not to and I've always had a very good rapport with the nursing staff. I think it's by using your sense of humour, trying not to complain and realising that you are just one of many that a very busy staff had to look after. I know the staff appreciate it.

The emotional pain goes by me NOT accepting that I ever had cancer. The way I get over it is by knowing that the fibroid that was taken out was a lump the size of a large orange with a hard coating on it. That hard coating hadn't allowed the nucleus of the growth to get out and attach to another part of my body. So, I figure because that growth was removed it was no longer within me. That was good enough for me to say, 'I don't have cancer.' That's why it was very important for me to ask the doctors every day, 'I really don't have cancer, do I?' The emotional pain was basically watching my husband and daughter and my mother realise what was going on, and me not being able to fully explain or be sure and positive in the early stages. It was pretty frightening. Quite often I'd ask my husband, 'Do you think I'll get over it?' And he'd say, 'Of course you will.'

A similar conviction that cancer would be successfully treated characterised Anne K's approach to pain. She has put much of the experience in the recesses of her mind.

It's so long ago now, I've closed the door on a lot of this. A lot of the time I probably went into automatic pilot. I'm very good at that in a crisis now. You get a little bit above it and just bear with it. There was no special technique for me but I know it was a lonely thing. I think any cancer patient will tell you that it's your problem and a lot of people become overwhelmed by it. It's your disease and it's up to you to take ownership of it. Never ever allow yourself to become a victim of the disease. You've got to control it, not let it control you. There were only a few moments when I felt swamped. I used to think, 'You're such an idiot. Why the hell do you bother?' Bang! I would go all the way down. I'd stay in that little black hole for a while then I'd think, 'This is no good' and climb my way up again. I think everybody has got the basic will to keep going.

> *On the days I was really bad, apart from going to aerobics—like an idiot—I'd get the make-up out and do the face up, and the hair, thinking, 'Bugger it! If I don't feel good, I'll look as good as I can.' You'd have to look twice to know I was ill because I became a master at covering it up. But that helped me to get on. Sometimes people would say, 'God! Look how thin you are! What's the matter with you? Are you anorexic?' I would say, 'No, I'm not. That's not the problem!' I never did tell people why I was so thin, except for very close friends.*

Tiny believed that she did not suffer a lot of emotional pain because

> *... as a family we can talk about it. It is a shared emotional problem, so it wasn't as hard on me alone. Everyone felt it, so we all helped.*

Even so, there were moments when she crumbled.

> *The first day that we knew that I got it was the toughest day. And then about a week after I first came out of hospital after the radiation therapy, I woke up suddenly one night and realised that I was paralysed. It hadn't clicked before. I was crying then. Before that I was too ill to realise that I was so sick, and then I was so tired. It must be worse when you're tired and you're in bed on your own. That is not a good time. But it goes every day better, just slowly. The doctor says it takes two years to get better so I know that it takes a long time, and I accept that.*

Although Ann T describes herself as a 'real worrier', who suffered several panic attacks in the year after she was diagnosed, physical and emotional pain at the time of her mastectomy were not an issue.

I don't think I had any. From the moment that I came out of that surgery, when I was in the recovery room and heard Stan saying, 'It's all gone', I never looked back. I always had a positive attitude. I'm not fluffing my own feathers because to me there was no other way to be. I just got on with it. I felt funny in the hospital with those girls who had the boob implants and the face lifts and what have you. I found that hilarious. Maybe humour was my escape? I know some people would have gone to pieces and to me it would have been quite normal to go to pieces. I thought I was a bit abnormal the way I was carrying on, but it saved me. I've had a few operations and every time I come out of an operation they give me one pethidine shot and that's all I need.

Mara's elation that the cancer had been removed was tempered by grief about the changes to her body.

The most upsetting thing was my own look. Even today, two-and-a-half years later, I don't want to look at myself in the mirror. I hate to look at myself. It's probably a funny thing to say but in a way it's easier without both breasts. I remember that week with one breast. I felt awful, like a deformed person. I had a cup size 36D, so I had reasonable breasts and I felt that I looked lopsided with only one. Therefore when my other breast was removed, I felt fine. Even without any implants or any prostheses I could wear my T-shirt and not worry about it. Right from the first day after the operation I felt elevated and very positive. I felt like the cancer had been there but it wasn't there any more—and up to now it seems this is true.

The thing that worried me most after my operation was that I found that there were sacks under my arms, really ugly-looking things. When they remove breasts I suppose they take a wedge and then when that wedge finishes under your arms there remains a lot of fatty tissue, like a flap hanging over.

This worried me immensely so I went to see my doctor. He said he could remove that so about three months after my mastectomy, I went in to hospital for about three days and he removed those pockets.

After they were removed I was OK although now I'm sorry I didn't go to a plastic surgeon. When a plastic surgeon does the operation, for aesthetical reasons they always follow the grain of the muscle and they stitch it up in a certain way so that stitches don't show. It heals nicely and the scar doesn't look unsightly. When the breast specialist removed that sack under my arms he cut straight through the muscle and sewed the skin back. Now, even after two years, those scars are still really red. The scarring is probably worse because I have diabetes so the scars don't heal very well, although my breast scars did. That is what a plastic surgeon explained to me. If I'd gone to her, she would have followed the grain. She also explained to me how the implants are made, she told me about silicone implants and about reconstructive surgery—how muscle is removed from different parts of your body and implanted into your breast. I wasn't keen on that even though I still think of it.

Within six months, I was pretty much back to feeling my old self. There is one strange thing though: before the operation I had a lot of shoulder problems and after the operation my shoulders were fine. They didn't hurt me any more. My GP told me it could be that I was carrying the burden of my breasts on my shoulders. Now the hurt is back again but I think it's the aging process.

Carmen also experienced emotional turmoil. Although she believed that she was handling chemotherapy well, she felt like creeping 'back into bed and staying there'.

Perhaps the cancer has been caused from the stress that I went through over the last few years. I nearly lost my house because of bushfires that went through the area. Then, two years later, we had a house fire. Every time I smelt smoke I went into a panic. That's more stressful than cancer.

A year ago I fell off a ladder and broke my ribs while I was cleaning my windows. The pain that I experienced from three broken ribs was much worse than any chemo I've been through. The only thing I've found with the chemo is the tiredness and the nausea and this ulcer. But I can handle all three of them.

The thing that has kept me going right through is that I do a lot of spiritual reading and my own form of meditation. Every time I go into the hospital I go into the chapel and I sit for a quarter of an hour. I have my quiet times at night when my husband's not home. That's what's helped me to put up with the sickness. Even before the sickness I had this religious belief that life hereafter is much better. The cancer has made me want eternal life more. I've got my Bible and some religious books. My faith has been my essence. If I didn't have that I would have given up.

There is something I don't understand: everybody is saying to me, 'Be positive. Think positive.' I don't know what they are trying to tell me. I don't understand what I've got to be positive about because I've got nothing to fight! I've got no battle. I'm accepting that I'm sick. I'm accepting that I've got cancer because the doctors have told me. Where's the battle? I've got no battle.

It would have helped me tremendously to have more understanding of what was being done to me by the health care people because I really don't know enough. I read through the booklets that they put out but I feel embarrassed to go and speak to the counsellors and I feel embarrassed to get someone to come up and speak to me. I would have liked to have spoken to someone my own age going through the same thing. I would love to go to a session where everybody lets loose and says their thing, somewhere where you know they are all going through the same sort of things.

This sense of isolation can rear its head even when visits to a hospital or clinic leave no doubt that there are many other people with cancer going through similar experiences. Kaye recalled how seemingly little things could feed a pessimism she did not want.

On the way to the clinic each day for radiotherapy we kept driving past a cemetery. This was very distressing in my state of mind so I had to ask my husband to go another route. In the waiting room of the clinic were people in various stages of treatment. Some had lost their hair. The atmosphere was very subdued and no-one talked very much. I think cancer is like that—it is a lonely disease. You feel that no-one else can know how you feel. No-one else can understand how scared you are. You long for someone to tell you, 'It will be all right. You will be all right.' That never comes. It is always, 'Wait and see. Ninety-nine per cent sure. There's always hope.' I seemed to feed on such optimistic words. I needed them. If I heard negative words, especially about someone dying of cancer, I would get depressed and negative myself. As time went by and I stayed in remission, these thoughts receded but to this day I still get worried and scared. I don't take cancer for granted.

The doctor once told me shortly after my tongue operation that I was lucky that the cancer had only been in my tongue. He explained that another of his patients with a similar cancer to mine had had to have her jaw removed. I felt lucky at the time, until it flared up again in my neck. That is when I realised fully the insidious way cancer can act. It just takes one rogue cell to get through and it starts all over again. I think that is why I became more frightened after the second operation, worrying if it was going to return, and about how long I was going to have: would it come back in six months or a year? How much time did I have with my family? Would I get to see my children grow up? After my neck operation I asked the doctor, 'When do you usually give the all-clear?' He replied, 'We like to get through three years.' At the end of the three years he changed this to five years. I went from weekly check-ups to monthly, then to six-monthly. After one such six-monthly check-up he said I only had to come back if I was worried about anything. He said he would always fit me in if I was worried about anything, and he always did.

Lynne also considered the most invidious pain was caused by the uncertainty of her prognosis.

There weren't very many times where I could say that I was in pain although I realised that by the time I was diagnosed I'd learnt to cope with an incredible amount of discomfort and a nagging pain that I'd built into my lifestyle. That was really the cancer eating away. The pain was the pain of the panic, of having a disease that—if it hadn't been caught at that stage—would have been much worse. I'd probably have had a time slapped on me by now.

Annie did have a 'time slapped on' soon after her diagnosis, although she later realised that this was based on statistical odds which meant little in real terms. Nevertheless—

There was a lot of emotional pain at the beginning. Now I suppose I'm used to it and I block it out a lot by getting involved with other things. Or I get angry. I get angry with incompetence, and I think that is part of my response. It's not to say that I'm perfect but I really don't want to waste time. There are a lot more pleasant things to do than put up with incompetence.

She has devised other strategies for the physical pain caused by her 'double jeopardy' of lymphoma and arthritis. Sometimes she can't figure out which symptom belongs to which condition, or which specialist she should consult. She also got 'fed up' with explaining all her latest symptoms twice over to different doctors.

My strategy now is I've got a sheet that I photocopied fifty times. It's got a front and a back aspect of the body and it's got a pain chart and descriptions of different kinds of pain. If I've got a lot of pain and I can't work out if it's arthritis or cancer then I fill in the chart with coloured pencils and do a pain chart. I hand this over to my two specialists and say: 'I can't be bothered explaining it. You work it out.' It's very difficult to describe pain, especially obscure pain that comes and goes. It's sharp one minute and dull the next and burning somewhere else so it gets hard to remember where the pain is. It's much easier for them and for me to draw it and it really works because they've got some physical thing they can pick up and look at. They're not dealing with vague verbal descriptions so I think it makes it easier for them to help me.

Sometimes the pain from the arthritis really does get me down because there's nothing that I can do about it. Normal analgesics don't really work. There are times when I can't sleep, I can't sit properly, I can't walk, I can't lie down because somewhere on my body is going to be sore from touching a surface. I'm totally uncomfortable all the time. That really does wear me down and I don't know what I can do about that except whinge! I've tried a whole range of things and some of them work. The arthritis loves sleeping on a sheepskin[1] but the lymphoma hates it because lymphoma hates being warm. You're very sensitive to heat so you sweat a lot. Lymphoma is like having a fever all the time because the lymph system is concerned with immunity, it thinks it's

---

1. Annie's latest remedy has been the addition of an egg-carton shaped sponge rubber mattress to her bed.

fighting all the time, so if you get too hot you pour with sweat. Some nights pain will wake me up one hour and then the sweats will wake me up the next hour, and on it goes.

I've worked out how to deal with having a disturbed sleep pattern and now that I'm working part-time it doesn't bother me. I take half a sleeping tablet once a week on Sunday nights. That will give me a four-hour sleep. The other nights I think it doesn't really matter. I fit my work in when I feel as though my head's clear. Fortunately I live alone so I can turn on the TV in my bedroom, or listen to the radio or read. I've been known to cook at two in the morning. I do what I feel like because I know I can exist on four or five hours' sleep. Even if I do that for a month, I know I will eventually sleep for six hours when my body really needs it. Although it doesn't happen often, if I sleep for a normal night from eleven until six or seven, it's just magic.

It's the same with physical pain.

I read an article somewhere that said the easiest way to cope with pain is to give into it, lie still and just let it ride. It's easier to do that than to fight against it because that wastes more energy. You can't do anything else but be with it.

Margaret P approached living with physical pain by taking analgesics.

I don't like pain and I don't suffer it if I don't have to. I don't see why I should. I suppose that if I have to kick and scream at least I know I'm still alive!

The incurable nature of her cancer has caused her the most grief.

It wasn't the fact that I had cancer that upset me, or that I might die early. It was the fact that I was never going to be totally cured from it, and that I would never be well again, never have much energy, no matter how long I lived. Then, when the lymphoma got more aggressive and was not responding to treatment, I felt the mental stress of physically rotting inside, because that's what I'm doing. Sometimes I feel like I should be wearing a bell because I have got a sense of something black and rotten growing all over me. Sometimes some people treat you like that.

When Beth reflected on her diagnosis and initial treatment, her focus was not upon physical pain but on anger, worry and grief—emotions which she learnt to ride through or with.

At first I was angry that it had taken so long to find out what was wrong with me. Then I was upset when they predicted that I only had four to six months to live because that meant I might never see my sons grow up and settle in careers and marriage—or see my grandbabies. I was sad for not being able to spend more time with John. I wanted us to grow old together. And I wanted the time to finish the PhD I'd always wanted to study for. But all through the early days, and some of the long nights since, I have been strengthened by a firm faith, a great family and some very dear friends. When the going got tough, those were the things that helped me through. Now, I'm thrilled that the doctor's predictions were wrong and that I might be around for a while to see at least some of my dreams come true.

Noelle's supportive network and strong spiritual life sustained her 'when the going got tough'. She learnt to work through past hurt and grief through meditation and self-exploration. Herbs, dietary controls and vitamin C injections assumed a therapeutic significance, and it was in relation to these that she expressed the most overt emotional pain—that of periodically doubting her own choices.

This has been a really awful week. I abused my body with the kinds of foods I've put in towards the end of last week. I went out to a couple of meals. One was a beautiful meat curry. Another was a Christmas dinner with a plum pudding and coffee afterwards. I didn't want to be unsociable because of my dietary requirements and I thoroughly enjoyed it all! The next morning my body was feeling very leaden because it is not used to that type of food now and everything appeared to accumulate so that I began feeling a lot of self doubt. That really surprised me because I felt that I was pretty well holding it all together. By Friday morning when I was preparing my teas and supplements I found myself thinking, 'Why am I taking this? What am I doing this for? It's not helping. I'm still getting lumps. It's not working.' That frightened me because I doubted what I've been doing up to this point and it was like the ball rolling and, gathering more doubts. I feel like I'm being tested and I don't like tests. I don't do very well with tests. Sometimes I feel I'm failing. I'm not doing the right things. The lumps are still coming and I know I'm not on top of it so I wanted to give up. That frightened me. It was very overwhelming.

Emotional pain crept up on Rae in a furtive manner which she came to recognise could be far more debilitating than the post-operative physical effects of bowel surgery. When she was sent home from hospital she was told that the Cancer Foundation would be the best place to get further information about bowel cancer, but she didn't follow up on that advice because she thought she could cope. It wasn't until she had been home for several months that she realised that she was becoming tense and needed someone to talk to. That didn't happen until she answered an article in her local paper calling for participants for this project.

That first afternoon meeting was like group therapy for me. It wasn't group therapy, it was just a group of women getting together talking about their problems, getting it out of their system and laughing about it. It was the best medicine for me. I really felt good coming away that day.

Looking back on the period after her operation, Rae now realises that she fell into a deep depression.

I don't know what the feeling was. It's not the worry of cancer; it's the worry of everything. It's almost like an aftershock, yet, because the crisis is over, you're supposed to be fine. People would always ask how I was feeling and I'd say that I was feeling fine because physically I was feeling very well. But inside, up in the brain, I was just about screaming and I wondered what was wrong because if physically I'm OK, mentally I should be fine too. Even now, six months after the operation, I'm feeling well, but I still have difficulty coping with what has happened.

Most of my experiences of cancer are with people who have died. No-one has actually survived. That's probably why I haven't been sleeping. Even though I might not be thinking about it, subconsciously there must be something there. I think a lot of women are like that; when they lie down at night, if they can't settle down and go straight to sleep, they worry over things. As you get older, I think it is also harder to get to sleep, although I've always been one of these people. I'll lie there and something that has happened that day will click in my mind and I start thinking about it, and it goes on and on. The next morning when I wake up I think how stupid it all was. There's no doubt that emotionally the whole experience of cancer is still getting me.

COPING WITH PAIN

- Pain is very difficult to describe. A simple pain chart can be made by photocopying the front and back aspects of a body outline, creating a colour coded pain chart, and colouring the parts of the body in the appropriate colour for the degree and kind of pain. This way, the doctors can see the pain, and you don't have to repeat your descriptions to different staff.
- Whenever Annie has to have a new treatment or her test results are not good or things are really painful, she thinks of things that could be worse. For her, the situation that is the 'ultimate worst' is being a refugee in a war torn country and having nowhere to escape to. As she says: 'Instead I am surrounded by my family and friends and massive amounts of support and help. I know that everyone is trying to do the absolute best for me and make sure that I am as comfortable as possible.'
- Whenever Kaye had to wait for results she decided that if they were bad she would be told immediately. If she had to wait for days then they must be all right.

SURVIVING TREATMENT

Surviving treatment is more than a matter of recovering a sense of physical wellbeing. In some circumstances, where treatment is on-going, the will and strength to keep going can be enhanced by having a break. Tiny found that she needed a proper holiday before she re-started treatment after a brief remission.

> I finished 'heavy duty' chemo four-and-a-half months ago and I've been looking good for the last three months. Although my white blood cell count is still very low, I had a two-and-a-half-week holiday with friends in Melbourne before starting this new Interferon treatment. The doctor said my holiday was more important than starting Interferon straight away because I've been sick for two years and I needed a holiday. That's probably why I'm feeling a lot better. I feel like I can go out and do something now. The lady I stayed with is also quite sick, so we relaxed and went on outings.

Even when treatment is of a more limited duration, recuperation can pose some challenges. Once the physical interventions are completed, contact with the medical system can decrease dramatically. There are many reasons to celebrate this transition, but it can also leave a sudden and potentially frightening void. Lynne described this, and the way she came through it.

> When I went home from the final treatment my body was in a state of shock. The substance injected into my body to protect my digestive system from radiation damage was a clay-like consistency that took over a week to excrete. I was unable to go to the toilet for days because, despite urgently wanting to, nothing happened. Here's a gruesome image—it took about three weeks for the 'clay' to move down the toilet bowl out of sight. I used to go and look at it in horror trying to visualise my bowel and the melted stump of my cervix. I was pretty off the planet trying to understand the changes in my body.
> For days after arriving back from hospital I had a splitting headache that nothing would shift. A neighbour came and gave me some painkillers that she'd used after a big operation. They made my dreams psychedelic but didn't shift the pain.
> I had been told that after the treatment I would be contacted in six weeks for a clinic appointment and thereafter

> would simply deal with my GP. After the intensity of the radiation treatment, it was a total anticlimax. I was hugely relieved to escape the hospital check-ups and processes but felt frightened by the suddenness of the end of the treatment. When I think about it now, I believe it's the swift change to looking after oneself after extensive interventions, with virtually no counselling, that causes this shock. I coped by travelling home to New Zealand to see friends, changing my diet, doing more meditation and giving myself lots of pleasurable treats. But all of these positive things were much harder work than they sound because I felt quite dead inside, violated and afraid. In the end these positive things took over. After about ten months I felt more alive than I've ever felt and absolutely determined to live the rest of my life consciously and with flair!
>
> After six weeks I went to the clinic very anxiously. I waited three hours to see a doctor and the whole check-up took just ten minutes. It was difficult relaxing enough to have a vaginal examination but they were reasonably patient and answered all of my questions. I made it a point after that to ask at least five questions, even if I already knew the answers. I wanted to establish a relationship with them—it seemed the least I could do when they got to be so personal with my parts! It also meant that I had to concentrate on my body's condition and not switch off in fear. I guess it is also about me learning to not be afraid and to take some control of my health.

Finding ways to deal with fear was something Kaye remembers contending with, particularly after her second operation. She suffered such bad attacks of anxiety that she sought help from her doctor, who prescribed medication which ensured that she would 'switch off fear'.

> I'd asked the doctor to give me something to keep my nerves down while I was under the radiotherapy. He gave me these

> tablets called Tryptanol. They calmed me down but I'd end up going to sleep. When I went back in to have a stitch out in my neck, I was feeling really down because of having to go through another small operation. The anaesthetist came in and asked if I'd been taking anything? I said, 'Tryptanol, for my nerves.' He said, 'Nerves! They're an antidepressant.' He took my blood pressure and it was right down low. I've a tendency to low blood pressure and it was even lower than usual. After that I stopped taking them because it obviously wasn't calming my nerves down—it was slowing me down!
>
> Half the time, if you don't know the name of the drugs you are taking, or they don't tell you, you could be taking something completely different to what you're thinking.

Kaye's decision not to sleep her anxieties away was one way of regaining a sense of control but learning how to live with the physical consequences of her life-saving operation has been an on-going exercise.

> The surgeon cut the scar so that it followed the fold of the neck so it wasn't too bad, although the scarring got worse for a while and stood out because the fluids built up in the chin. I was embarrassed about it back then but now I seem to feel worse and much more self-conscious, even though people say they don't notice it. I pull my hair over and wear high collars to hide it. My neck is very sensitive. If my husband wants to nuzzle me on the neck, he has to nuzzle me on the other side because the nerve endings are still so sensitive where I had the operation. I can't bump myself with a brush and it hurts and aches in cold weather. Also my right arm is weak. I can't lift it above shoulder height because a muscle was cut during the operation.

Ann T found surviving the physical effects of the mastectomy of her right breast was made easier by getting back to work.

> *I went to work a month after we got back home and that was probably the best therapy for my arm because you're supposed to exercise. I was putting mail into the boxes so it kept my arm moving. Now I've got full mobility in my arm. I'm very aware of lymphodema[2] which, if it happens, is probably the worst side-effect. Then you have to get a pressure garment that comes right up the arm and over the torso to hold it on. Now that I work for a health benefit fund I have noticed that a lot of people develop lymphodema in summer—that's when people come in for pressure garments. You have to be very aware of it.*

Carmen had major problems with infection around the site of her lumpectomy. Several months after the operation, she still had numbness around the suture line under.

> *One doctor said the numbness would go away in three months and another doctor said it would never go away so I'm not sure what will happen. But I've got good mobility. I can lift my arm quite high because I did exercises regularly although when I stretch it up it hurts along the inside. I don't know whether it's supposed to hurt. The scar where I had the lump removed still feels lumpy and quite hard. It's as if the lump is still there. I don't know if it's supposed to feel like that but I've started feeling pain so I think that maybe the feeling is coming back. I'll have to ask the doctor again. I have to keep asking him.*

She also had to come to grips with the discomfort caused by radiotherapy.

---

2. The accumulation of interstitial fluid as a result of obstruction of lymphatic vessels, disorders of lymp nodes, or surgical removal of lymph nodes for cancer.
Interstitial—any small gap or space in the structure of a tissue or organ, a crevice or interval between parts of the body.

All my skin peeled off my arm after the radiotherapy and that's just finished clearing up, thank God. It went dark brown, like a real tan. My husband was calling me two-tone! I haven't been wearing a proper bra, just these soft aerobic ones because when I had the radiotherapy the bra ripped all the skin from underneath my breast so I was all raw. But I finished radiotherapy about three weeks ago and all that burning has gone and it's just healed. It's still a little bit itchy, but not bad and I still have the cream they gave me. I was expecting the radiation to be ten times worse than it was. By the twentieth session it started to burn and then my nipple went really crispy. Then the skin came off that and it was really black and then it turned pink and it looked really ghastly. It's still tender under the skin.

Although Julie did not have to cope with radiotherapy burns, on chemotherapy she had to find ways to deal with the dry skin and thinned out, dry hair that accompanied her attacks of nausea, dry retching and vomiting. She tried to moisturise her 'flaky skin' by soaking in a bath laced with baby oil, although some days she was too ill to even make it into the shower. Once a week, she would treat herself to a trip to the hairdresser for a 'head massage, a shampoo and a set, and a treatment or colour whenever they'd advise it.' Julie considers that she was lucky.

Not losing my hair was a plus because I could think of nothing worse than looking in the mirror each day and being reminded that I've got cancer because I'm bald. After two operations I was as white as a wall. I couldn't stand the look of myself and I didn't want my family and friends to see how sick I was so I would get up at some ungodly hour of the morning, go to the loo and then I'd put tan make-up on. Then I'd try to do something with my hair, put a bit of lipstick on and some blush. Then everyone would say, 'Gee! You look good today!' You need to hear this because then you think, 'Yeah—and I don't feel too bad either.' If everyone was saying, 'God! You look awful,' I'm sure I would have felt even worse. I think make-up and feeling good is very important because, when you're used to being a big person, every time you look in the mirror you're reminded you have got cancer when all you see is a bald head, a pale face and a thin body. I can remember thinking: 'I'll never go on another diet and I'll never ever complain about how fat I am again' because my face looked so drawn.

Beth recalled how good she could make herself feel even when she knew she looked 'grey with bags under the eyes'. One time when she felt dreadful she had a work function to attend and she knew some people would expect her to arrive looking 'skinny and half-dead'. Determined not to look like she felt, she 'put on the make-up, did the hair, and put the brightest things on'. She had taken the advice of the Cancer Foundation and been to a program called 'Look Good, Feel Better'.

They get about eight to ten women who have cancer together and ask you what your colours are. They have all these beauticians there, because your skin changes; my skin went very dry and patchy and my eyes watered for months, just continual twenty-four-hour-a-day watering and they got all red and split from the chemo. My mouth got ulcers and my lips cracked. So they have these beauticians come and they tell you how to do your make-up for your skin. They have wigs and scarves and all that sort of stuff. I was the only one with hair.

Wigs, beanies and scarves can help shield a bald head, and gentle oils or lanolins can assist dried or burnt skin. Many women find make-up a useful tool for disguising the ravages of treatment. Something more substantial is required after a mastectomy. Ann T was grateful that her cancer was in a part of her body which could be easily operated upon. Even so, adapting to her changed body image took time as well as support from her partner and some good tips from the woman who fitted her prosthesis.

> *After the operation my biggest fear was having the bandage off and trying to face looking down—having one breast and not the other. My husband stayed with me and held my hand the whole time the doctor was taking the bandage off. I think because I was building a big thing out of it, it was a real anti-climax! It was just a straight line and I looked like a boy on one side and me on the other! The only time I ever got teary was after we came home from hospital. There was a lingerie fashion show on the tellie and without thinking my friend said to me: 'Aren't they beautiful?' I cracked up. I was thinking, 'Will I ever be able to wear those again?' Mind you, I could if I had a reconstruction but I don't have the time to have it. It's not necessary to me at the moment and I'm grateful that I didn't rush in and have an implant. I may not have had a silicone one anyway because I know that for people with mastectomies, there are different implants, different types of reconstruction that can be taken from your own body, from muscle tissue, from the back or from the stomach. I am thinking about that now because I've put on a bit of weight all around my waist but I never sit down and think, 'Oh God, I'll have to have this reconstruction.' Never.*
>
> *The hardest thing was trying to dress. Where we were living is very, very hot so it was mainly nice T-shirts or whatever. At that stage because the scar was so new, I had to keep a bra on and you couldn't hide yourself under shirts and jumpers. I always wore a skimpy bikini but that wouldn't do any more. I had to get a particular kind of bikini from a shop in Perth. It's like an aerobics top, or a crop top. I still get them. I find they are more comfortable than bathers because if you've got a*

prosthesis in the bathers, you haven't got anything to hold up around the breast area so they sag. It's not very comfortable and doesn't look very nice.

Mara loved to swim, and it was her desire to get on with activities she shared with her family which forced her to get a prosthesis fitted. Even then, she needed encouragement. 'It was almost like I was expecting that my breasts would grow back naturally again, like a nail grows or your skin grows!' Her observations about the prosthesis fitting indicate just how important it can be to enhancing a woman's dignity and sense of normality. Both are important aspects of surviving a form of treatment which has removed one of the most culturally dominant symbols of femininity and motherhood.

I didn't order my prosthesis until a month after I walked out of hospital, and even then my daughter pushed me. She said, 'You listen, Mum. Summer's coming and we're going to Rottnest Island. You have to have a swim. You have to have your prosthesis fitted.' Finally I went to a place that was recommended but I didn't like the set-up of the shop: the assistant wasn't helpful, it was cramped and looked more like a warehouse. It was not restful and there didn't seem to be any privacy. That's the main point. I didn't want to bare myself in there.

We went to a shop in the city, a little hidden shop right up at the top of an arcade, and just going in there felt private. The woman there was trained. She fitted me with the prosthesis, did pockets on my bra, helped me to find the proper bathers, advised me how to claim from my health insurance company to get a refund and delivered everything to my home within two days before I went on holiday. She fitted me very sensitively. She knew the right way to approach it. You're very touchy about such an intimate and private thing. You need the highest standard and to feel that you're treated like a special person. If you go behind the curtain anybody can walk in, pull the curtain, and you're there with no breasts.

One thing she said sticks with me: 'Once you dress yourself and wear your prosthesis, be it bathers, or dress or T-shirt, nobody has to know. You don't have to say anything to anybody because it's not noticeable. Only tell people that you want to know. No-one else has to know that you have had your breast removed.' It was important because you find that you are living with the image of normality. She also gave me some fine merino wool to put next to my skin because the scars were still fresh and the wool has lanolin in it which helps the healing process.

Unlike Mara and Ann T, Carmen had a lumpectomy and therefore has not had to adjust to life without breasts. However, her treatment involved surgery which left scarring, as well as chemotherapy and radiotherapy. Altogether they took a toll on her sense of physical and emotional wellbeing.

In the booklet I read it said you may get ulcers in your mouth from chemo, but it didn't say you can get them in the oesophagus, which is where I have got them. I've gone off tasty food and I have come to hate cooking. I always used to like satay and bolognaise sauces but now I can't eat anything that's got any type of flavour in it at all because the minute I eat it I get this terrible chest pain. The first time it happened I thought I was having a heart attack.

Margaret W found the removal of her stomach left her with practical problems digesting food.

They'd taken the whole stomach and I asked, 'How am I going to eat? What happens when I eat? Is there a cavity there, and the food drops straight down to the intestines?' The doctor's description was too complicated for me, but he explained it to my son and there is definitely no stomach there. The food must go straight into the duodenum or small intestine. The doctor said I was to eat a little food every two hours, and never eat too much. But everything I ate left a nasty acid taste in my mouth.

At night it's terrible, although it doesn't keep me awake. That's one of the good things—I sleep well at night. But if I do wake up I can hardly open my mouth. I have to smack my lips together to get the saliva working. That eases it until I get back to sleep again. They told me to prop my bed up by putting a brick under the head of my bed but I can't sleep like that because I slide down. You just get used to it and put up with it. That's all you can do.

Anne K's bone marrow transplant left her body vulnerable to infection.

When you have a bone marrow transplant, you are susceptible to herpes simplex[3] for the first six months. They're airborne viruses and if you pick them up, you can get a dreadful dose. You can get it in your eye and there is a good chance of losing your sight. Or you can get a huge dose of shingles, which is sort of an adult form of chicken pox. So to prevent these infections they give you gamma globulin intravenously every three months until they think your fledgling system is strong enough to take whatever is airborne. I had to be very careful about avoiding any type of infection. I didn't use public transport. I didn't go anywhere much. If I was going shopping, I went in the car, did the shopping and came home. I was extremely careful. It was another isolating thing but it was simply a temporary condition.

---

3. Cold sores.

LIVING ON DRUGS

For many people with cancer, surgery or an intense blast of radiotherapy or regimen of chemotherapy will draw treatment to a conclusion. This was the case for several women in this group. But those whose cancers required extended periods of drug therapy have had to deal with varied, and often unpredictable, physical and psychological effects. All the women in this group have, to different degrees, accepted the consequences of medication as a 'trade-off' for managing their cancers, but this has not always been easy. One had to make a decision about continuing her chemotherapy drugs while her husband was encouraging her not to take them. He believed they were making her sick and would kill her faster than her cancer. She had to 'battle on two fronts'.

Uncertainty about the effects of drugs is compounded by the mythology surrounding cancer. Even doctors cannot predict exactly how an individual will cope with medication. As Margaret P put it, 'Not only are there a hundred odd different cancers, there are a hundred and one different reactions to every different treatment.' Mara experienced a drying up of her body secretions while taking the anti-hormone drug Tamoxifen.

> *Other than the dryness it's hard to distinguish what is a side effect from Tamoxifen and what is part of an aging process. I'm now sixty-three and I have aches and pains so I think these bone problems are more likely to be arthritis than anything else. But does Tamoxifen aggravate arthritis? Does it make dryness in your bones so that it hurts you moving them around? Maybe the normal lubrication is not there? You never know.*

Annie is reluctant to take anything but minimal medication, although she now has a pharmacopoeia in her kitchen cupboard and admits there are some drugs which she accepts as essential if she is to get on with life.

Living on drugs is a real issue, especially when you're not used to it. The one thing that I really hate is prednisolone, which is the basis of a lot of chemotherapy. I've been on heavy doses for too long and so every time I go near it now the reactions are immediate: I get hair on my face; I get this huge stomach; I get pains in my legs; I go back to all the symptoms I had at the end of six months of high dosages of chemo. I get fat and feel awful so I hate going on it.

I find it diffficult to take analgesics because I'm really wary of them. It's silly, but I've been brought up with the idea that drugs like analgesics are addictive or the longer you take them, the less effective they are. When I was nursing, thirty years ago, that is what we were taught—so now it is really hard to stop that way of thinking. That can become a real problem when you're supposed to be on pain control because I think, 'I haven't got any pain! What's the point of taking pain-killers?'—which of course defeats the whole purpose of pain control. I'm really strict about sleeping tablets and only take at the most one whole one a week and nothing in between. But I really don't like taking anything—especially analgesics. I think I'll cope with the pain somehow until it gets too much and then I give in.

It is extremely rare for dependence to develop when analgesics are taken for pain relief, including opiates such as morphine, and resistance does not develop to a particular analgesic. Nor do changes in pain level have any relationship to the length of time someone has been on painkillers. Even so, like Annie, Marinomoana has developed a cautious approach to the use of pain control medication, but for different reasons. After years on various regimes of radiotherapy and chemotherapy, for the last few years she has 'only' had to take Panadeine Forte or MS Contin, a morphine sulphate drug used for the chronic, severe pain of cancer.

I am still getting painful muscle spasms. The trouble is the spasm is not in any direct area. It'll be like there will be a pin-point on top of my nose or a pin-point through the middle of my arm. Then my hands will go silly, wobbling all over the place. Sometimes it's my right leg. Apparently it's the nerve endings so the MS Contin is to relax those. I don't use MS Contin unless it's severe because it makes me a bit nauseous and I don't like Panadeine Forte because for some reason it sets my sinus flowing and I get a runny nose! Anyway, when you are taking MS Contin you don't want any other stuff. Usually I just have a couple of glasses of wine and that calms me down!

Like Annie, Margaret P has had extensive periods on the cortisone drug prednisolone. While it has helped to inhibit the growth of tumours, it was not without a price.

Prednisolone can cause diabetes and I've now got a touch of that. I had to have three toenails removed and they took a long time to heal. I've also had hypertension and a lot of facial hair from prednisolone, and had to have my entire face waxed about three times one year. I also got withdrawal symptoms when I went off prednisolone after several years of having to take it on and off, even though they cut me down slowly over a few months each time.

In the eight years since Margaret was diagnosed she has become accustomed to living with drugs. Complete with side-effects, they are an integral part of her life with low-grade lymphoma.

Chemo is chance. It is a gamble. They don't know what's going to happen, how each individual's going to react. The biggest problem for most people on chemo is the white cell count and I've had all sorts of infections. The trouble is, the longer you've had low-grade lymphoma, the less antibiotics work. Bit by bit, they all stop working. I'm allergic to penicillin which doesn't help and when I got pneumonia a year or so ago, I was in hospital for twelve days before they tried the old Erythromycin.[4] In twenty-four hours my temperature went in a straight line from 39.4 to 37 degrees.

At one stage of chemo treatment I lost about ten per cent of my hair, in clumps in the shower or on my pillow at night. That was awful but then it stopped. My oncologist says that sometimes people become resistant if, like me, they've had chemo for a long time, but that you can never predict what will happen next. On heaps of occasions my lips have peeled and once I took my false teeth out and brought an entire length of skin with them. Funnily my nails have got stronger on chemo, although they are rather woody, like an old person's nails. A lot of these chemo drugs can cause kidney damage so you have to drink a lot—fluids, not alcohol. If necessary, they measure your urine output, testing it all the time so they stop instantly if you're coming up with any blood in your urine. Indigestion is another long-term effect of a lot of these heavy chemos.

I've been through all the anti-nausea drugs. Personally, I found lorazepam is the best. It knocks you out and one of the side-effects is short-term memory loss but who gives a shit! There was one famous day I couldn't remember my name for a full second. That really did surprise me. The thing that gets to me has been the effects of all these drugs on my thinking. I can't think as clearly and I am used to having a good memory so it affects me badly. It's partly stress, partly drugs and partly the illness itself. But my memory is not as good. I concentrate more on my illness than on other things, although after I got cancer, I got my TEE and a degree in psychology. I couldn't do that now.

Margaret was able to study in the first years after diagnosis because

---

[4]. An antibiotic.

she was still able to organise her life around treatment. As her lymphoma has become more aggressive, this has been harder. This is a prospect which concerns Annie.

> *I am a very organised person, so organising my life around treatment is like an extension of my normal personality! I have to be organised if I know I've got to spend thirty-six hours flat on my back. When I have treatment I ring around my friends and say, 'We are in a bit of a crisis. We need to roster. Can you help?' I'll get one friend to come in for coffee or lunch, and another to give me tea and someone else to tuck me in at night! I have a tray with Milo and the coffee stuff ready. Whoever leaves here last makes sure everything I need is around the bed and brings the thermos so I've got hot water to make a drink during the night. You've got to be organised. I get worried sometimes that when I'm no longer able to do the organising, the whole system will fall flat. But as long as I'm able to get to a phone I'll be fine.*

The incurable nature of low-grade lymphoma means that both Margaret P and Annie face the prospect of being drug dependent for the rest of their lives. Anne K's myeloid leukaemia was kept under control with drugs for four years before it became chronic, and a bone marrow transplant was performed.

> *I was on drugs from the day that I was diagnosed. I would be on oral chemo until my white cell count would drop back to normal. Then it would take a period of time for that to build up again, back on the drugs again. So it was an intermittent thing right up until the transplant and then afterwards I had to have the anti-rejection drugs like the cyclosporin, which is damned unpleasant. That blows your face up. I had prednisolone as well for quite a long time and all sorts of other bits and pieces but you come down*

> when it looks like you're not going to reject the transplant. Gradually they wean you off and now it's been over two years clear without drugs.

While Anne K's treatment necessitated a slow withdrawal from drugs, in other cases the end of treatment can be sudden, and this can cause particular kinds of insecurities, as Julie explained.

> When I was on my seventh intravenous chemo treatment, I said to my oncologist, 'Can this be the last one?' He said he would let me know that night. He did say yes and I was so thrilled, but at the same time I was very insecure because I knew I only had tablets. Then when I actually finished the tablet form of chemo I felt even more insecure. I was so pleased to get off everything because even the tablet form made me quite ill. It was like it was all building up in the system. But I had the feeling of nothing to hang onto, nothing to help me. I almost needed counselling because I had finished the chemo. I let them know about that and they said that it's not really uncommon because chemo becomes a security blanket. Going through my mind was, 'I'm having this because it's killing off the bad cells,' and I'd psyched myself right into this, and when it was no more, I thought, 'Are those cells growing again? What if they are?' I couldn't wait for my next check-up so that I could hear that I was really all right.

Some drugs are highly aggressive and some people question whether the cost of taking them doesn't outweigh the benefits. Carmen didn't have any doubts.

> I'll take them if the doctor says I have to. I reckon if drugs are going to keep you alive, then take them. You have to live with them and accept it.

Others are ambivalent. Tiny did not like taking and having injections and explored non-medical ways to counteract the effect of her drugs.

> *When I came out of hospital the first time I was given a lot of tablets. Some of them I need to take but a lot of them I have to take because my tummy was upset. I put those away and only took what I had to take. I think that was a good thing to do because when you take too many tablets, the one is not always good with the other one. My skin is good, maybe because of herbal teas and vegetable juices. I do a lot with the herbs and vegetables we grow. I do it to help myself. I think it's a great help to my healing process and is the reason I have been feeling so good. I try everything because it's not going to do any harm. I don't know if it's going to get worse if I don't do it, so I might as well do it and see what happens.*

CONSIDERING COMPLEMENTARY THERAPIES

Several women in this group used herbs and vitamins as complementary therapy. Other alternatives or supplements to the 'medical model' of cancer treatments included acupuncture and massage for physical pain control, meditation, aromatherapy and special diets.

Tiny trusted her doctors enough to believe that the medications they gave her were crucial to her life chances. She also believed that she could aid her own healing process by using diet and vitamin supplements to strengthen her constitution. As her whole family had always drunk herbal teas and eaten homegrown, unsprayed vegetables this was already part of her normal approach to diet. However, she discovered that some of the things she had assumed would be good healing agents were incompatible with her condition.

> *I started reading books on cancer which said I had to drink four litres a day to wash the chemo away. So I drink a litre of*

carrot juice and litre of orange juice every day and then herbal teas which are good for the bloodstream. I don't know whether that helped or not, but you'll never know so you just try.

I also went to see a GP who is interested in alternative medicine. This doctor is good because the concern is for positive thinking and meditation, low-stress diets, proper vitamins as well as conventional medicine. I think that is a very good thing because when you take some herbal tablets like vitamin C or A you don't know if it is good with the tablets from the doctor. It might be bad for you. If you are going to take alternative medicine as well as the medicine your doctor gives you it is important to go and see someone who knows what they're doing. This doctor said that in my case with the blood the way it is, it's not a good thing to take a lot of beta-carotene, as well as calcium. I thought these would be a good thing to do because of the bone marrow disease in the blood, but I now know that if I get too much of it, it will make it worse. This doctor is going to do a blood sample to tell me exactly what my blood needs so I can use the right supplements.

I think that it worked for me. It has given me hope and made me positive. The other doctors keep saying that myeloma can suddenly take off and that's always in my mind, especially as they have said that I will never get my blood count down near zero—that it will never go down below thirty. This alternative doctor is saying, 'You can do it' and has told me of another patient with myeloma who has got her blood count down so low that the myeloma can't be traced any more. This gives me hope that I might live normally.

The importance of hope, and taking action to help herself, was something Kaye discovered. Once the key stages of her medical treatment had been completed she considered that a complementary treatment was essential for her peace of mind.

The doctors tell you to go home, put your feet up and don't do anything else except maybe take lots of different medication. I didn't even have that because I didn't have anything to take after the radiation. It was always in the back of my mind that I wanted to do or take something so that I could feel like I was helping myself. I think you get to the stage where you're willing to try anything.

I went through one alternative therapy and some of it was really radical. This man did hair analysis and said he'd cured himself of cancer and that he'd been clear for twenty odd years. There were all these different other people who swore by it. He made it out like the cancer fed on certain things that you ate so you had to cut all that out and starve it. I started to think of it like that. There it was, this little thing inside me that was hungry, and so whatever I was putting in there, if it liked it, it was eating away. If it didn't like it, I'd starve it.

Would you believe that I never saw this guy? I sent off a sample of my hair and was sent back a big sheet of what was lacking in my body. By the time I'd finished adding up all that was on the page, like folic acid and this and that, it was quite expensive. But I thought, 'If that's what I need I'll take it.' Besides that I got a health sheet. One side had what you don't eat and the other, which was a lot shorter, told you what you could eat. It was a very healthy vegetarian diet with lots of fruit, vegetables and nuts. I could not eat any red meat, not even fish or chicken except a little bit towards the end. You were allowed nothing out of an animal—no butter, no milk.

It was very drastic and you had to detoxify your body first. You made up this mixture, like a soup made from all the tops of the vegies—all the green parts, not the vegies themselves. I had a hard time finding those because they chop them off before they sell them. Then there was a mixture I had to drink made from a small amount of hydrogen peroxide. I don't know what that was supposed to do but it tasted vile. I can't believe that I went on it, but it did help me to put my cancer in perspective. It was a good way of thinking about it and I was on it for a fair while but I became so terribly tired.

I know the doctors shrug it off and say that if you're in remission it's not because you've gone on a diet or something. But I thought it didn't do me any harm. I was happy on it, so why not? You're actually doing something for yourself. It cost a lot for all the vitamins but I really paid for it watching other people eat all the stuff that I loved, like cakes and cream. I found that was absolute agony so as the years went by I started eating a bit of this and a bit of that and gradually slipped back again. Now, I eat practically anything. I shouldn't because I've still got it in my mind that cancer might be caused by, or feed off, what you eat.

Lynne sought non-medical therapy soon after diagnosis. A qualified masseuse and naturopath, she was a firm believer in their therapeutic value, although the acute nature of her disease left her in no doubt that radiotherapy offered the best chance of recovery. However, she discovered that she had to wait four weeks before radiotherapy could begin, despite the advanced nature of her cervical cancer.

It was probably this situation as much as my personal attitude to health that took me off immediately to find a herbalist, dietary advice and a meditation regime that would help me through. I wanted to battle the cancer on as many fronts as possible. I went immediately to a herbalist whom I've continued to use. He was brilliant and I do believe that the herbs and the emotional support that I got from him got me through the radiation because it was a terrible experience. I also adjusted my diet in a very radical way, I went swimming every day and I did lots and lots of meditation and visualisation. All of those things made it possible to go through the medical treatment without too much drama.

Noelle's only medical options were surgery and the possibility of participating in an experimental program to see how melanoma responded to Interferon, which she declined. She decided quite early on that her best chances lay with maintaining her good health and boosting her own immune system. Her attempts to do this became the most significant aspect of her treatment so her experience of therapies to complement surgical removal of tumours is included in full. Her exploration started when she was browsing in a bookshop just after she was diagnosed.

> *While I was looking, this book by Dr Ruth Cilento,* Heal Cancer: Choose Your Own Survival Plan, *leapt out at me. It was as though I was meant to buy the book. Cilento comes from a renowned family of medical practitioners. Her mother was pushing for the use of vitamins in the forties and was considered a bit of a crank and a quack. Cilento has basically taken over where her mother left off. She herself was once a cancer patient so she has used the treatments in her book on herself. She has also researched the values of vitamins and a history of different alternative treatments from all over the world. This book contains a discourse on each of those, focusing on the success rates. She is not pushing her own ideas although she argues that if you follow the nutritional plan and the vitamin supplements she recommends it can ease the side-effects for people who are taking chemotherapy and radiation treatment. They are able to come through the treatment with minor discomforts and disability. At no time does she actually downgrade the orthodox treatment because she discusses the reasons for it but she does point out the 'fors' and 'againsts'. All the way through she reinforces the choices that we have.*
>
> *I felt that some of Cilento's suggestions were the way for me to go because it gives you choices. For example, it mentioned a German doctor called Gerson who expounded the benefits of raw calves' liver mixed with fresh orange juice because of all*

the vitamins and minerals within the calves liver. It sounds absolutely horrendous. Fresh calves' liver is very hard to obtain and the stuff you find in the butcher shop is frozen solid. With the thawing out you lose all the goodness. Actually I had read about the Gerson's treatment in another book by a chap who had hairy cell leukaemia, but the whole idea of drinking raw calves' liver juice was too horrible for me.

So, through a friend of a friend I was given the name of a naturopath. I took my book and went along and said I would like to follow some of the things in this book, not all of them. Now I am pursuing a regime of fresh fruits and vegetables. I stopped eating red meat over twenty years ago although I did eat a little chicken and fish. Under this regime I have increased my fish intake and decreased my dairy products, which includes cheese, which I love. For a while I was very rigid but now I don't see that a little of what I fancy can hurt me every now and then. You've got to treat yourself. I take vitamin supplements and, in the morning and in the evening, a herbal tea which is a blend of four different types of herbs. It's classified as an elimination diet: I jokingly say we've eliminated everything that I like to eat and the stuff I am allowed to eat, I eliminate out the other end!

One good thing about the diet is that it's given me more energy. I haven't had the flu for I don't know how long. I used to suffer from throat infections and urinary tract infections. I don't know what they are now! I'm always surprised when I do get sick. I had a virus a while back that made me so low for two days that I took myself to bed. By the third day I was starting to feel better, by the fourth day I was much better and on the fifth day I was feeling really good. The naturopath seems to think if I hadn't have been on my diet and supplements I would have been much sicker because my partner, who is a junk food addict, got the same virus and was ill for a fortnight. I took that as positive.

Normally I use the time when I am preparing my herbal teas and all my supplements as a meditation technique. I bring all my treatments together and then I sit down and play some music and meditate on my treatments to make it a positive thing. Before I learnt to do this it was a negative thing of shoving this stuff into me, getting it out of the way and thinking of it as a nuisance. So I tried to turn it around. Meditation has put a whole focus and a clarity in my life that I didn't have before. I was looking to meditation to bring a little calmness and stillness into my life. I simply hoped it would stop my mind from going all over the place and being very erratic but I've had some wonderful experiences from meditation.

Because of meditation I have dealt with things from my past things, like the separation from my ex-husband eleven years ago. I had been quite convinced I had laid that to rest but meditation brought things to the surface and allowed me to let go of the hurt and sadness. Once it started it was like a dam bursting and I was bawling my eyes out but eventually the flow slowed to a trickle, and then I was just sitting. I didn't feel like a wrung out dish rag. Instead there was a lightness there, as though something had been drawn out and the pain I had been denying had gone. I had forgiven. I had let go.

My naturopath also suggested that maybe I should try vitamin C injections because the lumps were increasing in number and I didn't appear to be holding my own. She gave me the name of a GP who is not opposed to other types of treatment as long as they are not harmful and have been of benefit to other patients. For example this medical practitioner suggested that I might like to try the shark cartilage treatment. Sharks appear to be the only creatures on earth that do not grow tumours so they dry and powderise the shark cartilage. This has to be mixed with something like fruit juice and you take a gram of shark cartilage per kilogram of body weight. I think it is supposed to cut the blood supply to the tumour so that the tumour shrinks and dies because it is not being fed.

They have had some success—some people's tumours have shrunk and disappeared. It was recommended that I take a five month course. I presume if it hasn't worked in the five months it isn't going to work. But it is extremely expensive. A ten day treatment for a fifty kilo person used to be $290, although I think it has come down in price to $250 because more people are trying the treatment. I don't weigh fifty kilos so I'd have been looking at $5,500 for a five month treatment. I couldn't afford it.

The vitamin C injections work out at twenty-six dollars per treatment after Medicare has refunded in part. That is the short-fall which I have to pay. It seems that vitamin C is entrenched enough in the system for Medicare to recognise it although it won't recognise shark cartilage or any of the supplements that I'm taking. Each treatment works out at 140ml which you have in five syringes of thirty-five millilitres each, although I'm not sure what percentage of vitamin C they use to make up the thirty-five millilitres. It is quite a thick viscous substance so it flows a lot easier into the veins if it is warm. The doctor or one of the qualified staff puts the line in and then they leave it up to the patient to actually administer it into the body, although they normally come back to change the syringes.

It is an expensive treatment as it is but it would be really expensive if they had to have somebody there injecting it into you—especially when there can be as many as six people in the room at any one time. There is a bell in the room and if you require any assistance, like changing the syringes over, you ring for help.

At the start of the treatment you must have a beaker of water with glucose in it, I think because your blood sugars

> drop. *After that you drink water because the treatment makes you very thirsty. You sit in a chair with a pillow across your lap and the arm extended straight out. It must be kept straight at all times because if you bend the arm the needle will pierce through the vein into the tissue. I bent my arm one day when I was leaning over to get a drink of water. It is excruciating getting vitamin C in the tissue. It stings.*
>
> *Vitamin C treatment is not aimed at a cure. It increases the size of the blood cells and strengthens them so you get more oxygen. The more oxygen you have flowing through the blood stream, the cleaner it keeps the blood so it is more able to get rid of the toxins and helps to heal scar tissue. People on chemo who I've spoken to while having the injections think it is wonderful because it either lessens or gets rid of chemo side-effects, like nausea.*
>
> *I am very aware of my body now. I know exactly what I should or shouldn't be doing, like eating the wrong foods. At the time you think, 'What the heck? It won't matter.' But it does, especially if you do it twice in one day and then have a coffee on top of it.*

Noelle used these combinations of meditation, diet and vitamin C injections until shortly before her death in 1995. They were a crucial part of her experience of cancer because

> *... by doing this I feel I've got some sort of control. There is no other treatment for me and I feel that I should be doing something, even if it's just the fact of making me feel good. That in itself has got to be of benefit.*

A sense of control and active participation in treatment, rather than rejection of medical treatments for cancer, is characteristic of the women in this group who sought complementary therapies. As Marinomoana observed, these therapies could also provide additional sources of moral and physical support. Although she has never used a lot of herbal treatments because she doesn't like them, eats whatever she likes and continues smoking and drinking, she has found benefit in some natural therapies practised by her mother-in-law.

> *When I have bad bouts of muscle spasms my mother-in-law is able to calm me and the spasms down through stress release. That's very important for me because my stress levels go high very quickly and I tend to ignore things, and that makes the stress worse. I think if you are more relaxed you must be getting better. She does 'Touch for Health' which is like an acupressure—acupuncture without the needles. She locates the appropriate pressure points and massages those. I don't really like that because my husband and dad have to hold my feet to keep me still. It makes me crack up. I giggle and fall off the table.*
>
> *When I was having chemo and radiotherapy I'd go straight over to see her and she'd give me herbal tablets and teas for strengthening my body so that it could cope with all the stuff that was being done to it. She also uses the 'one brain theory' which believes that there is no distinction between the mind and the body. That's really good because it's holistic and it gives me the feeling that I'm doing something. When you're in hospital, they're doing things to you. I think naturopathy is a lot more caring, although that might be because she's my mother-in-law. I don't know any others. But she asks questions that are relevant to me. She wants to know how I'm feeling, what's going on and then she'll tell me what she's found. Naturopaths are better than psychologists actually!*

Beth also found the healing interests and skills of non-medical friends a great source of support.

> *You can use your mind to help you be more relaxed, to get*

through the pain, to be more peaceful and more accepting, or—on the other hand—more demanding about having your needs met and being prepared to go for the things that you want to do.

Thus she has focused upon

. . . the things I can do in myself because I think, while it's not all in the mind, the mind is a very powerful thing. I have a friend who does massage, reflexology, acupuncture and Chinese traditional medicine. She massages my feet and I love that. Another friend who does aromatherapy thought aromatherapy massage might help me feel relaxed and at ease, and it does. I don't know that I have reflexology or aromatherapy because it's going to fix me. I have it because it makes me feel great. I don't want to be running off here, there and everywhere getting help from other people because I think I have got that strength in me. But if people come to me, as these two special friends have, offering to help, then I am glad. I really appreciate their support in making the time and effort for me.

She has also used facilities offered by the Cancer Support Association who had

. . . a beautiful property where they had support groups and rooms where you could go and stay for a break. One day every month they had volunteers in who did massage, reflexology and that kind of thing. I used to go in for a massage because I get very sore and it was good to get out and meet people and come home relaxed and comfortable.

Other than that, she hasn't

. . . had any burning desire to race off and find alternative

treatments like apricot kernels or special injections, nor have I tried special diets. I had a lot of immune problems some years ago and I lived on cortisone for a long time. I got to the point where I was grasping at straws and tried almost anything anyone suggested—sometimes with disastrous results. I ended up in hospital with carotene poisoning from too many carrots and sulphur burns from too many sulphur baths. As a consequence I'm now very wary.

Although Ann T always felt very positive about the success of a mastectomy and a regime of chemotherapy, she also recalls that

. . . there were always times in the first year that I used to get panic attacks. I'd freeze up and I could not sleep. I needed something so I went to my doctor and said, 'Any chance of giving me a few sleeping tablets?' But doctors don't like giving you sleeping tablets and I didn't want to go onto tranquillisers. The girls in his surgery were very good and they told me there was a man coming to town to do a course in the 'de Silva Method' of positive awareness. The de Silva Method is just one method of positive awareness and it's really a way of living your life, of helping your state of mind to cope with anything that's worrying or upsetting you. There's a lot of things that we worry about that we can't do anything about.

I thought the course was terrific. It relaxed me so much and it did teach me to meditate and, although I didn't keep it up, it does help me when I get panic attacks. I was a real worrier. This is one of the things that may be a reason for my breast cancer. We don't know but that was the only thing I could put it down to really and I suppose I did blame myself and I still probably do. I think, 'OK. Breast cancer may be hereditary but if it's caused by stress I'm not going to do it to the other one.' When I first did the de Silva course your outlay was about $400. It's probably far more now but to go back *and do reviews only costs about thirty dollars, so I want to do it again soon. It definitely did help me an awful lot because I think when you're going through something like this you can let the 'what if?' get to you and really bring you down. That course did make me very much aware of what I was doing myself.*

She has continued to 'dabble' in a range of stress management techniques and ways of maintaining good health.

I started looking at diet a lot more. My one downfall is I love the ol' wine, but you have to have some vices! If you did everything perfectly it would drive you mad!

Other women in the group chose not to pursue complementary therapies for a range of different reasons. Margaret W did try 'some things from the nature shop' to stop the acid taste after her stomach was removed but she found that they tasted so horrible that she couldn't swallow them. She also considered trying acupuncture to relieve a painful spasm in her foot, probably caused by poor circulation, but found that an elastic bandage helped more. Mara also toyed with the idea of some complementary therapies and was intrigued when she heard

... people talk about herbalists, naturopaths and Chinese medicine. Many times I wanted to go and talk to somebody but because I don't have educated information, just hearsay from people, I didn't do anything. In my own garden I have a lot of herbs and when I make a cup of tea I always drop a few leaves of mint or marjoram or thyme. I have a big book of herbs from my own country in Croatian language which my mother and grandmother used to use in the olden days. Home medicine. I have read that book and a lot of times I wonder if any of this would help. But except for having herbal tea, that

is about all I have ever ventured into. I am curious because sometimes I think that those people can help a more natural aging process, to slow it down. If you have bone aches or arthritis then they are there to help you. But for something drastic and dramatic like cancer, I don't think it's a big possibility that taking different herbs or doing different manipulative exercise will help.

In contrast, Carmen didn't think of trying any complementary therapies because she already used meditation, ate very little meat and liked vegetables and salads. She believed that—

. . . you should eat all the five groups. I don't believe in diets or trying to get thin. I do aerobics to tone my body. I've got good hair, good skin and good nails so what I'm eating must be good although maybe I don't eat enough. I don't think I need to go to any health farm. I believe that you should eat a little bit of everything. I'm not a diety person.

Julie also had always done 'the right things' by following a low fat diet with plenty of fresh fruit and vegetables, and she had given up smoking years before. After she was diagnosed she thought about the diets of raw vegetables and remembers 'wanting to thumb through every book in a health food shop looking for solutions, looking for answers, or maybe some magic potion.' Although there was none she

. . . ate very cautiously for a while there, and thought about going to see a naturopath or a herbalist. But I didn't know where to start and I'm very cautious because I know that there's a lot of quacks out there that are in it for a money-making game. I work hard for my money, and I thought I've got to put my trust in somebody. I could relate to the doctors I had, and that was fine. Had I not been able to relate, I think

> *I would have been out there looking for somebody that I could have trusted.*

Like Julie, Margaret P had a medical doctor whom she trusted, and this contributed to her faith in the treatments she was being offered. Although she had decided long ago that if she 'had to live on carrot juice' she 'would rather die', she knew many people who had used alternative treatments.

> *I went to visit one of them the week before she died. Her left arm was livid, solid purple from her wrist up to her biceps. I've never seen that before. Right up to the last she'd been having vitamin C injections given by some alternative with the name of doctor. This woman was not only terminal, she was on her last legs. She wanted to try anything that might do her any good. That's alternative medicine. They took a lot of money off her. Maybe there are some people who can help with side-effects, and if it makes you feel good, like your placebo, well why the hell not? But I would strongly advise anybody going into it to make sure they are not paying out large amounts of money for something which is useless or may even be harmful. If it is complementary, and not alternative, all they are going to do is cost lots of money, and make people a bit comfier. But it does not want to be instead of conventional treatment, it wants to be as well as. Then everyone will claim that it was their treatment, not the other that succeeded! As a person with cancer, you can't care about that, you've got to put yourself first. But no, I don't consider complementary therapies. I've no faith in them.*

Annie also lacks faith in most complementary therapies although she acknowledges that they provide 'supportive care' for some people. Once she discovered that she had cancer she 'switched immediately into the medical model and conventional treatment'. She found it objectionable when well-meaning people insisted that she should follow rigid dietary or meditation programs.

I'd like to know the definition of meditation. I use tapestry and craft work as meditation and I think of it as just a space where I can sit quietly. I'm not very good at sitting quietly without doing something because I find that sitting and gazing at my navel is a complete and utter waste of time. I have never toyed with carrot juice. Unless something has got a common sense basis, forget it. I became very adverse to new age stuff because so much of it is a con although I know it helps some people. But I get annoyed when I hear about people paying $700 for a carrot juice extractor because it goes anticlockwise instead of clockwise, or people eating totally vegetarian diets when you need a well-balanced diet and an adequate amount of protein. I don't think it's the time to go on dramatic diets.

I think that when people haven't got support from the medical profession or from their friends, then they go looking for a support mechanism, and they will find it in alternative therapies because they are paying big bickies for it. You can get all the support in the world if you pay for it. I had a friend who used to pay $100 a session to get hooked up to some machine that was supposed to do electrical pulses. I guess because she had come to the end of all medical treatment and this was some sort of treatment it helped her. But it makes me very angry that people are making money out of this need, when people with cancer aren't in a position to be paying out. I went to a lecture once by a woman who had come out to Perth from the American Cancer Association. She was talking about alternative therapies and said that out of any profession, the medical profession will latch onto something if it will cure people, whether it's a diet, a drug or whatever, because that's their whole game. That is part of the reason that they are not too good at looking after death

> *and dying—because they've been trained to cure. If there's something that will cure someone, then they will use it and you won't have to pay for it through the nose.*

As with all aspects of the experience of cancer, there are no categorical rights and wrongs about the ways in which complementary therapies can be used. Some therapies offer people a degree of personalised care, a sense of control and an opportunity to participate in their own treatment in ways which the medical profession sometimes finds hard to duplicate. Those women who undertook rigorous adaptations of their diet, or who chose herbal mixtures and vitamin supplements or treatments, did so with the conviction that these helped their bodies deal with the rigours of tough medical treatments. The same is true of the various methods to relieve the emotional and psychological pressure which can accompany cancer. For others the whole notion of alternative treatments was a waste of time. Anne K, who opted for conventional treatment and 'never used any other therapies', summed the situation up.

> *All I could do was keep my mind on getting through that day and the next day. I don't knock any of those other alternatives. Perhaps a lot of them work but I decided I was going to have to go through the system and I would do it in the most positive way I could. People deal with these things in their own way. Everyone is different and you do what you have to to get through.*

7

FAMILY, FRIENDS AND FELLOW TRAVELLERS

A DIAGNOSIS OF CANCER STARTS FROM THE POINT OF IMPACT AND spreads outwards in concentric circles, creating waves which wash over a surprisingly large number of people. Just as the experience of cancer is unique for the person at the centre of the 'ripple', so are the ways in which other people respond. While these women came from diverse socio-economic and familial situations, all were mothers. The impact of their diagnosis on their children was of paramount importance, but they all became aware of the ways in which their experience of cancer challenged other relationships. Some relationships were weakened to the point of breaking; others were strengthened. Nearly all were changed in some fundamental ways. New friendships were formed, often with other people with cancer—fellow travellers who shared an understanding of the ways in which cancer could transform relationships. While none of the women in the group wanted to skate over or ignore issues they believed fundamental to their experiences of cancer, neither did they want to 'damage' or embarrass those they love. Where there has been any prospect of doing this, anonymity has been opted for.

FAMILY—PARTNERS, PARENTS AND CHILDREN

No matter how common the incidence of cancer, few of the women ever seriously contemplated that it might happen to them. Often, a woman newly diagnosed with cancer was left alone to tell family members that the domestic status quo had suddenly changed. Annie found herself in this position because she didn't take anyone with her to the doctor the day she was told.

She 'honestly didn't expect to have cancer'. She found herself in the middle of 'a major prickle bush', trying to 'deal with the shock of diagnosis and then tell everybody'. On reflection, she considered that the one thing that was 'totally lacking is any sort of support in telling family' about the diagnosis and the prognosis.

> *Who can tell your family for you? It is the biggest thing that's going to affect your kids and your parents and whoever else, and there you are left to deal with the diagnosis, knowing that this is going to be the most painful thing to your kids, and you have to tell and deal with it on your own. There doesn't appear to be any support available for doing that. I don't know what can be done. I don't know whether doctors are trained to meet with the kids. I'm sure if you asked medicos to do it then they would. But, the thing is then you've got to ask them: it's not something that's considered automatically. It's left to the person who has just been hit with a brick wall. You know that you're causing pain to people around you while you're trying to assimilate any information that has been given to you. It's just too much and there is nobody there to help you. Nobody has ever asked me how my kids are going or how they are accepting my diagnosis. No-one has asked me how my parents are coping. That is really difficult.*

The women in this group came from diverse socio-economic and ethnic backgrounds, so there was no uniformity of experience in the ways their diagnoses of cancer affected their family relationships. Apart from cancer, the only thing they shared was that they were all mothers, so the impact of their diagnosis on their children was of primary importance. Even here, generalisations are impossible because these 'children' ranged from babies through to adults, some with families of their own. But it wasn't only children whom these women cared for: elderly parents, partners and, in many cases, siblings and in-laws came into the orbit of these women's lives. Some of the older women in the group did not have to confront the grief of a parent distressed at the prospect that their daughter might not outlive them. One woman was widowed, others were separated or divorced from their children's fathers, others became so later. Still others remained happily married despite the pressures their diagnosis placed on family relationships. The web of women's relationships is not easy to unravel.

The issue of 'to tell or not to tell' was particularly difficult when young children were involved. While professionals generally advise that it is 'better to let your children know at an early stage of diagnosis' (Lowenthal, 1990, pp. 103–104), several women in this group decided against this course of action, at least until treatment made some explanation of their mother's condition unavoidable. For Anne K this time came four years after diagnosis; that time had given her sons more time to grow up without the fear of losing her.

> *The kids didn't know. I didn't tell them until the very last minute before I was going for my transplant. I had organised everything with the teachers at the school, although I told them at the very last minute as well. They were very good to the boys, very supportive.*

Marinomoana and her husband also chose not to tell their two boys because 'they were too young', although she acknowledged that 'this didn't mean that they didn't know there was something on'. She found this decision difficult but necessary because they 'didn't want to smother them like there was something wrong'. Children tend to be sensitive to subtle changes in their parents' behaviour.

Kaye and her husband

> *... didn't tell the children much because they were only four*

and six years old. They knew in their childish ways that something had gone wrong but I would just say to them that I had something bad and the doctor took it out. They would ask if I was better now and I would say 'Yes.' As long as nothing much was going on, and mum wasn't going away, they went back into their normal mode. If we started to talk about it around them it was about 'that thing'. Some of my friends and relations said, 'Shouldn't you tell them? What happens if it comes back again or you die?' I said, 'I'll cross that bridge when it comes. They are so young, why put that on their young shoulders? They'll have all that worry for nothing.'

Despite other people's doubts about the wisdom of this course of action, Kaye has had no regrets.

It wasn't until my daughter was twelve that she asked, 'Exactly what was wrong with you, Mum?' I told her and she was quite surprised. I said, 'I thought you'd woken up to it. We talked about some things'. She said: 'I sort of woke up to it but I wasn't too sure.' That saved all those years of worry because even when I actually came out and told her, for about a week she was following me around, even at that age. All of a sudden she thought I was going to disappear. She realised how bad it had been and she wanted to cling.

If I'd put that on their shoulders when they were really young they would have been petrified that something was going to happen to me all day and every day. I didn't want that to happen. I wanted life to be as normal as possible. If it had come to the stage where I had to go back in again, or I'd become terminal and only been given a certain amount of time to live, I would have had to rethink how to prepare them. While there was still hope and while I was doing reasonably well, I didn't see any need to worry them.

While this approach worked for Kaye's family, Lynne's totally different tactics worked equally for hers.

My kids have been brought up in this atmosphere of people who talk really straight to them and so I didn't hold a lot back. I talked about how frightened I was and about the implications of the treatment I was having—the fact that I would be likely to be bitchy and exhausted, and that I didn't have much energy. I told them what I understood about how this cancer might develop, and what its possible causes were. I actually did quite a lot of talking about sex with the children. It was important to talk about that because cervical cancer is generally regarded as a kind of sexually transmitted, viral-based disease and it is that aspect that people get heeby jeebies about. They think, 'My God! Cervical cancer! That's what whores get!' Cervical cancer has got a different kind of stigma than breast cancer, where women are victimised in the most primal sort of way.

It was amusing in a way because in the hospital when I was told about cervical cancer's connections with the herpes virus, they didn't want me to talk about my sexuality. This is a real problem for lesbians who are diagnosed with cervical cancer. A number of times the conversation would end with, 'We know that you've done it with a man at least once.' Actually I've done it more than that and I don't believe that any of them have actually transmitted this disease to me.

I think that there are lots of aspects of that kind of diagnosis that need some really careful thinking about. There's all sorts of funny implications and I talked to my kids about all of that. In a strange way it opened up all sorts of other areas of intimacy as well, not just about coping or about fear of dying, but also about the way that we live our lives in a very day-to-day sense. It was an extraordinary experience. They weren't nicer or more freaked-out or more traumatised children because I had cancer but the bonds between us grew. They're still frightened of me getting sick again and I have come to terms with the fact that I can't dispel that fear for them. I mean it's there for me too now.

Where there were young children to consider, it was not always just a matter of 'to tell or not to tell'. Sometimes there was no way treatment could be undergone without a child being aware of the changes taking place in a mother's life. There was a natural anxiety about how a child might react when treatment, no matter how essential, was disfiguring. Ann T was concerned about her son's reaction to her mastectomy but found life was much easier for both of them once his curiosity was satisfied.

We've always been quite happy to go around home without our clothes on. Nothing like that embarrasses us but after the operation we were all staying in one room at our friend's house. I was trying to shield my son from my mastectomy by turning around when I took my bra off until he asked, 'Let's see, Mum.' I said, 'Are you sure? It's quite a big scar.' He said, 'Yeah.' He was eight at the time. I turned around. He said, 'Oh, it's not that bad.' From that day on it didn't worry me really.

With breast cancer, the issue of how a mastectomy might affect children was not the only concern. The genetic link caused especial concern for a woman with daughters. Mara found that she worried about her daughters and three grand-daughters, wondering what chance they had with a hereditary history of breast cancer. She has tried to combat her fear by talking with her GP 'about genetic and dietary connections and environmental influences' and participating in a university research project about breast cancer. By doing this she discovered that 'there are quite a few factors that can influence breast cancer'. This left her a little reassured because she felt that at least when it came to diet, her Croatian heritage meant her daughters had grown up on a diet low in fats, rich in 'vegetables, fibrous things and oils' with small servings of meat served as an accompaniment rather than the central ingredient of a meal. There is nothing more she can do about their genetic inheritance except hope.

The decision whether to tell younger children, and how much to expose them to the effects of treatment, was a personal matter. The same applied to choosing who else in the immediate family should be told. Rae recalled how tempted she was to try to protect her family by not telling anyone except her husband.

> *I may be an over-protective mum at times, for when I was first diagnosed with cancer it went through my mind, 'I don't want the kids to know. I just want "this thing" taken out without them having to worry.' Of course I realised that this was selfish of me. They are grown-up responsible adults with children of their own. They had to know.*

This urge to protect her family extended well beyond that early stage. Even after treatment was completed she tried to hide her feelings 'so as not to make the family upset'. Later she reflected

> *... maybe that was the wrong thing because they were hurting as well. I thought I could hurt for all of them, and that I could hide that hurt. But you can't do that. They need to be told your feelings. They've got to feel it as well. It gets down to communication. You should say, 'How do you feel about it? How are we going to cope with it? What are we going to do now?' You can get through it that way, through strength in numbers.*

Rae was not the only woman who realised that this desire to 'protect' family members could be counter-productive. Despite the best of efforts, family members had to deal with the situation as best they could and, as Noelle found, being properly informed could provide their best chances of confronting the situation.

> *For quite a while I shielded my mother because I knew she wouldn't handle it, but then I realised I was doing her a dis-service because by not knowing the truth she was expecting all sorts of horrendous things. I was also doing myself a dis-service because my lying to her was putting a great emotional strain on me as well and I didn't need that. So I made a pact with my mother: I'm now up front with my mum. She is the first to know when new lumps come up and then if she falls in a heap, I'm afraid she falls in a heap. She will deal with it in the best way she can. She has got the support of my eldest brother and her next door neighbours.*

The desire to 'protect' family could be particularly acute when they could not be present to absorb the shock. Tiny, as well as several other women in this group, had migrated to Western Australia, leaving siblings and in-laws back in her country of origin. She explained the reasons she didn't tell them at first, the difficulty of explaining exactly how she was faring and how the distance weighed on her heavily at times.

> *I have got a big family in Holland, and so has my husband. At first I didn't tell them exactly what was happening because one of my sisters had just died and my other sister was very worried. I felt like I needed to protect them a little bit. It is really hard to talk about it because they cannot see me and they don't know what it is, and I cannot see how they react when I try to explain. It is not so easy to talk about sickness on the phone. When I say, 'I'm feeling all right' they don't know how it really is. The most difficult thing with my family is the distance between us. I'd love to go to Holland for a visit,*

but the doctor says, 'No, not this year.' So we have to wait another year.

Marinomoana faced similar problems of distance. She and her partner decided not to tell anyone else in their family, at first because they needed time to deal with her prognosis on their own. Her continued reluctance to inform them was also based on her understanding of how her family would react. She reflected:

My husband's family have been wonderful but it was a year before we told his parents and that only came out because my husband got angry and yelled at his father. He told him in anger. Now they're here at the drop of a hat. It's hard for them because they're not only losing their son's wife but the daughter, 'cos my husband is an only child. We are their family.

When I went to tell my father, I found out he was very sick so I thought I'd better not. That was the year before he died so I never told him. I still haven't told my mother. She lives in New Zealand, and half my family are on the Eastern seaboard. I've got ten brothers and sisters. Only one brother knows: he was living with us at the time of treatment so he had to be told. He's coped quite well but he's sworn to secrecy. Actually I did tell one sister-in-law when I was back home, and her reaction told me I shouldn't tell anyone else. She cried and cried. That's to be expected, I understand that, but every time she saw me, she'd burst into tears and my mother would start asking: 'What's wrong?'

I'm afraid of my family's inability to deal with my illness. It was bad enough when my father died: five years on they still can't get over it. I'm scared of their reaction because I know they'd be here, the whole lot of them and I don't want that because I'm well. My brother says every now and then he thinks he's going to blurt it out and a few years ago I said, 'I

> *don't mind if you do end up telling them.' In fact, I think it might be easier coming from him. If I tell them they'll think, 'Here goes the show pony again! She could not just have an ordinary sickness. No! She's got a terminal one!' That's what they are like!*

For most other women in the group, the possibility of not telling older children or adult family members did not arise. While older children, partners or parents should have had a greater understanding of the possible implications of cancer than little children, they often had just as much fear, so the issue became one of how to deal constructively with their responses. One woman was left in no doubt that 'the word cancer' affected her son more than herself.

> *He's very tense about his mother having cancer and he is my biggest worry because he's had a nervous breakdown. He panics and finds difficulty in coping.*

Another woman found that her whole family, including her young adult children, greeted her diagnosis with 'total non-acceptance'. Their initial response was understandable, if not particularly helpful. For them it was a case of, 'Oh don't be so silly—it can't be!' The pressure of her family's inability to come to terms with her prognosis eventually became so pressing that she asked her GP to explain to her parents the implications of her prognosis. That proved to be ineffective so she made an appointment for her parents to visit a counsellor, hoping that disinterested, professional information might help them understand the situation more clearly. Gradually, her family came to understand that this diagnosis was indeed a serious matter which would affect them all.

Family reluctance to accept a diagnosis was a common response although it took varied forms. One woman described how her 'whole family' responded exactly like she did—they 'buried their heads in the sand'. This had unfortunate consequences because they couldn't understand that she could no longer fulfil the domestic duties she had always undertaken. Their initial unwillingness to lighten her load left her feeling rejected, a 'hurt' which she had to come to terms with at the same time as she confronted her own fears. She 'learnt to cope' with her family when she

> ... *read a book called* Dealing with Cancer in the Family *which said how some families don't want to accept it: that's their way of coping. Once I read that it put me at ease. Another thing helped me. A woman from the student welfare council at my daughter's school came to visit me while I was at home. I told her that I felt terrible about my daughter and that my biggest worry was how she would fare without me. She said, 'Don't worry. I was nine years old and my mother died instantly in a car accident. She did everything for me and I survived. Look at me now. I am successful. Maybe it was the best thing that could have happened to me because it made me do things for myself.' That took away the pain. My father died when I was eighteen months old so I realised that although I never had a father, I had survived.*

Even where family members' reactions showed they comprehended the implications of the diagnosis, their ways of dealing with this could also lead to feelings of rejection. One woman recalled that she 'felt really left out' when her family were first told of her diagnosis. She could see them all outside her ward, crying together. But they would not cry in front of her. Perhaps hiding their tears was their way of trying to be strong for her, but she 'wanted to see how much they cared'. Another woman had almost the opposite problem: one elderly member of her family showed so much care that she felt she was 'being wrapped up in cotton wool'. While she appreciated the motivation, being 'molly-coddled' could get frustrating because she still needed 'that independence'.

Songs *of* Strength

Clearly, some families experienced difficulty finding the right balance of care and independence, or sustaining the balance over a long haul. One woman, who has had extended periods of treatment over several years, reflected upon the impact this had had on her daughters.

> *After all these years of being ill, my daughter has more than had enough. I am not allowed to mention my health except quickly, in passing. I am told there is nothing wrong with me and I will live for ever. If I get upset about a friend dying, she says, 'That is nothing to do with me.' She can no longer cope with being on the edge and has gone into denial, and yet she does 90 per cent of the housework and all the gardening as long as nothing is said. My other daughter is OK, but I rarely see her. I get my chemo fortnightly and I watch the other patients who are almost all accompanied by relatives or friends. I am always alone. I struggle home on the train often feeling envious of how easy it is when you have help. Neither of my daughters visits me when I am in hospital. My daughters have had to get on with their own lives. I do understand but it is hard and I feel awful saying it.*

This woman has come to the conclusion that

> *... it's no good talking to anyone who has not had cancer. You can't talk to your own rellies. Nobody can. I've not known anybody who has totally felt that their relatives had been what they would have liked them to have been over the cancer. Some of them are good, but they don't understand. They don't know what you feel like. I have an enormous need to talk and I need to be able to talk to somebody who understands, or at least somebody that will non-judgementally listen. We all get depressed or worried or fed up occasionally. We get all kinds of negative emotions. You have to talk to somebody and it seems*

to be fairly common that many families just can't cope. In my case I have a death sentence, but for my family it's a life sentence.

Other women found their immediate families to be their chief source of support and hope. Mara found that her husband and adult daughters provided enormous practical and moral support, while the presence of her grandchildren gave her joy, even if her daughters were anxious that they might be too much for her.

My daughter from Sydney came with her two boys and stayed with me for a month after the operation to help me with washing, cooking and doing strenuous things. My four little grandchildren cheered me up. I wanted to play with them and even started lifting them up on my arms straight after the operation. My daughters would freeze, saying, 'Don't do that! You'll damage something.' I never felt that I could damage anything by lifting my grandchildren. They were my best therapy.

Rae also found her seven grandchildren an important source of strength. At times there was no remedy quite like having them 'come to me, put their arms around me, hug and kiss me and say, "Grandma, I love you." ' For her, this has come to symbolise 'what families are all about.' Although her instinct was to shield her family from her emotional pain, she was grateful that

... we have always been a close family, so I was fortunate that they wanted to talk about it and help see me through. After my operation, my kids wouldn't let me do anything for quite a while, which was nice, and the support and love I received from my mum, brothers and their families has been fabulous. They cannot do enough for me. Through our tears and laughter I feel we have become closer. God has been good to me.

Tiny also found that

> ... as a family we have pulled together more than we used to. We talk about everything—not just my illness but how I am feeling, what I want and need. It is very important, not just for me but for the whole family. We have learned a lot from this. A lot of people like to go to a group to talk about it more, but I've got my family and friends to talk to and that has been enough for me.

Julie has no doubt that her experience of cancer was made more tolerable by the support she received from her husband and daughter. Her observations of this time reflect the contrary wishes which could arise when an arduous regime of treatment led to wanting support on one hand and wishing everyone else, particularly children, well out of it on the other. She also hinted at the sensitivity needed to understand how ghastly it could be for a young person to see and hear the dramatic effects of chemotherapy on their mother.

> The three of us bonded very closely together to get through this saga. At one stage my daughter was starting to go off the tracks: she thought that if she wasn't at home she didn't have to see Mum sick all the time. I would've liked her home sometimes when I was on chemo but then I thought she's only seventeen and I can't put her through this. I'd be sick for a full week: I couldn't move, I couldn't eat, I couldn't do anything so there was not much point in anyone staying home really. After a while my family got to know that I was all right, and it was just the treatment that made me sick. It was disappointing for them. For three weeks I'd climb up to nearly the top rung of the ladder and then I'd come down to the bottom rung again. I had chemo for about eighteen months, so it was pretty rugged on all of us. I still cannot stand to remain in bed in my bedroom when nobody else is in the house

because it reminds me of when I had the chemo and how sick I was.

As Julie suggested, no matter how supportive a family, in the final analysis treatment has to be undergone alone. Intensive bouts of treatment can be debilitating and ways have to be found to ensure that households keep functioning and that dependants are cared for. Many of these women had to reorganise their lives so that family responsibilities were met even though their physical and emotional resources were low. Lynne had a supportive network and she was able to focus upon her own needs while her partner took care of running the household.

My partner and I had actually decided to live separately just before I was diagnosed. When I found out what the treatment was I said to her, 'I really would like it if you would come and live back in the house because I'm not going to be able to get through this with the children.' I was right and it was her support that got me through all the practical stuff because there were some weeks during that period of treatment where I didn't remember what happened in the day. I was completely out of it. I slept a lot but that's not what I'm talking about. I'm talking about not being conscious really, feeling a way that I've never felt before, even when I was pregnant. I felt that I was my body and my body was in crisis and I needed to be there with it, or as it, every second of the day as a way of getting through.

There wasn't any choice because the treatment was horrendous. It produces a cocoon effect. Frankly, I couldn't care whether the washing got done. I never felt like eating anything. The children's fights just slid off me. My moods were fairly profound but people were supportive and careful of me. I really couldn't function on a practical level. I think if I had chosen to stay on my own, I would have probably paid for

> some practical support. I went to the clinic for the treatment every day, and I was seeing women who caught a bus to get there, or who had small children with them whom they had to get other people to look after in the waiting room. My situation was so different and I felt almost guilty because of it: if I'd been catching a bus from the outer suburbs every day for five weeks, with a stack of kids at home and possibly an unsupportive partner, my life would have been very different. As it was, I found it very difficult to cope even with the kind of privilege and support that I had.

Even if children or a partner were there to help with practical matters, or to 'hold your hand' and 'encourage you through' the procedures, the immediate experience was not theirs. When family members were not able to 'be there for you', for whatever reasons, then the loneliness of treatment was made more stark. Anne K accepted this right from the start.

> My husband made it quite clear that I had to deal with this illness on my own. It was probably his way of coping because he was starting off a business. This is not easy when you move to a new area, let alone a new country. I realise now that my leukaemia was something he couldn't even begin to think about because it meant that I would be a different person and he wouldn't be able to cope with that. To be fair to my ex, at the time he was working a ten to twelve hour day most days. He was physically tired when he got home, and then he would have more to do. He assumed that I could do things on my own, probably because I very quickly accepted my lot. He presumed that I was OK, that I was managing just fine. In a sense I brought a lot of that on myself by saying, 'OK. I accept that you can't deal with this. I'll deal with it.' When it came to the actual transplant, he was more involved and spent quite a lot of time visiting me in hospital.

As Anne K's experience suggests, there was something about the 'toughness' of most intensive cancer treatments which made an impact on everyone, even those who had been unwilling to accept that they were necessary. One woman found that although initially her husband wouldn't believe the doctors, he eventually came to understand her situation with more sympathy. At first, he would 'really shout' at her:

> 'How do they know you've got it? Why are they taking out your glands? They might be good glands! That's totally unnecessary.' I had to say to him, 'It's a precaution.' Eventually it turned around. When my husband saw me with the nausea I think he started realising that there was something wrong. Now he brings me a drink and makes the bed.

This woman's marriage has lasted the distance. Other partnerships have not been as resilient. Margaret P's marriage foundered. Years later she observed

> My ex-husband once said to me it would have been all right if I had died within six or nine months. That would have been all right, but not to keep going on like this. He couldn't handle it. I'm one of those who has got divorced since I got cancer.

For other women, their experience of cancer simply strengthened partnerships that were already strong. Rae considers that

> ... since I've had the bowel operation, my husband and I have been a lot closer. It was a big shock to him and although he kept a stiff upper lip, I think he was thinking the worst. He broke down in the hospital when we were told that the cancer had been caught in the very early stages. He was howling his

eyes out in pure relief. I didn't. I was telling him not to worry, that it was all over. When I came home it was nice to be spoilt. I wasn't allowed to do anything. He's a good provider and he can cook and everything like that. He's good that way and he's been a great support.

Likewise, Kaye's husband was her most consistent source of practical and emotional support.

My husband did most of the running around, paying the bills, doing everything while I was recuperating. Up until that time, I'd done it all. He was good. He stuck by me and took over, even with the kids. My daughter used to laugh because he'd try and plait her hair or put it up in a pony tail for her to go to school. She'd come up and say to me, 'Dad tried to do my hair this morning!' A lot of other men would have said, 'Here, Mum, or here, sister-in-law, you have the kids because I can't do it.' But no, he always would do everything for the kids.

Emotionally, in front of me, my husband was always a rock. One of my sisters-in-law said to me that the closest he came to breaking down was when he said, 'I can't imagine life without her. If I have anything to do with it there's no way in the world that she's going to go.' But to me he would never say anything like that because I had enough worries. Every time I was down he would put me back on a positive note. I fed off that. If he'd been negative and if he'd been more emotional in front of me, or gone down with me, I don't think I could have coped but every time I broke down he would be there saying, 'You've gone so far and you haven't had any worries. Come on, don't be silly.' Quite a few people I've spoken to through the years have told me of stories where the husband has been the one who has broken. In actual fact, a lot of them have walked away and left their wives because they can't handle it.

Marinomoana's husband could and did handle it. His ability to see things as they were, accept them, talk about them and get on with the business of living was an obvious source of delight and encouragement, even when things were at their bleakest.

My husband is very perceptive. He sees things and he is strong. That is just the way he is. I chose him very well! There are some things that I do and he'll just look at me like 'what are you doing?' Our communication comes naturally. Like if I say, 'I'm well' but I'm not really, he'll say, 'No you're not. Don't bunk!' That actually allows me to be honest about times when I don't feel too good. He has this strength about him and this boosts me up because I think I can be strong like him. My husband is strong because he is strong, he is not just strong for me. He knew that if I should die at any time that he would be the one left to bring up our boys. We constantly talk about that even now because we need to make sure plans are made for the boys. That worry is taken away. He doesn't just cope, he does things, and he does this because he loves us.

The ability to 'be with' a loved one with cancer rather than 'being strong for them' was a subtle but crucial distinction. One woman described how her partner returned home from a support group for the partners of people with cancer perplexed by their attitude. He told her that he didn't want to attend that group again because he felt that

... those people think they are being strong for their partners. Their partners are already strong. Can't they get that through their heads? Their partners are living with cancer! We're just watching.

The stresses of 'being with' and watching a loved one throughout the experience of cancer should never be underestimated. This was something Noelle became intensely aware of as her melanoma multiplied.

> *My partner has brought peace into my life but I do worry about him. He's the strong silent type who doesn't express what he's feeling and that bothers me. I've got him to prop me up, but what about him? Where does he go?*

Partners, like the women themselves, found their own ways through the maze but it was all too easy to forget that they might also need 'a holiday' or 'release' from the situation. This was particularly the case when other events in life compounded the stress—and most people who have experienced cancer would testify, there's never a right time for a diagnosis of cancer. It took Ann T some time before she 'computed' that her husband had had a rough trot.

> *Although my husband was marvellous while I was having treatment and after—he was there for me—when it was over he said one thing which I regretted afterwards. I'm not saying he did anything wrong; I know he was frightened. He said, 'You're over it now. It's gone. Just forget about it and get on. Don't consider yourself a victim of cancer.' I think maybe he was trying to put a block on it. He had been going through his own hell at that time. First there was my mastectomy. Then, the day I had my first chemotherapy dose, his dad died in Ireland and then within six months my brother died, all within six months. So at that time, I kind of put it all behind me as if it was just another illness. I didn't think of it as 'cancer', it was just like I'd had something wrong and it was now gone.*
>
> *We've had our barneys—not half—and there was one awful time when I was still on chemotherapy and not feeling too good. It was just after we got back to home from Perth and my husband went out for the paper at ten o'clock in the*

morning and didn't come home. He'd gone straight up to the club and got as drunk as a skunk. I couldn't understand it at the time and I thought, 'This is it. This is so selfish. We're getting divorced.' Here I was dying and he wasn't thinking of me. I think one of my friends finally said to me, 'Get a hold of yourself for Jesus' sake! He's been through hell too!' I thought afterwards it must have been his release from the pressure of the two months that we had in Perth, but I couldn't see it at the time. When I thought of it later, I was the selfish one.

Marinomoana became more aware of the importance of finding ways to relieve the pressure on her partner after she and her husband spent a weekend at a retreat for carers and for people with cancer in the hills outside Perth. Three of her friends, people she had met at a support group, had gone there together after the deaths of two other members of the group.

It was so lovely to be alive and out where you see so many things living. What was funny about that particular weekend was that the spouses kept meeting and having little discussion groups. We would joke and say, 'They are conspiring against us' but what they were doing was drowning their sorrows with each other. They needed that. There's very little support for the carers. When you're living with someone who has cancer—it doesn't matter what kind of cancer—it's hard and it takes a special person to hang in there. A lot of people don't cope. I have seen marriages break up especially when one spouse has a long-term illness. That was a good weekend away, we enjoyed ourselves and drank heaps of alcohol.

Although a woman's diagnosis of cancer and subsequent treatment affected her immediate family most intimately, it could also have a profound impact on her extended family. Even those who had migrated to Australia, leaving relatives in their country of origin, found that their families made great efforts to show how much they were thinking of them despite the distances that separated them. Tiny was in regular telephone contact with her family in Holland, while Anne K had 'lots of letters, lots of phone calls' and found her family kept her—

> ... *up to date with everything that was going on. They did all that they could. My donor was from my family. They all trooped in en masse to have their blood screened and tested for compatibility. It was nice to know that I had a good chance of getting a compatible donor. They were a bit far away being in another country but they were all very supportive. However, my sister came out on a working holiday just before the transplant. She was incredibly supportive both during the transplant procedure and afterwards. We talked for hours and that helped to keep me sane. She was there for both the children and me.*

This kind of practical support from relatives living far away could not only be literally life-saving, as in Anne K's case, but could boost morale significantly. Ann T remembers how her family in Ireland gave her—

> ... *tremendous support with phone calls, cards and letters. Then, six months later, out of the blue, my sister came out to see for herself how I was doing. That was a great surprise and did me the world of good.*

Most of the women in this group had relatives who lived closer by and several were touched by the ways in which they reached out to offer assistance. Rae cherishes the memory of an unexpected visit from some relations.

> *Soon after I came out of hospital my sister-in-law and my niece called around. When I look back on it, I think it was meant to*

be because I was here on my own and I'd had an upsetting day—I'd been concerned. They believe in spiritualism and my sister-in-law laid her hands on my head, and my niece sat on the floor and held my legs. They didn't say a word. It was the healing of hands. It was a wonderful experience for me because I felt the inner strength there, these two not saying a word, just moving their hands over my legs, my arms and my shoulders. The tension and concern went away. I felt so good after it. Something had been lifted. Something was there to give me inner strength.

This sense of family members being there when they were most needed was something Kaye came to appreciate fully. She had an extremely sympathetic family who found practical ways to help.

They were all great. I was very tired and run down and they were very supportive in looking after me or taking me anywhere I wanted to go, especially when I was on the radiotherapy. We got out of the fish and chip shop in Mandurah after my neck operation because I was too ill and it wasn't fair on our partners. That meant my husband was in between jobs for a while so he could run me up and down to Perth while I was attending the clinic for radiotherapy. We didn't know what the future was going to hold so we moved in with my father-in-law in East Fremantle. The whole lot of us squashed into one room while we were looking for a place. When I came out of hospital we went to Homeswest to see if they could help us out with a house. Luckily, one had just come up so we moved in and the children started going to the school down the road. That wasn't too bad.

When my husband went back to work as a metal worker, the family would come over to see if I wanted anything. My mother-in-law couldn't do enough for me: the housework, the washing, looking after the kids, anything. My brother couldn't do enough for me either: when I first got cancer of the tongue I came across a book that went through how to recognise the symptoms and know how your body changes when you're getting cancer. At first I couldn't read it because I'd think I had practically everything that was in there! Like they say, don't read a medical book. But this book was quite thick and I said I was going to get it photocopied. He took it away and photocopied it all for me. It would have cost him a fortune. Then when I mentioned I would have to buy a juicer to go on a juice diet, he turned up on the doorstep the next day with a juicer. I was very lucky. Half the time, I would catch them watching me as if I was going to have a relapse and a lot of times they didn't know whether to talk about it or not, or how to bring the subject up.

Unfortunately, not all extended families found ways to 'talk about the subject'. One woman found that her siblings coped by 'running'. This was a particularly sensitive issue but an important one because little attention gets paid to the feelings of siblings in situations like this—and they, like everyone else in the drama that surrounds cancer—have their roles in the support networks.

I tried to put myself in my siblings' position. I realised that it wasn't easy, and that the easy way out for all of them was to be too busy to drop by to see how I was going. They didn't want to see this painful, pale, thin person but even the cards and flowers were conspicuous by their absence. I went through all my cards later because the cards and the flowers got me through. The support from my mates was tremendous but there was not one card from my immediate family. There were flowers from Mum but the rest of the family couldn't cope. I won't say it didn't hurt but they're all back now—not close, but we are all on good terms.

FAMILY, FRIENDS AND FELLOW TRAVELLERS 315

This woman was not the only one who discovered that her diagnosis heightened her sensitivity to the nuances of family relationships. Sometimes these nuances were highlighted by the idiosyncratic ways in which a family member might approach a cancer crisis. One woman had to learn how to accommodate a family member, whom she loved dearly, but whose whole approach was incompatible with hers. She was

> ... one of these people who doesn't accept things at face value: if she is told something then she must look it up, she has to find out for herself. When I was first diagnosed she was there hovering in the background saying, 'Have you been here? Have you asked this? Have you done that?' If my answer was 'No' then she would want to know why and she would get agitated and quite angry. I found it difficult at times to go and visit because I knew I was going to be bombarded with questions. That was a need of hers, not my need. Once I accepted that, it wasn't a problem.

Noelle was grateful that her family rallied around and 'provided a huge buffer zone' of support for her. Even so she was aware that

> ... there is a part of me as well that asks, 'Would I be getting as much attention if this thing hadn't happened to me?' The devil creeps in every now and again but that's just the cynical dark side of me. Like my brother recently gave me a birthday party. We never celebrate birthdays in our family but he rang me up before I went away on holidays and said he wanted to put on a birthday party especially for me. Straight away I thought, 'Oh my God! What ever for?' It was to be all the immediate family for this party and the more I thought about it the less I liked the idea. I was thinking it was for all the wrong reasons and I was calling it 'the just in case party'. I could imagine everybody saying, 'we must have photographs,

just in case—this may be the last time all of us are together.'

But it wasn't for the wrong reasons. And I was actually the one who made them take some photographs! They were horrified but I thought blow it! So we got the four children with the two estranged parents on either end ... When my brother got up and said he wanted to say something I thought 'Oh my God! Here it comes! The long and teary speeches!' He simply said how much he loved his sisters and wished my partner all the best. It's not until there's a crisis that people are given the opportunity to put their best side forward, and then it comes out in all its glory. It's not a put-on thing. It's genuine. It's from the heart and it's always been there but there hasn't been a need to express it all the time. We get too wound up in everyday life, I think, too busy with day-to-day living.

FRIENDS—WIN SOME, LOSE SOME

As Noelle observed, there's nothing quite like a life-threatening illness to encourage reassessment of aspects of life that are often taken for granted. Relationships with friends came into that category. Although some women found that a few of their friends were suddenly 'too busy with day-to-day living' to make room for them, many made new friends and discovered unfathomed depths of friendship. Few of the women were left in any doubt that their diagnosis had profound effects upon their relationships with friends and colleagues.

Some, like Lynne, were surprised at the people who offered support, and the 'constancy of that support'. Although she considered that it was 'having people to talk to, people who were basically affirming of me' that got her through, it did not take her long to realise that the way friends and workmates reacted to her diagnosis was unpredictable.

I had a lot of emotional support from friends, some from work which surprised me because university really is a most barbaric and competitive place. There were men at work, for instance, who took the opportunity to talk to me about their mothers or wives having cancer and there were other people at work who haven't spoken to me since—maybe in case they catch something! Some of them actually asked, 'Is it catching?' Mostly people were really supportive. They found out that I was drinking carrot juice so they went and bought me a juicer and I had all these flowers and positive expressions of interest in my wellbeing. Sometimes I wondered whether they had ulterior motives in being so interested in my sickness. In all the time I'd been here, this level of interest had never happened before so I thought: 'Is it because I'm about to die?' Maybe they could see my contract coming to an end sooner than they thought! Anyway, overall it was quite decent. I think cancer actually marshals people together, very often out of fear because people want to believe that you can survive it.

The mixture of support and discomfort which could be expressed by work colleagues was something Julie learnt to deal with quickly when she realised that even the best of intentions could sometimes backfire. At times like this she found humour the best defence, although this could be emotionally draining.

Some of my closer workmates did ask outright, 'Are you going to be all right?' 'What did the doctors say?' 'You didn't lose your hair, did you?' A lot of my workmates were good but in every work group you get a few who make real boo-boos and you have to find excuses for them. I think they were just ignorant: they're still my buddies—they sent me flowers, their name was on the card, I'll forgive 'em. You have to be quite strong actually. People don't know how to ask questions. They don't want to say the word 'cancer'.

Although overall Ann T 'felt much closer to people after her mastectomy' and found that her experience enhanced her appreciation of 'just what people could do for you', she experienced this same ambivalence—expressions of goodwill mingled with uneasiness. Like Julie, she tackled this head-on. When she returned home after her mastectomy she was

> ... *frightfully spoilt. Within a week all the unions in town had sent me a big bouquet of flowers and I was given fruit and chocolates. It was magic. People were OK doing that but a lot of people were frightened to face me. They didn't know what to say. I just got in there, among them, and I think that broke it a bit. A lot of it was up to yourself to do things and join in because people are frightened to include you. I was glad I was in a small town because there were friends there that did understand and always made sure I was part of things. I'll always be grateful to the friends who looked after my husband and son when I was in hospital, and me after I came out. I can't say enough about the way they helped.*

While it was perhaps not surprising that friends 'outside the inner-circle' sometimes blundered, this uncertainty about how or whether to broach the topic of cancer could be something even close friends suffered from. Beth recalled that

> ... *there were only two people I had trouble talking to about my cancer. They were two male friends and colleagues and a few days before surgery we met for a meal—something we did quite often. But this time it was hard to know what to say or how to express what we were feeling. They told me afterwards that they called it the 'last supper', but I'm glad to say we've had many suppers since then!*

Kaye found that although her very close friends stuck by her, some of them 'didn't know how to talk about it'. However, she found that if she raised the subject, 'they didn't feel uncomfortable, or give the impression that they didn't want to hear'. Another woman found that it was mostly 'people of her mother's generation—people in their seventies and eighties' who were 'absolutely hopeless' at handling the topic of cancer. They would say

> *'Aren't you being brave?' and 'Isn't it a sad thing?' It drives me to distraction. I used to go and have morning teas when she brought in her mob but now I don't want to be in a social situation with them. Maybe it is because they are reaching stages in their lives when they have to confront death and dying so when someone younger comes along it raises a whole lot of stuff and they try to gloss over it by saying 'Aren't you brave?' I find that really difficult because if it was my age group I'd say, 'Bullshit! You'd do the same thing. You haven't got much of a choice.' But my age group—people in their forties and fifties—seem much better able to deal with it and I don't know why. Perhaps we're all more aware of improvements in medicine, treatments, services and so on. Whatever, there is certainly a difference in the way the different generations deal with cancer.*

Generational or not, there was no doubt that some people found it difficult to express their concern in appropriate ways. Indeed, it could be hard for friends to know what the most appropriate forms of support might be. Rae's friends found the right mark for her.

> *It was a real concern for friends when they found out I had bowel cancer. There was nothing much anybody could do, but the cards and letters of support that I got were a great help. In a sense it was lovely because there were so many very caring people who would do anything they could to help.*

For many women, especially when they were in the throes of treatment, cards and letters were an effective way of showing concern.

While Carmen was 'absolutely overwhelmed with friendship from everybody at work and at church', and gratified because she had 'never realised that people cared so much' for her, she gradually realised that in her own interest she had to take the initiative and tell friends what not to do.

> *My phone rang non-stop and I found that really was disturbing. They don't know whether you're on the toilet, in the shower or in a deep sleep. Sometimes you haven't slept all night and you've just been able to get to sleep. We don't have a phone in the bedroom and it's terrible having to get out of bed for the phone when you are really sick. It's not that I was ungrateful but eventually I had to say to my friends, 'Can you phone me in the night at six o'clock because I need to sleep during the day.'*

She found that

> *. . . the people that helped the most were the ones who didn't speak so much! They sent me a letter with some nice words rather than phoning up. That tells you that they care and that they're feeling for you because they took the time to write a letter, get a stamp and post it. I found it meant so much more.*
>   *Other friends came and brought me food or a book. It's the practical things that you need help with. Friends from my church group would bring a cooked chicken, soup, casseroles and pikelets and even if I couldn't eat it the family could and at least I didn't have to supply them with their meals. If somebody came and said let me hang up your washing, wash the dishes or make the beds that's a big help although I personally don't like people in my house doing my cleaning up. I'm very uncomfortable about that. You've really got to be careful who you say can come into your house although that was the kind of help I needed more than anything else.*

Anne K agreed that when it came to

> ... the practical day-to-day things, it would have been good to have someone come in and put the washing out. Support from my husband and friends would have made life a bit easier just by sharing the load, but that didn't happen. People are busy with their own lives.

She recalled that she had a couple of very close friends who were supportive, although—

> ... in the end it boiled down to one close friend because the other was leaving the country. I lost most of our mutual friends throughout the ordeal. They went one by one because they couldn't cope with it. It was very tough going because you feel a sense of isolation. You think: 'I've got this thing that no-one else has. My future is uncertain. My friends can't cope with it, so how am I going to cope with it?' This is where the day-to-day basis comes into it. At some point, I just shut down and only thought about getting up tomorrow: 'I'm going to get through tomorrow and then, whatever the following day brings, I'll get through that.' I have an old maxim that I always stand by. 'No condition is permanent.' My kids are sick of listening to me say it, but this is what I firmly believed and that gave me the strength to carry on. That was my driving force. I cut everyone else out except the one close friend I had. If I got really down I could talk to her. She would come over and, if she found me in a mess, she would roll her sleeves up and have more done in twenty minutes than all the phone calls could ever do for me. She was just fantastic and I am profoundly grateful for her on-going support and friendship.

Anne K was not the only woman to find out that some friends couldn't last the distance. Most came to the conclusion that, although painful, in many ways their loss simply 'sorted out the wheat from the chaff' Although Marinomoana discovered that she had 'some really great friends', she 'lost some people who we thought were friends, but weren't'. Annie had a similar experience. She considers that her

> ... *friends are the mainstay of the whole caboodle and you certainly know who your friends are. I'd say I've lost about one third of my friends. Actually, it's a bit of a relief because I figured out that I was the one who was maintaining those friendships and they really were not all that fantastic.*

Lynne found that what she considered her 'extended family' of women whom she'd 'been lovers or friends with was really called into question' by her having cancer 'because it brought up lots of fears for other women about their own lives'. She lost friends she never expected she would lose 'because they couldn't cope with the idea of cancer'. Marinomoana found that while some of her friends coped by pulling out all the stops to help, others withdrew and got gloomy. She recalled—

> *Sometimes friends would come over to cheer my husband up and he'd end up having to cheer them up because they'd get themselves so sad! We found some wonderful gems among people that we've known: people who've stood by us and ferried me and the kids all over the place. There were other friends who couldn't cope. One woman asked me why I didn't look after my children better, why my home wasn't cleaner and why was I always so slack. I was really in a down time, so I turned around and told her. She's never spoken to me since. She saw my husband soon after that and told him she couldn't cope. I thought: 'That's strange! She couldn't cope and it's ME who has the tumours!'*

Margaret P summed up the changes in her friendships.

> *When you are in any kind of trouble you find out who your friends are. Some of your friends that were just friends become better friends, while some people can't handle it and avoid you when you get cancer. It's as though you are ringing an unclean bell, because some people react like they are scared they are going to catch it. A lot of people will ask you how you are but will only want you to tell them everything is fine. People who can't cope with the pain keep away from you. You might have known them for years. I reckon a lot of people have an attention deficit disorder when it comes to cancer! With some people, I know I've worn out the welcome mat because I'm supposed to always be smiling and happy and brave and biting the bullet but I can't do that, especially over the long term. I'm going out kicking and screaming.*

But even women who didn't believe in 'kicking and screaming' or telling people exactly how they felt could be surprised how quickly erstwhile friends and acquaintances 'dropped them'. Margaret W had emigrated from England to Western Australia, but she had first spent many years in the Eastern States. Without rancour, but with the straight-forwardness which characterised her whole approach to her situation, she observed that she hadn't

> *... made many true friends in Western Australia, not so many as I made in New South Wales. I'm a little disappointed in the women's association that I've been involved with. After all I've done for them, only a few women from the local branch bother to ring me up or come to see me. You would think that it would be part of their philosophy.*

Other women were more fortunate. Tiny was given both moral and practical help by friends from the Dutch community and from her church. She also found that she made new friends.

> We haven't lost any friends. I think that some friends are closer than they were and even acquaintances who weren't really good friends come to see how I am. This is good, especially when we can't go anywhere because I am not feeling so good. You don't feel that you like to go to other people but still, they come to visit anyway. We are Catholic, and the priest and the church here are very supportive. When I need some help I can get the help from there, even if it is just someone coming over for a talk. That has been very good. And we have gained a lot of friends through the hospital—other people who are sick who I can talk to.

Beth also had great support from her church and felt impelled to rekindle 'some great friendships with a group of old church friends from twenty-five years ago'. Friends 'were often her sanity in all the drama', and she was amazed by the ways people found to express their care.

> Some just rushed up and gave me a big hug, one or two cried and others tapped me on the shoulder and said: 'I hope it's OK'. Some didn't really know how to handle it, or me, and they are the people you have to let go. One friend said: 'Don't exclude me' when she felt I was not allowing her the closeness she wanted nor letting her support me enough. Another lady that I'm really fond of surprised me when she sent me a card that said: 'I hope you are OK', but she never called or came to visit. Then, twice, in the mail came tapes of music that she thought I might enjoy, accompanied by beautiful notes. That thrilled me to bits. People have different ways of expressing themselves and their friendships.

Beth also made friends in unexpected circumstances.

> I rang a menopause group and a member who lives nearby

called with the information. We chatted for a while and then she said, 'When you need to go to chemo, I'd like to go with you.' I was embarrassed because I'd never asked anyone for anything and needing help made me feel vulnerable. But I accepted and I'm glad I did because she takes me to chemo each week. She's become a wonderful friend and I look forward to our time together. We still have coffee or lunch even now I'm not having chemo, and that is a special time with a special friend who I might never have met.

Noelle interpreted this idea of special time as 'quality time' and came to believe that her time with everybody

... should be quality time. If it's not going to be quality then why bother with it? I think 'quality time' is a tired cliché but to me it means being somewhere or with a person that gives me joy and happiness. That doesn't mean it has to be for x-amount of time. It can be the briefest of moments when someone has done something very spontaneous for another person. Like yesterday a little guardian angel button hole arrived for me in the mail totally out of the blue. It was sent by a friend of my sister's who I had only met on very odd occasions. All it had with it was a note saying 'from Kerry's friend Ann'. That's what I call quality. To me that means Ann's friendship to my sister means a lot to her, so by doing me that kindness she is really doing something for my sister through me. Since I've had cancer I've found that people do these beautiful things and it's because they want to do them not because they think they have to. This has given me recognition of the goodness that is in people and how people feel about other people in their lives. I may never have experienced it—or I may have experienced it in a different form and not have recognised it for what it really is.

For Noelle, the experience of cancer finetuned an awareness of the interconnections between people. In the process, she came to appreciate that amongst the finest gifts friends could give one another was that of mutual acceptance. This was something she believed passionately: it was fundamental to the way she nurtured her friendships and lived her life.

> *I've got a magnificent group of friends who are so supportive. I've numerous friends I ring up and say, 'I'm having a terrible day. I feel like shit!' I can scream down the telephone and it's acceptable. My friends have always been important to me and I love them all in different ways. They are very much individuals and come from all walks of lives and their different life experiences makes them very unique people. Each one of them gives something to me and by each individual giving a little bit of this and a little bit of that, it brings it into a whole. But I never realised how much I meant to them and this has given them the opportunity to show me that what I felt for them is reciprocal. That's absolutely marvellous and probably my biggest learning experience.*
>
> *It's a beautiful feeling. I know a lot of people will say you're sick, soppy and sentimental and I've had sessions with friends when I've said to them, 'I love you very much' and they say, 'Oh shit! Don't start that! You're making me cry.' Maybe subconsciously we know what these friendships give to us but we take it as read. These are the things that should be said. We don't have to go around all the time saying 'I love you. You mean a lot to me' but I really think every now and again you do have to take a person and hold them and say: 'There is meaning to my life because you're my friend.' We don't do it. We shy away from it and we leave it so damn late.*

FAMILY, FRIENDS AND FELLOW TRAVELLERS

FELLOW TRAVELLERS—OTHER PEOPLE WITH CANCER

While discussing the impact her diagnosis had on her relationships with other people, Lynne observed that it had made her acutely aware of 'how prevalent cancer is'. It made her face the possibility that a number of her 'friends might die of cancer', just as her mother had done. This heightened awareness of the number of other people who have, or are, or will, experience some form of cancer is perhaps inevitable simply by virtue of attendance at clinics and hospitals for treatment. But as Beth observed, she didn't need to attend these in order to meet other people whose lives had been affected by cancer.

> *I haven't made a point of going off to meet people with cancer but I have found that I seem to be meeting more people with cancer. Maybe I'm just more aware of it—you know how when you buy something unusual, like a white MG, then all you seem to notice is white MGs everywhere! For example, I went to visit a friend whose Mum has just been diagnosed with lung cancer and I spent an hour listening to her because she needed to talk to someone. On the way home, I popped into a local shop and the lady's husband has got bowel cancer and she also wanted to talk. At work I have met up with two women who have cancer and so we ring each other occasionally and meet for coffee. Even though the contact is limited I feel a closeness and an affinity with these fellow travellers because we all share a similar experience and we can relate to what each other is feeling or going through. If people know that you have cancer I guess they approach you because they need someone to talk to and they know you will understand. And if you look healthy and as if you're doing all right they find that even more positive.*

Rae became conscious that

> *Cancer is still a no-no and a lot of people don't like to hear*

> *too much about it even though it is coming out on TV and in the papers more. You start talking and they try to change the subject. People will say 'it's good to see you' and 'how are you feeling?' but they have never asked what it was like. I would never talk about it unless anybody asked but you've got to talk about it, and it is better to talk about it to someone that is experienced because they can understand. Anybody who has been told they have got a cancer has got to talk about it—they've got to let it all out. They say cancer is an eating thing: just by not talking about, it will eat you up inside. I don't think it really matters who you talk to as long as you don't bottle it up inside.*

As Rae suggested, while friends or acquaintances may be ambivalent in their approach to discussing cancer, people who have experienced cancer often exhibited an empathy which enabled uninhibited exchange. Julie described how her experience had equipped her with new communication skills.

> *Having cancer has taught me a lot about dealing with other patients that have been diagnosed. I'm not frightened to go up and say: 'Oh heavens! Where? What are they doing for you? What chemotherapy are you on?' Before I may not have wanted to speak the word cancer and I wouldn't have known what to ask because you really don't know what people have to go through. I didn't know what chemo was all about and nobody seemed to want to talk about it. Now, I don't mind talking about it—as long as it's not all the time. It's always at the back of my mind but work and family make my life very busy and I don't have time to dwell.*

Open interaction with another woman of similar age who understood her circumstances was what Carmen felt she lacked as she moved through her initial treatment.

I needed to speak to somebody in the same predicament as me because you can't keep all these confused feelings cooped inside. The best thing is to find a good listener who will sit down and listen to your point, listen to how you feel, everything that's going through your mind. You need to talk about it and you need to hear what other people have gone through. I wanted to ask someone how they felt when their hair dropped out and how they coped with the nausea. It was really wonderful when the person from the Cancer Foundation came to the ward because I didn't expect anybody to come. Up till now I haven't come across anybody my age with breast cancer. Even the people I have seen while having the chemo and the radiotherapy treatment are all old. I've only seen one lady at the clinic who is about my age.

No matter how much support could be gained from discussions with another person with cancer, Carmen discovered that it could be a mixed blessing. While she was in hospital, she met a woman with a totally different kind of cancer. She recalled how

... this woman's attitude gave me a horrible shock. When she first spoke to me she said, 'I've already arranged my funeral and everything.' I hadn't been thinking of myself as ever getting to that really bad stage and really, to be quite honest, I wasn't interested. I was trying to say no but she just kept going on.

The simple act of meeting another person who has cancer did not automatically bond people: a great deal depended upon whether the ways in which they understood and integrated their experiences were compatible at the time. Nevertheless, many of the women were adamant that fellow travellers often develop a real camaraderie. Noelle discovered that this happened despite her initial resistance to mixing with other people with cancer.

> When I went for my first two treatments of vitamin C I got a very strong negative feeling because all of a sudden I was put into the patient category. I hadn't seen myself in that role but there I was with five other people, all giving ourselves intravenous injections of vitamin C. Now I see it as a social event because everyone feels good about what they are doing there and the vibes are really good. You get to see the same people and find out what is happening in their lives: some are having good days, some are having bad days and they are all very supportive. They'll ask after you and wish you well if you're going for surgery. People will bring in books or pamphlets they have read and it's not always about cancer. People will talk about movies they've seen or bring in recipes. It is a general exchange of things and that surprised me because I had these very negative feelings about being a patient in a clinic.

Although Kaye had great support from her family and friends, she still found that

> ... when I met other people with cancer I felt like there was someone there that knew what I went through. With friends and relatives, and even people in the street, even though they would turn around and say: 'I know what you're going through' or 'I can imagine what you're going through'—they can't.
>
> You have to have cancer to know what another cancer patient is going through. If someone has an operation like an appendix, or just a normal operation, that's traumatic enough. Cancer is like a death word. When you meet someone that's had it and they've been through all that trauma, you can associate with them because you know that here's someone who really knows the way you are feeling. Friends and relatives give you so much support but unless they've been there, they can't

know. At the time I was diagnosed my main point of contact with other cancer patients was on the wards where I had the operations and the radiotherapy clinic. Since then, I haven't met a great number of people with cancer although my father-in-law's wife got breast cancer so we occasionally talk about it.

Most of the women in this group decided against joining a cancer support group. Some, like Julie, even decided against contacting the Cancer Foundation because she felt that doing either was an admission that she had cancer.

It might be ridiculous and maybe the [Cancer Foundation or a support group] could have done wonders for me, I don't know. It's just something I chose not to do. Having workmates—I just got through that way.

Anne K did not take up the suggestion that she seek 'group counselling' for similar reasons.

I wouldn't allow myself to do that because they were sick people and I wasn't. I had an unwillingness to admit I was ill and I thought: I can't be around sick people now. I don't want to be visually aware of someone who is ill because it's too hard trying to hold myself together.

This desire not to be surrounded by 'sick people' was something Mara understood well.

I didn't want to go to the Cancer Support people. Some people said that cancer patients live longer if they join the support group but I thought that if I got there I would listen to other people's stories and it would be depressing to revolve around cancer. I did not want to make cancer the centrepoint of my life, or listen to other people's stories. Even when friends of mine come to visit and say things like: 'I know a lady who had a breast cancer operation years back and she's still alive. I know how she was crying. She was so upset and then her husband died and she is still alive.' But then you meet other people who die. I have another two friends who died from breast cancer. People tell you things of other people's experience and I hated it. I just didn't want to listen to other people's experiences. I wanted to push it into the background.

But while Mara had no desire to join a formal support group, she was appreciative of the practical advice and moral support she received from hospital visitors from the Cancer Foundation. She considered this kind of contact with fellow travellers to be good sense.

The lady who came to see me from cancer support clinic rang me in hospital after my first operation, before I knew that I had to have my second breast removed, and said she would come and visit me. But then the doctor came with the diagnosis and I decided to remove the other breast. This woman had only one breast missing and now I have two so I wanted to talk to someone who had a bilateral mastectomy. So the people from cancer support clinic arranged another lady to come and visit me. This woman was about forty-five when she had a bilateral mastectomy. She was really good. She came in a T-shirt and I was so glad because that was my worry—to see how the prostheses looked when I was wearing a T-shirt. It doesn't look artificial. It feels so natural. She talked to me quite a while and even after coming out of hospital she rang me regularly for a year.

Regardless of the fact that Mara decided against attending a breast cancer support group, she was well aware that she might have benefited from the support of other women, especially after the most intense phase of her treatment was over. She felt that her doctor, who had a lot of time for her before and during the operation, didn't have time to talk with her once the immediate crisis was over.

> *That's really annoying because I have a lot of questions to ask but then I forget, even when I write them down, because I see that he's in a hurry to get the other patients in. I would like to find out more about what symptoms could be indicative of something going wrong because it worries me that I didn't have any pain or any lumps when they discovered the cancer. And if I feel the same now, who is to tell that I don't have it somewhere else and still don't have to feel anything distinctly wrong? That worries me because the doctor says to me, 'You're fine, you don't have any pain.' I said, 'I didn't have any pain even before the operation when my cancer was there. So how am I sure?' I would love to find out a little bit more. They teach us how to examine our breasts for lumps so, now that my breasts have been removed, why don't they tell me what to look for? That's probably one reason I should go to the cancer support group. They will probably have more answers than the doctor. But every case is different. That's why I'm avoiding other people who talk about breast cancer because I know my case is my case and nothing to do with other people's cases.*

In contrast, two of the women who had breast cancer thought that they probably would have attended a support group if one had been accessible. Carmen was told about the breast cancer support group by the woman from the Cancer Foundation who visited her in hospital. She explained:

> *I did want to go to their meetings to mix with more people that have breast cancer but I'm really a terrible driver and I don't like being on the road. I think it is a good idea to mix with*

other people but because we live right up in the northern suburbs there's no local support group. Everything that is available is out of my jurisdiction in areas where I don't go.

Like many rural women, Ann T had to find her own support mechanisms because there were none available. Even when she did have access to a support group, it was not designed to cater for women in the paid workforce.

If I had been in Perth I would probably have gone to a support group after my mastectomy, but because we lived so far away there wasn't any support and there was no-one else in town that I knew who had had cancer. If I needed to talk I would talk to one of the girls in the medical centre. A year later we left because there was a lot of strife in the town. There'd been strikes and a lot of people left and new people coming in and it was like a big division in the town. So, the more our friends left, the more I said to my husband, 'I don't really want to be here any more.' Plus I thought Geraldton might be nearer some support and that it would be easier to get down to Perth. When we got to Geraldton I got in touch with a lady who was in the mastectomy support group. She gave me her card but I never got in touch with her again. I was working full-time and it was very hard to go to the meetings because they were always at eleven o'clock in the morning.

Although Ann T couldn't attend support groups, her work helped her find ways of reaching out to other women with breast cancer.

If anybody with breast cancer ever came into the private health insurance company where I worked, I always tried to help. One girl who my sister knows was diagnosed a few years behind me and is always saying how much I helped her. I'm glad I did but I didn't do it consciously. We were just swapping stories and that helped—just talking.

Marinomoana attended three support groups before she decided that they weren't a useful strategy for her because they began to reinforce the notion that cancer equalled death.

The support groups were good but I saw fifteen people die. How many people have seen that many deaths in their lives? The first group I belonged to was attached to the hospital and was good fun. Privately, we called ourselves 'the sombre corpse'. It was really horrible when you think of the name but we found it funny. One of the rules we made was no spouses. It was a time for us to feel sorry about ourselves within our own time 'cos you don't do that with your family. This was a time and place where we could whinge about everything. The sad thing was that the group started getting smaller because the people were dying. It was traumatic for me because I should have been popping off before the other members of the group but they were all coming in wheelchairs and here I was still doing well. One of my friends in that group was a wonderful man and when his wife came and told me that he had died the previous day, I was so upset that I didn't know what to do. My GP and psychologist thought that if I went into another group, it might help me get over the death of my friend because I was feeling guilty about being alive! The second group was all right but they died too and it was depressing for me watching people no longer coming. It wasn't until the third group that I realised this was getting to be a bit of a cycle and I'd better get out before anyone died. I'm a bit of a slow learner!

Although Annie has never joined a support group, it didn't take her long to realise that friendships with other people with cancer could be a mixed blessing, and not only because watching their death could be a difficult reminder of the uncertainty of her own prognosis.

> *Fellow travellers are great. I think everybody should have one. How many you have depends on how much you can deal with because the trouble with some fellow travellers is that they go and die on you. When I first started at the clinic I made friends with quite a few people but now I'm very wary and I limit it to one at a time because I find I develop very intimate relationships with fellow travellers. They become immediately close. It's like a meeting of soul mates when you immediately recognise a friend. It becomes double that because you're in such a similar situation and it really is traumatic when they do die. Then again, there are some fellow travellers who get cured. Then I get really angry because they're past their five year clearance, they're off and away and I'm left dealing with it. I feel as though that bond is sort of broken because they're now OK and I'm still left here. I can get really bitchy! 'How dare you get better! How dare you!'*

Like Annie, Margaret P has an incurable cancer, and has become conscious of the differences which set people with chronic systemic cancers apart from those with treatable forms. Although she considered all fellow travellers to be 'peers' she felt a special bond with people like herself who

> *... are having so much treatment and for a long period. If you can regard cancer as an acute problem, which for most people it is, they either get cured, or they die within the period, say the first year for instance. But I've got no hope. All I have to look forward to is dying slowly. I've met quite a few other people with cancer—people who were in the same stage as me—especially when I started needing more treatment. We all clicked. Staying in hospital and going through similar stuff,*

you get really close. But then I lost three friends in a month and a few weeks later another friend died. It really knocked me for six, especially as their rellies didn't tell me so I didn't know for several weeks. They died faster than I was expecting even though they had been struggling up and down for a long time. It upset me because I keep seeing me like that. I keep saying I'll survive, I always survive, but the trouble is, I won't. You can't ever get away from it. It's more than a monkey on your shoulder. It's your entire life, which is why we talk about it so much! Cancer can make you feel really alone and I think cancer patients may sometimes be a bit exclusive when we get together. It is possible that other people understand some aspects better than I think they do but because they haven't been through it, I don't believe them!

The experience of these women suggested that most of them found some form of contact with fellow travellers beneficial. Apart from the odd exception, even those who wanted nothing to do with other 'sick people' acknowledged that they found solidarity with fellow travellers which no other social network could duplicate. Even Julie, who flatly refused to seek out a support group, acknowledged that she could

... feel a bonding between survivors of cancer. A person that hadn't experienced cancer could walk in and try to offer some advice. It would be like water pouring off a duck's back: what the hell would they know about it? But with somebody that's actually been through the experience of being told they've got cancer, somebody that's been through the experience of chemotherapy and the traumatic effects it has, you immediately feel this is a positive thing! This person is alive and kicking, and able to tell me that she's got over it. That is what I wanted the minute I was diagnosed: where are those people that have survived? I wanted desperately to talk to somebody

who has had cancer. The nurses were no good because they didn't understand what I'd just been told. They could guess all they like, but you really have to experience the actual shock of being told you've got cancer to understand.

Despite Marinomoana's decision not to continue attendance at any support group, she would agree with Julie. She has remained a firm believer in the value of contact with fellow travellers because

... it is good to talk to someone who is going through what you're going through. It may not be the same, but you share the same feelings, the same anxiety and fear and it is good to know that it is normal. Talking with someone who has been through a similar experience can give you information about how to keep control for yourself, how to empower yourself, how to keep your self-esteem. Self-esteem is important because that can go really quickly if you start thinking: what did I do wrong to get this? You can believe that somehow you are an evil person and that God doesn't love you. That is crap.

8
How Cancer Changes Perspectives

THE ANXIETY, FEAR AND POTENTIAL LOSS OF SELF-ESTEEM WHICH MARinomoana identified were understandable responses to having her world turned upside down. She was not the only one who experienced variations on these themes. Whatever their prognoses, all these women have had to learn to live with cancer. While this meant that their lives would never be the same again, each one of them nevertheless found a new axis which allowed their world to keep revolving. In the process, many found they had to make considerable adjustments to such fundamental components of life as sexuality and humour. Both could be deeply affected by the physical and emotional changes which cancer could induce. And there's nothing quite like a diagnosis of cancer to heighten awareness of human mortality and provide a certain urgency for getting on with the business of living. In the process of working through issues of dying, many of these women discovered their primary challenge was creating a quality life despite the restrictions cancer placed upon them. While death comes to us all in time, each woman, in her own unique way, came to the conclusion that the most important thing was making the most of the time she had.

SEXUALITY
Most serious illnesses temporarily dampen interest in sex, if only because certain bodily and psychological functions go into shut-down

while the system attempts to rectify the damage. In the case of many cancers, this process can be exacerbated by the nature of the disease; many of these women have described the feeling that their bodies were being invaded and violated, firstly by the cancer and secondly by the treatments which they underwent to destroy or control the disease.

All of these women were 'biologically mature' when they were diagnosed, thus there was a greater risk that chemotherapy, in particular, was likely to cause infertility and early menopause.[1] But whether their treatment consisted of surgery, radiotherapy or chemotherapy, or some combination of these, there was some impact on their sexuality as they dealt with loss of libido, tiredness, varying degrees of physical disability or pain, or psychological withdrawal from intimacy as they focused attention on their own body's need for space. For some women this was a temporary state which they were able to work through after the shock of diagnosis had settled or after they had recuperated from the emotional and physical impact of treatment. Even so, considerable readjustments were needed. For others, the effects of cancer on their sense of sexuality has been more permanent and dramatic.

Many women chose not to discuss this issue; some areas of our personal relationships remain sacrosanct. However, this need for privacy highlights one of the key problems identified by several women who were prepared to discuss the impact cancer had on their sexuality; their own reticence about discussing issues of sexuality with their doctors and the reluctance of many professionals to raise the subject. This could be the case even where the women had sought information which gave them warning that treatment would affect their sexuality. Annie pondered upon this issue after she realised that her treatment had induced menopause.

---

1. Lowenthal (1990, p. 85) notes that: 'The more intensive the chemotherapy, and the older the patient at the time of receiving it, the more likely the occurrence of infertility . . . Many women who receive chemotherapy in their late thirties and forties commonly find that it brings on an early menopause, with all the usual symptoms associated with the change of life, such as cessation of menstrual periods and hot flushes.'

I don't know how many other women are told that if they have chemotherapy, or radiotherapy in certain parts of their body, or even if they have an oophorectomy[2] that they would be going straight into menopause. Not one person told me. Not once has anything to do with sexuality been discussed with me by anyone. I sort of knew that this was what's going to happen, but there was no discussion of it, no preparation that 'this is probably what will happen, and have you thought about menopause before? Would you like a bit of literature?' It was as though you didn't really need to know. It's like this invasion of the body—again.

With natural menopause it's gradual and you can accommodate it. It's just part of living. But when it's physically done to you, it's very sudden. I believe that if you have intervention to cause sudden menopause then it's going to perhaps be more violent, more extreme, than if you did it naturally. You have the hot sweats and all the menopause symptoms and, although it might be a shorter period of time that you have them, they're much more pronounced at the time. I didn't have the mood swings that I've read about but I was on so many drugs at the time, who knows. But it would be really interesting to know how many women, or men for that matter, are affected.

As a nurse, Beth was also intellectually aware that treatment would have certain ramifications. She recognised that there would be

> ... *the emotional issues of scarring or instant menopause and hormone disruption after surgery, the loss of sensuality during radiation or chemotherapy, and the need for increased warmth and closeness with a special person. There are also the practical issues, such as the need to improvise when normal sex isn't possible, which lubricants to use, the need for some people*

---

2. Removal of an ovary.

to have mechanical vaginal stretching, and the appropriateness of Hormone Replacement Therapy.

Yet, despite the importance of sex and sexuality, and especially the way it is affected by treatment, she found 'minimal talk about these issues' because 'many people are embarrassed to raise them'.

We all appreciate those doctors and nurses who are prepared to talk with us rather than us having to ask or read about these issues in a book—if we can find one.

Such doctors do exist. Julie's gynaecologist warned her that she would have to be abstinent for several months and was quite happy to discuss any issues she wanted to raise. Even so, she was worried by the fact that she'd had a hysterectomy and a removal of all the organs. Despite discussions with her doctor: 'I wasn't quite sure whether I was going to grow a beard or what.' Mara also felt able to discuss sexuality with one of her doctors. Her GP was a 'lady doctor' who discussed sexuality with her in detail.

She was always enquiring: 'How's your husband taking it?' He was fine: it didn't worry him very much. But I really lost my drive. I wasn't interested in sex at all.

Margaret P recalled how, after her diagnosis she and her husband

. . . had several weeks of intense sexual activity—as if to reassure ourselves that we were still alive. But since I have been on heavy chemo—three years now—I have had a non-existent libido, so it's just as well I am divorced!

Likewise, after prolonged periods of treatment, Annie has found that 'there is no such thing' as sexuality in her life.

> As far as I'm concerned prednisolone has ruined anything to do with sex—I'm a sexless being, I'm afraid, because of my body changes. It was such a shock to have this really barrel shaped body with skinny arms and legs but it hasn't been a problem. I suppose I shy away from the potential of a new relationship because some people are so scared of cancer. I mean, how do you confront it? 'I've got cancer and a few other things . . .' or, 'I've got a shelf life. Take it or leave it.' I've given up even thinking that there might be a potential in something. I live alone and I've lived alone for eight years and I don't get lonely any more so it's not a problem. I've got a lot of friends and I don't need a sexual relationship. In fact, it would be added baggage that I don't need. All those games . . .

Issues of sex and sexuality can recede in importance because of the physical and emotional energy required to undergo long-term treatment and maintain other aspects of life. Anne K also described this phenomenon.

> It was all I could do to survive. I was too busy getting on with things throughout, until the very end after the transplant, when you've lost all body hair and your face is blowing out and your mouth is pulled down from the mouth ulcers. All transplant patients get graft versus host disease which affects the skin and all the mucosal linings. You don't exactly feel like Mrs Universe. Sex and sexuality disappeared because I felt like an empty husk. I felt a bit androgynous and sexless.

Even when the cancer was more acute, and the treatment shorter, the effects on feelings of sexuality could be just as devastating. While the very act of having radiation rods inserted caused feelings of numbness, alienation and violation, Lynne had no doubts that this was made worse by the silence from her medical professionals. They could not approach the topic of sexuality with a woman who was not heterosexual. This 'wall of silence' left Lynne unable to voice her concerns.

> *I can remember driving home with my lover after the radiation rod episode and feeling numb and withdrawn. She was very warm and worked hard to support and love me despite how in shock I was. I didn't want to be touched and even struggled to have my kids cuddle with me. I didn't feel human. The alienation from my body was like what some women feel when they are raped—alienated, isolated, trapped in a personal horror, ostracised and filthy. For a couple of years I felt as though my sexuality had been irradiated as well. I couldn't enjoy sex, felt afraid of my body and pessimistic about my physical wellbeing. I had little self-esteem despite continuing to work full-time, care for people with HIV/AIDs and be a parent to my kids. The sexual part of my relationship ended and it was very traumatic trying to work out whether it was because of the relationship or my treatment. At times I thought losing intimacy was worse than having cancer.*
>
> *The process was made worse by not being able to talk about my sexuality with the medical people I consulted. They simply didn't want to know that I was not a heterosexual. I believe that 'straight' women are counselled about easing back into sexual relations, prescribed hormonal creams so that their vaginas don't tear and so on. Although I have always been completely 'out' about my sexuality, after the treatment I felt emotionally unable to encounter the wall of silence in the clinic consultations. When I think about it now, I wish I had begun my treatment with a gay and lesbian-friendly doctor—or at least one who wasn't homophobic, with whom I could have talked freely. This is one thing about my experience I would have liked to do differently. There is little information written for lesbian*

women about cervical cancer. It needs to be written. Lesbian women, especially those with children, often live in family relationships and with kinship arrangements and expectations that may be different from heterosexual women. My lover for example was not considered to be a family member and therefore entitled to be with me when I was told my diagnosis, despite her being listed as my next of kin and my asking for her. Treatment for cervical cancer inevitably affects how women think and feel about their sexuality and medics need to deal with this holistically.

Lynne was left very much on her own, reliant on herself, her friends and her family, to find 'holistic' ways to heal her battered body and psyche.

Treatments can cause physical changes which make sex difficult or uncomfortable. In addition to losing interest in sex, Mara found that there was 'one aggravating thing' about taking tamoxifen. Although she understood the need to take it because her breast cancer was

... hormonally oriented by oestrogen and the tamoxifen suppresses oestrogen, it is not a wonder drug and there are side effects. All my wet areas like my nose, my mouth and my vagina are very dry and very sensitive. In the morning I wake up and my throat is very dry. It could be from tamoxifen or it could be because of diabetes. I am more inclined to think of tamoxifen because it's connected to the oestrogen. I never had problems with my hormonal imbalance during my menopause—no hot flushes and everything was functioning fine. My oestrogen level was really high because my periods stopped in my mid-50s which is reasonably late. The change of life did not affect me but now the dryness of those areas affects me in the way that I can't have normal sex with my husband.

Ann T and her husband were able to discuss the impact of her cancer openly. As a consequence, it didn't worry her and her husband at all, even in their sex life. She found ways to 'get around these things' by dressing as nicely as she could, wearing 'nice sexy little tops—little chemise things, not fitted'. She also found that a light-hearted approach went a long way.

> *My remaining breast seemed to get really big quite suddenly after the mastectomy, so I had this big prosthesis as well. I looked like I had a fine pair and I remember going to the pool in my new two-piece when I first got home. There was a bikie and his wife down the one end and he actually said to his wife, 'Gee, she's got a fine pair of boobs.' He was one of the new people in town and he didn't know who I was. She said to me later, 'I didn't have the heart to tell him!' I said, 'Thanks!'*

Although Ann T and her husband have had no problems adjusting to her mastectomy, she has considered the possibility of a reconstruction. However, she has come to the conclusion that she hasn't got the time at present

> *... because it's a big, long drawn out process. I've often thought that if anything did happen to my marriage, it would be the first thing I would do because I don't know whether somebody would accept me the way I am. My father died very young and my mother never re-married but it's always there—the 'what if?' My brother-in-law and my brother died very young. I don't want to be left on my own and I think that would be the one thing that would make me go and have a breast reconstruction done.*

The women found they relied on their partner's sensitivity and caring to nurture their bruised sensuality back to life. This could be particularly difficult with gynaecological cancers where treatment affected crucial reproductive and sexual organs. Beth recalled that around the time of her diagnosis and initial treatment she 'didn't know the meaning of the word sex'. She did have the presence of mind to

> ... ask the doctor what the situation would be after surgery. He said they try to leave you with enough vagina to allow intercourse. I am fortunate that my partner is a very caring and resourceful man, but it is hard because sex is an important part of a relationship. I think many women can manage better with warmth and touching and caring even without sex, whereas for many men, sex is the way they express their warmth and caring so if that is lost they lose an important means of expression. So for each to understand how the other will be feeling, sexuality is something that needs to be discussed with both partners when one of them has been diagnosed with cancer.

Noelle and her partner found numerous ways to express their physical intimacy—an aspect of their relationship which she cherished. She spoke of the importance of doing things together.

> My partner is a loving supporting partner, a very tactile person. This is very special to me because, although I didn't realise until I met him, part of what I was missing in my life was the touching—and I don't mean in a sexual way. I mean a hand placed on a shoulder, an arm around you, a hand being held. This is what I needed. This is what had been missing all those years before I met him. As far as I'm concerned a good cuddle is as good as sex any time. We have a marvellous relationship, very physical in all senses. We hike together; we scuba dive together; we do all sorts of outdoors things which I've always liked but never had the opportunity to do. Our relationship was

also physical in the sexual sense but the things that have happened to me recently have put a dampener on that. The physical scarring hasn't left any impression on my sense of sexuality because I came to my partner not only emotionally scarred but physically scarred from two large abdominal operations when I was a young woman.[3] *The scars all these operations have left look terrible but I'm not a vain person so that has not been the problem. The groin dissection meant that they have taken out a huge area of my groin so any sort of pressure causes me great pain afterwards—it feels like someone has been stabbing me for days afterwards. Even lifting my leg to get into a pair of knickers is quite difficult at times so having my legs spread causes problems. The missionary fashion can be very painful because nerve endings have been cut. I can slap the top part of my thigh and it feels like it's dead. That whole side of my body has been weakened so I have to be very careful. We laugh and say, 'We've got to find a way of doing it with my legs stuck together!'*

HUMOUR

There is an old adage that humour is the best medicine, but the poet Shelley managed to sum up the true pathos which often accompanies humour when he observed that, 'Our sincerest laughter with some pain is fraught'.[4] Just as Noelle found that humour was the best way to 'manage' the changes in her physical ability to enjoy sex, so other women in this group used laughter as a method of acknowledging and dealing with the more painful changes cancer wrought in their lives. As Margaret P observed:

---

3. As a young woman Noelle had a loop incorrectly inserted which caused a miscarriage six months into a pregnancy. The loop couldn't be found so she was 'opened up from the navel right down to the pubic line'. Then she fell pregnant twelve months later and had a traumatic birth by caesarean section.

4. Percy Bysshe Shelley, 'To a Skylark' (1819).

There's been many a time when I have laughed and cried together. Perhaps it's a survival technique—but it might just be a twisted sense of humour.

Humour offered most of the women a crucial emotional outlet when their circumstances threatened to overwhelm them. For some women, such as Tiny, illness dampened humour.

We haven't found that there's been a lot of humour in my illness, especially when I was very ill. When I have been better, then we can have a good old laugh. In hospital you could have a bit of fun with some of the patients and a lot of the nurses joke around, especially the night staff. They know how you are feeling.

Kaye couldn't see much humour in her situation at the time of her operations and radiotherapy. On reflection she realises that her husband used laughter to keep her optimistic.

My husband kept my spirits up and tried to joke a bit to make me feel better. If I moped he would say something like, 'Stop going on about it! You'll make yourself sick!' I thought he was being hard but if he had been morbid with me, I would have been even worse. You're morbid enough yourself but half the time if people say, 'I feel terrible for you' then you end up feeling worse. If they turn around and say, 'Come on! Cheer up!' then you start to feel a bit better. Anybody that can keep your spirits up or make you feel better with jokes or encouragement can help you have an 'up day' rather than a 'down day'.

Over fourteen years she has developed the capacity to laugh about incidents which were dreadful at the time.

After my neck operation I couldn't move very well. I was very tired but the nurses got me out of bed the next day to make my bed up and asked me if I would like to sit in a chair. I thought it was a good idea even though I had all the drains with me and the chair was a fair way away from the bed. They said they'd come back in a few minutes to see how I was going, and then they closed the door. I couldn't stay awake and I was trying to keep my head straight because of the operation, but I kept nodding off. All I wanted to do was go back to bed but I felt so weak in my legs that I was scared I'd fall if I tried to get there by myself and, of course, the bell was by the bed so I couldn't reach it. All I could think of was: 'Where are you? please come back.' It seemed like ages before they came and I was nearly in tears because I was so tired and worried about my neck because I couldn't support it. I can look back and laugh now. I must have been silly because I should have asked for the bell; I knew I was down the corridor, away from the work station but I didn't realise they were going to leave me for so long, or that it would be so exhausting just sitting in a chair.

Another woman who couldn't find much to laugh about in her treatment or prognosis could see the humour in the way her son was able to use her diagnosis to get 'out of a few scrapes!' He had

... started a new job two days after I had the operation. The day that he got the job he had signed up to do a course and it all proved too much for him so he asked for a deferral and he blamed me! He said, 'My Mother's got cancer.' In the meantime I had hardly seen him! There was another time my husband used it to get off work early saying that he had to take me to the hospital even though he hadn't taken me once.

Most of the group seemed to find retrospective humour in odd situations. Beth remembers being in a coffee shop in a busy shopping centre one day when

> ... *all of a sudden these tears started pouring down my face and my husband asked what the matter was. I said, 'How dare all these people be walking along as if nothing is happening in the world. This earth-shattering thing is happening to me and they're not even taking any notice!' For a while, I wouldn't buy any clothes in case I didn't get the use out of them. My husband said, 'That's all right. If you don't get any wear out of them, we'll take them back and trade them!' Then I broke my glasses and I wouldn't buy a new pair until I had my CT scan. My husband said, 'Even if you're going to die, you want to look good, so go and get some glasses.' But I wouldn't spend the money until I had the results. The day I got my CT scan result I went straight to the shops and shopped until I couldn't carry any more! I think things like that are funny now.*

Ann T found that some friends could show quite touching degrees of unnecessary sensitivity which gave her plenty of light relief. One of the funniest incidents happened when she was

> ... *coming home from Perth on the bus. A friend of ours met us at the turn-off, on the highway between Onslow and Karratha. He's a lovely guy, although sometimes a wee bit crude, and he and his wife had just had a new baby. I asked how the baby was. 'Oh! She's great!' he says, 'I've just left her screaming her tits off!' It went right over my head and I didn't think anything of it because that's the way he is but for weeks after he kept saying to my husband, 'Why did I come out with that?' Even to this day he's embarrassed, just over something he said.*

Embarrassment could come in many forms. Mara used humour to navigate one episode when, while on a family holiday at a beachside caravan park, she went to the communal showers.

I hung my bathers on the hook inside the door and one of the prostheses slipped out of the pocket in the bra and fell into a drain which ran right through all the showers. I wrapped myself in a towel and I was screaming out, 'I've lost my prosthesis!' The showers were all full and so the water was running fast down the drain, carrying my prosthesis with it. One boob following the line of the drain! Nobody reacted fast enough to catch it so it went right through the hole at the end and disappeared. Wrapped in my towel, I ran to my daughter in the caravan and said, 'Oh my God! I lost my prosthesis right into the drain and it's gone. It cost $220.' She said, 'I'll go and ask the man. He probably has a filter somewhere to drain out all the hairs and yucky stuff.' He went and found it, and proudly carried it into me saying, 'I found your prosthesis.' It was embarrassing but it was so funny.

Mara's prostheses became the subject of good-humoured family jesting, all of which helped her adjust to a new body image. She still laughs about another incident when her daughter and grand-children were visiting from the Eastern States.

Their youngest son was still having bottles and my daughter bought two new bottle teats. The little boy threw them into the garden and my daughter was looking everywhere for them. In the end I found them and I came in saying, 'Look what I've found ... two tits! Just what I want!' My daughter says, 'That's not tits, Mum, that's the TEAT for the top of the bottle!' That is what I said, but with my accent it sounds the same. We laughed for days after that because 'two tits' WAS just what I wanted!

Several women found that their sense of humour became somewhat unacceptable: their understanding of the world had been transformed in ways which made taboo subjects highly accessible, while common concerns became irrelevant. Anne K described how, during the period when 'survival' dominated her life, humour and cynicism became intertwined.

> *My sense of humour became very grim. I was a bit cynical about almost everything as well. I used to wonder why people were running around like chooks with their heads cut off because the things they worried about seemed so insignificant. Two years ago if someone had said to me, 'I'm living for a leather suite', I'd have said, 'What? I am living for living's sake!' But that only lasts for a short time. You soon get back to where you were before. It's the human condition.*

Several women found that their sense of humour changed quite radically, but that they could only express this openly with fellow travellers. Beth recalls her first meeting with this group of women as a turning point because, recently diagnosed and not long out of surgery, she had not found much to laugh about. Only a week before her first dose of chemotherapy, and feeling like 'the new kid on the block', she found a group of women who

> *. . . were talking about these horrendous things—and I laughed! One person was telling us about having a bone biopsy. She was in agony, but the doctors drilling through the bones were saying, 'Don't make a noise. You're upsetting everyone!' She replied, 'It's not everyone who's having their bones drilled!' It was horrible but we all laughed. One woman locked herself in the loo and wouldn't have a bone biopsy until they gave her some pain-killer. We laughed when she told us. So she should! When I came home from that meeting my husband asked how it went and when I said I hadn't laughed*

so much for a long time, he wanted to know what we laughed about. When I told him he looked horrified. I think that your humour does become very black.

Although Beth wasn't aware that her sense of humour had changed after her diagnosis, she has found that

> ... people tell me it has. I find myself making a lot of quips like, 'It's a filthy disease but it grows on you.' You think different things are funny but I think that it's been very good to laugh. As a group of women with cancer, we laugh a lot over really macabre things like death and illness and our frailties. Maybe it's a survival technique because if you don't laugh, you cry. Some people think that because you've got this deadly disease, you have always got to be serious. You can't take everything serious all the time—it gets too depressing. The only good thing I could think to come out of cancer was that I would probably get slim and beautiful for a while on chemo, but blow me, I didn't get slim and beautiful! I put on weight with the chemo! You've got to have a sense of humour.

Marinomoana's sense of humour—shared by her partner—has kept her optimistic. She is aware that it has changed, and that sometimes friends cannot appreciate the joke. Her sense of humour 'became a deadpan, really warped sense of humour', and it 'became easier to crack jokes about dying'.

> We were with some friends after a New Year's Eve party, all really jolly. We drove past a funeral home and my husband turns around to me and goes, 'Oh, hon—what about that place?' I said, 'Yeah, we must take that name down and go and have a look at the caskets.' All of our friends went quiet because they didn't understand that I enjoy it: when you're living with cancer and the possibility of death all the

time, it's like a cold shoulder. My relationship with my husband has survived because we share that sense of humour about it all. A lot of people got very 'ooh' because he'll make some crack like, 'Keep that up and I hope you die soon!' We'd kill ourselves laughing while everyone else is looking very wary.

Annie summed up the ways in which humour could act as a buffer, a vital mechanism which most fellow travellers understand but which other people can find difficult to accommodate. She uses humour to get through those long nights when the lymphoma sweats or the 'spondy burns'[5] make sleep impossible.

I lie there some nights thinking about who I could donate my diseased organs to. 'Umm—it's a shame Hitler's dead: he could have done with my chemoed-out kidneys. Same with Stalin—wouldn't have minded giving him my heart, completely surrounded as it is with tumours. Pity Pol Pot has just popped off—he could have had my lymphoma-invaded liver, or my lungs, ruined as they are from years of smoking. Ah—Idi Amin has yet to go the way of most tyrants—he can have the lot! And I'll give him my inflamed spine to boot!' Of course, occasionally I come a lot closer to home . . .

Annie has found 'an incredible amount to laugh about'. Humour has become

. . . a way of dealing with the disease process with like-people. You can't really do that with people who aren't fellow travellers because you offend them. People get very shocked very easily because it's black trench-humour. Even many health care staff get quite taken aback. Perhaps what you're doing is threatening people's mortality by being so open and blunt about life-threatening diseases.

---

5. Pain caused by inflammation of the spine.

While many of these women have discovered that cancer does not necessarily equal death, all have confronted the possiblity of not living out their 'three score years and ten'. In the process they have become aware of how precious life is—but that doesn't mean that there is no humour in the inescapable and natural transition to death.

WORKING THROUGH THE ISSUES OF DYING
Marinomoana was blunt about the issue of dying. Although she could joke about it, and felt its presence as a 'cold shoulder', she chose to

> *... ignore the issue of dying, totally, because I know I have already made liars of the doctors! Anyway, I am only thirty-eight so I'm just starting because life begins at forty!*

Many of these women have discovered that working through issues of dying, much like dealing with the business of living, is full of contradictions. When a diagnosis of cancer has made an awareness of death inescapable, shock can accompany acceptance, fearlessness can link hands with a refusal to believe that 'death will be the next great adventure', anger about the pain being caused to loved ones can marry sorrow at the prospect of tasks left unaccomplished. Above them all presides acknowledgement that we are all mortal, and that how we live our lives is ultimately far more important than how we die. The journey through this paradoxical maze to such a conclusion is a highly personal one.

While all people diagnosed with cancer confront the possibility of 'imminent death' if treatment is unable to arrest the spread of disease, people with incurable cancers 'know that they have been given a shelf life'. As Annie observed, this means that 'there is no situation quite like an incurable illness'. She has found that, while friends have been quite willing to ask what her prognosis is, many have difficulty dealing with an honest reply.

I tell them that the average life-expectancy is six to ten years, but that that doesn't mean much. Still, it means I know that I am likely to die from this illness sooner rather than later. I've been surprised how often people will reply: 'Oh! But we are all dying. And I might get knocked over by a bus tomorrow!' I know that their response is largely out of an embarrassed attempt to empathise with me, but they can't. It's impossible because I've already been hit by the bus and it didn't kill me instantly! Instead it's a long slow process—which doesn't mean that it's morbid because it doesn't take long before you realise that you don't actually die till you stop breathing and your heart stops.

Margaret P, too, has become aware of the difficulty people have when she is up-front about her shortened life expectancy.

The most common response from anyone if you say you are going to die (usually when they have asked) is, 'Oh! But we're all going to die!' What a cancer patient understands by this response is that their reality is denied. In effect they are being told their early death is unimportant and that they are no worse off than anyone else. But of course they are and they know it.

People use this response partly to try and make the listener feel better—which it doesn't—and partly to distance themselves from any possible emotional outburst—to protect themselves. The way to help legitimise the person with cancer's emotions is to admit that the situation is rotten and allow the person to admit their fear or anger or whatever they feel. Patients should not have to feel bad about crying, nor should they have to remain quiet just to protect the listener.

Anne K had a characteristically straight-forward approach to the issue.

I didn't work through the idea of dying, but I had no fear of it. We've all got to die sometime: we all know we will—that's the only certainty in life. I didn't plan for it because that would be admitting that I possibly wasn't going to make it and that would have been a contradiction in terms. I never ever thought like that. Death doesn't particularly worry me. I may die of another form of cancer or I may get run over by a bus. The only difference this experience made is that I have made a will which I wouldn't have done previously, and that's mainly for my children's sake. The actual process of dying doesn't worry me because it really doesn't matter.

Consideration of children was one of the major concerns for all of these women. As Ann T commented, this was particularly painful if they were still young.

I think the worst thing when you have got kids is the fear of leaving them behind. That was a fear just before my operation: that I was going to die before I could get to see my son grown up. After the operation it never entered my head.

Kaye shared this sentiment, although the course of her cancer meant that she could not dispose of her fear quite so rapidly.

In the beginning, I thought about dying and wondered how long I had. In fact it wasn't a question of 'will I die?' it was 'when will I die?' All I was looking for was someone to turn around and say, 'You are not going to die.' Of course they won't say that. I was told I had a ninety-nine per cent chance that they had taken it all out so all I could do was wait and see. Nobody was able to say, 'Don't worry about it. You're not terminal. You're not going to die.' You keep looking for that reassurance and it doesn't come so your mind just keeps going,

'Why me? Will I be here next year? How long do I have with the kids? Will I see my kids grow up? Will they be able to handle it?'

I sent up all these prayers: 'Please give me another year. At least wait until the kids are older and they can understand a bit more before you take me.' I think everybody goes through that, especially the 'why me?' I was thinking of all the things I haven't done and all the places I hadn't been. I knew that my time could be up any time and I was very aware of all the time I'd wasted going along in a little rut. It does give you a sense of mortality. I think that's why I chased alternative things like putting myself on a special diet and inquiring about the Tronado machine. It was, 'What the heck! I may as well try everything.'

Tiny also tried complementary therapies in the knowledge that her prognosis was not promising. She went through so many periods of acute sickness that the prospect of dying from myeloma was, at times, inescapable. Much of her thinking was done in the quiet times.

When I was very sick, I thought about dying but I didn't tell anyone. My sister in Holland died of cancer one year before I was diagnosed. Like me, she had lost a lot of weight and it was not long till she died. The fact that my sister had died was a very difficult thing to put out of my mind. That was the trouble. I remembered phoning her a couple of weeks before she died and she said she was too tired to even watch TV. I got too tired as well at one time, so I thought, 'Yes, I'm too tired for that as well now. Am I going to make it?' I was so tired when I had to get up in the morning I put my clothes on and the pain went right through my back. Then I would think, 'This is it.' But it would only last a few days and I would start picking up. When I put a bit of weight on I'd think, 'Now I am going better.' But I am less afraid of dying. I don't think you go until your time has come; you won't die until you're ready. I was very close at one time, but we all decided that I wasn't ready yet.

This sense of 'not being ready' or not feeling that the time was nigh was also experienced by Margaret W. Despite her age, and deteriorating health which kept her largely confined at home, she didn't feel she was 'going to die yet'. In fact she told everybody that

... when the weather gets cooler I'm going to start playing football and they're all coming to watch me! I don't think about dying and I don't try to work out what happens when you die. I don't like watching or listening to programs on television or the radio about dying or about people coming back from the dead. It makes me shudder. To be honest, I would rather be like this than crippled with arthritis. The only difference is that cancer can be a killer and that might worry me if I was younger—I don't know. When you get to eighty-four you know you are going to die. I might have lived to be ninety-two, and I might still be alive to be ninety-two despite my cancer. I want to live to see the year 2000. I wish to goodness I could eat a little bit more comfortably, get a bit more energy and not be so exhausted all the time. There's so much food that won't go down. Those are the biggest problems, not thinking about dying.

I have never been very religious although I do believe in a creator and I do have a relationship with God. Every night my one prayer is, 'Please, God, stay close to my son and help with his problems. Stay close to me and help me with my difficulties. Help us both to stay close to you and take care of us through the night.' I don't believe in asking God to do things for me. You don't need to be always asking if you trust and I think that's what God wants from us—trust and love for each other. I am sure that I get a lot of help through God. Shortly after my last operation I had a spiritual experience. I was sitting here looking through the window, feeling depressed and wondering what was going to happen. Suddenly the whole room seemed to be alight. It was a brilliant light, and a very, very clear voice within me said, 'Don't worry, Margaret, everything is going to be all right.'

Rae's strong relationship with God has supported her through the testing times. The knowledge that she has lived long enough to see her children well established has helped her face the possibility of dying from cancer, but it has been a trial even with that sense of a life fulfilled and an abiding faith.

Initially, if anybody says you've got cancer, the first thing you think of is that you are going to die within the next couple of weeks. That's an automatic thing. I felt that I was ready to die, although I didn't want to, of course. The shocks aren't as bad when you are older because you know of people, maybe in your own age group, or who have been younger, who have had things happen and have gone so quickly. You seem to accept it more if you are older. My heart goes out to younger people with cancer who have children, and to parents who have children with cancer. It hurts so much to see them, and hear about them. I feel for them because when you have children you want to see your kids grow up and have a life of their own. I'm not quite up to the three score years and ten but I've seen my family grow up and they are all happy, so I am happy because at least I know that they can cope and look after themselves. That's the biggest thing. Now I would like to see the grandies grow up, but that's borrowed time. If it is my turn to die, I've got the faith to believe that God is calling me and I am ready to go home. I know if I'm so sick that nothing could be done for me, I am willing to just let God take over. But it is a big ordeal. Nobody wants to die, even though every one of us has to die one day or other. To some people death is the final thing, but I don't believe that. I have a strong faith in God and I do believe that there is life after death and that I will see my friends and family again one day.

Carmen shared this belief in life after death, but the shock of diagnosis and the possiblity of early death was acute.

The thought of dying never entered my head because I'm only forty-six. I was planning my next long service leave and thinking of living out a relaxing retirement life. This diagnosis hit me like a thunderbolt and stopped me in my tracks. It has made me realise that I am very vulnerable and that I can die at any moment. I'm not scared to die although I don't want to die suffering. I don't think anybody wants to suffer. But on the other hand I keep saying, 'They took my lumps out and the chemo is taking care of all the runaway cells. In three months that will be finished so maybe I won't have cancer any more.' So, along the way I say I don't care if I die and then I say I haven't got cancer any more. I am confused at the moment, I really am. I don't know what I am trying to say to myself.

The one thing that has pulled me through everything is my faith. If I didn't have my Catholic religion and everybody else praying for me, I'd be lost. I feel the greatest comfort knowing that people are praying for me but the funny thing is that I'm not praying for myself. I don't know why but I feel as though I shouldn't be asking God a favour to cure me. When I am having the nausea from chemo, I pray: I ask God to take it away and when it does go, I say thank you. But I don't believe in miracles. I think if you're diagnosed early, the doctors can fix it, and if they don't, it's finished. But the whole experience has made me rethink my life: what I have done and what I should do. It has made me more religious and I feel my faith is stronger and that I have a better relationship with God. It has made me prepare better for my eventual death, whether it be sooner or later. This is one of the good things about cancer: you get the opportunity to improve yourself. I think I am one of the lucky ones because I have a chance to prepare myself for death. Some people do not get this superb opportunity of preparing to face God.

Even with her profound faith, Carmen's gratitude for the 'opportunity of preparing to face God' took some circuitous routes as she muddled through her contradictory feelings about the possibility of 'imminent death' and the impact that would have on her family.

My first reaction when I was diagnosed was, 'I'm going to die! My poor daughter.' I felt pain at the thought that my daughter was only sixteen and that if I died it would upset her studies. I didn't worry about my son because he's twenty-two. He's left home and he'll be able to cope. My husband had always teased me that he was going to trade me in for a younger model, so even though I knew it was a joke I still felt it would give him the opportunity to get married again.

Confronting the prospect of death included sorting out practical tasks such as making wills or tidying up papers and possessions, as well as considering the impact death might have on loved ones. Mara recalled that she

... thought of dying and looked through my papers and sorted things out. I also looked through the history essays which I did at university and thought how sad because I would like them to be published some day and I didn't think that could happen. I thought about a lot of things that I wanted to do and thought I wouldn't be able to do. That's mainly what I was sad about. I don't think my husband ever faced the

possibility. He always turned to humour when I mentioned that I might die before him, because he is eleven years older than me. He says, 'You're crazy! You're not going to do that to me, are you?' He thinks by the law of nature he's the first one to go! We never really discussed what he would do but I sometimes jokingly say, 'You will marry somebody and you'll be OK.' He says, 'No. I don't think I will.' We have been married forty-two years.

She also decided that there was a key issue that she needed to discuss with her adult daughters.

Before I went to hospital I sat down with my daughters and said to them, 'I'll tell this only once and then we won't mention it again. I want to tell you that if anything happens and I start deteriorating and I die, please never feel guilty.' I said this because it's silly how we burden ourselves with guilty feelings. I nursed my mother for three months before she died and today I still feel guilty that I didn't do everything possible. I moved a bed into her room; I stayed there day and night; I didn't go anywhere; I gave her glasses of water; I washed her; I changed her bedding and her clothes; all the intimate things I did for her and I still feel that I didn't do enough. But she had lost the will of living and I think that I didn't go to Croatia soon enough—that I left it till the end. If I had gone earlier we could have brought her spirit back up, and with medication she could have lasted much longer and had a good quality life. That's why I wanted to tell my daughers, 'If I die, please don't feel guilty for anything. I don't think about how unruly you were during your teen years. Don't ever feel guilty that you did something wrong. With your children you give me my pleasure.' I wouldn't like them to live the way I felt for my mother.

The importance of discussing issues of dying with other family members was something that Rae acknowledged, although she admitted that she

> ... never even mentioned the possibility of dying to my family because it all happened so fast, although it was the family I thought of most. You always think of who you would leave behind and how they'd cope. I know my kids would cope very well and so would my husband. I thought most about the effect it would have on my mum if I should die before her. She would be fine, but it would be a big ordeal for her. I've heard there are people who refuse to talk about death to their families and I think that's sad when you know that it is imminent. You should talk about what you want because it makes the healing afterwards a lot easier for your family.

Talking with family and friends requires a certain 'preparedness' and this can sometimes seem to sit uneasily with an unwillingness to accept that death may be hanging around the corner. Beth explained the way she has approached this.

> I think, because I am still here, that I'm probably not going to go yet but I have kind of prepared. I want to stay at home as long as I can. Then it's up to the family. I don't particularly need to be at home to die. I'm happy to go somewhere else for that last bit because I've seen people die in excruciating agony. I don't want that. I'd rather be given extra morphine and allowed to drift away. As soon as I stop having any pleasure or any use, I want to go. I don't want to die although part of me accepts that I'm going to die sometime. I could get run over by a bus. Faith is part of my life, so it will be part of my death as well. We all have a belief in something and I think our beliefs become more important at a time of crisis.
> Some people live on their anger, some on their friends, some

on their faith in God, or in doctors, or in alternative treatments such as apricot kernels. I've been helped by my beliefs and by my family and friends. If anything my faith has been strengthened. I've said 'Why me?' and all those things, but it's never made me question my faith. I know I haven't done all the right things in my life and I know I've got things to sort out before my time is up. I've thought about death but I don't think anybody accepts it until it gets close. I think that's good because if you get too accepting of it you might almost be wishing for it to happen.

I think I've got a healthy respect for death although I won't know how I'm going to handle it until it happens. This is the first time I've had cancer. I'm not good at it. I haven't practised and people will have to put up with the mistakes I make. It'll be the same with dying—it will be the first time. In the meantime, I think I've got to get on with making the most of the life I've got.

Getting on with 'the life she had left' was what Noelle decided to do.

I have always believed that the power is within us to help ourselves, whether it's to totally heal ourselves or to come to an acceptance of what's happening and to deal with it the best way we know how. I know I'm going to die but whether melanoma is going to kill me or whether I am going to die from heart disease, I'd like to think that when my time comes I'll die with dignity. I want to do it my way. I'm not frightened of dying. Dying is the easy part! It's the living that can be difficult because cancer doesn't just affect the person who has got the cancer: it affects everybody who means something to you. I'm finding it very hard to accept what it does to the people I love.

This week has been very difficult in that way and I was so low that by Saturday night my partner was asking, 'What can I do? Tell me.' There isn't anything anyone can do except be there and hold me when I am frightened. After that I realised I have been trying too hard—for all the right reasons. Maybe my expectations of what I am able to do in terms of self-healing have been too high. I'm not superwoman. I'm just another human being with fears and failings. I also want to make it easy on the people around me. I know my cancer is causing them grief and I want to be able to lessen it a bit. I know everyone has to deal with death and dying in their own way, just as they have to live their lives in their own way. So this is my life. I've got to live it and I want to do it right! It may sound silly but if I'm going to die then I want to do it well. I feel if I can live whatever is left of my life with dignity and without fear, then maybe that will ease my death for the people I love.

LEARNING TO SURVIVE

Working through issues of dying is part of learning how to survive—whatever the prognosis. Lynne identified this as a central issue when she observed that cancer

> *... may kill you but the real point is how are you going to live until then. That was something that came out of my mother's dying. She'd reached this point where she said: 'I don't want to think of myself as dying. I feel fine about dying but I'm not going to talk about it all the time. I'm not even going to prepare for it because I want to live every moment until I die.' That really impressed me and that was something I learnt again when I was diagnosed, even though it wasn't as extreme as her cancer.*

Learning how 'to live every moment' often meant coming to grips with on-going contact with the medical profession and Beth came to the conclusion that a crucial starting point was

> ... being able to out-manoeuvre and survive the health system. That's the first step and there are so many obstacles that if you can survive those you can survive anything.

Marinomoana has decided that, brain tumour or not, she will survive as long as she is interested and engaged in the world around her, even though her specialists have decided that her brain tumour is 'very definitely terminal', and that 'it's just a matter of when'.

> *I reckon that will probably be when I get fed up with everything! I've asked them, 'Couldn't it be that you've made a mistake? Maybe it's not cancer? Maybe it's just some blocks in my head?' They have said it doesn't work like that but I know it's not following the usual track of brain tumours because I've already exceeded well beyond the five years. The usual track of brain tumours is early death. Now, when I see any of the staff who have looked after me when I'm at the hospital for some other reason, it's funny because their mouths drop and their eyes go wide! I cheerfully say, 'Yes. I'm still alive!' Creeps! I don't like that negativity from the health care system. It's like, 'We've told you you're going to die. Do it and stop making us liars!' Some people actually comply with them but I like making them liars!*

Doctors also gave Tiny a pretty tight time frame. She decided that the best way to approach her prognosis was to learn as much as she could about myeloma from her specialists, and then have the audacity to believe that they might be wrong.

> *The best way to survive is to ask your doctor exactly what's going on. At first they didn't tell me a lot about the disease,*

just how long they thought I had because of my age group. But you've got to understand how the disease works and how the recovery process works. You have got to know what is happening to you. And you have to think positive. Then you can make it. When you think positive you do things for yourself with the herbs and you don't listen to other people as much, especially doctors who say you've only got so long to live. Don't listen to that—make up your own mind whether you're going to live through it. The doctors think I had only got two years to live. It's been over two years now and I'm feeling better.

But 'surviving and manoeuvring around the medical system' did not just entail healthy scepticism about a poor prognosis. Sometimes, the problem could be one of dealing with an overly optimistic initial prognosis, given with the best of intentions. Mara found this when she counselled a cousin who had also been diagnosed with breast cancer.

I rang her and we talked over the phone for quite a while. I told her how I felt and she said she felt much better after that. She asked me to visit her in hospital and she had such a good outlook that I felt proud because that was my first counselling after my cancer. It made my cousin feel good that she had such a positive outlook so freshly after the operation. When she went home she was told that she would not need any more treatment but at her next visit to the doctor he told her she needed chemotherapy because her cancer was a fast-growing one. She said, 'Why didn't you give me a little indication that I should have expected that?' He could have done it because then she wouldn't have been so shocked that she needed chemotherapy. Doctors quickly come out and say the positive but they should always in-build some negative possibilities because it's always like that: cancer can go one way or the other and it is better to be prepared.

For women with incurable cancers, manoeuvring around the medical system became a way of life. But even for those with treatable cancers, surviving initial medical intervention was only stage one. Rae had to learn how to deal with repeated check-ups. Although she was feeling physically fine, about a month after her operation she suffered from a kind of psychological after shock which she couldn't identify. When she tried to talk to her doctor about it she found that he only asked—

... if I had any family problems. A few things had gone wrong for us and, although they sorted themselves out, they really got me down for a while. The doctor put me on some tablets to make me relax a bit, but he didn't ask if I was having problems with the cancer. It was as though because they had caught it early and, because physically I was fine, there shouldn't be any other problems. You've virtually got to tell the doctor you've got a problem; they can't see it. They are always so busy. As soon as they get you out of the appointment, they are into another appointment and another problem.

Although she admitted that her heightened vulnerability and fear of a recurrence of melanoma had possibly made her 'go overboard in thinking about cancer', she felt increasingly dissatisfied with the way her plastic surgeon treated her whenever she went for check-ups.

I've been going to my plastic surgeon every four months but it was stupid because I'm in there for thirty seconds and all he does is check the glands in my neck. Not another word. It's a waste of money and I worry that another melanoma might be coming up somewhere else and he is not checking me out. He is a good surgeon but I didn't feel comfortable. Even if he could sit down with me for five minutes when I feel I need to talk or if he could give me support and say 'everything is fine'.

One day I was really furious after visiting him. I usually try to make an early morning appointment because he's so busy. This particular morning I could only get an appointment at half past eleven. There were two women before me and they were going to have a face lift. They were in there with him for a good half an hour, and when they came out they were being so pampered: they both wanted to go to hospital at the same time and blah, blah, blah. I was furious because he only had to see me for thirty seconds and yet he took these other women in first. I had to sit there and listen to all the laughing and carry on, and that got me down. They wanted to get their faces done! I've had this uncomfortable feeling with him ever since.

Rae was 'getting so up-tight' with this specialist that she made an appointment to see a dermatologist who had been recommended as very good for checking out cancer. He took the time to examine her carefully and gave her advice about how to proceed.

He said, 'There's nothing to worry about. There's one little thing which we'll watch but because your melanoma was in the second stage, I should only have to see you once a year. I will ask for the pathology report. Next time you see your surgeon tell him you have been to see me, that you live closer to me and that it would be more convenient for you to consult me.'

A bit of time and the freedom to express her fears and have them heard without being brushed aside was what Rae needed. Lynne stressed exactly the same need to be treated as an intelligent person with real concerns. She has now found just such a professional.

When I go for check-ups now I am able to talk with my doctor about anything that concerns me, or her. But this is in a smaller hospital and in a different country. For example she asks if I want information about hormone replacement treatment and I say 'no thanks'. She asks what vitamin and mineral supplements I'm taking and whether I'm doing specific things to handle my stress levels at work. And—this is especially remarkable—she calls me 'doctor' at least once during our session. It's a little ritual we have, after she said, 'Why wouldn't I call you doctor? You've studied for your philosophy degree much longer than I have for my medical one.' This is in stark contrast to the way in which my premature menopause (caused by the radiation treatment) and general health status was handled initially. The doctors would not listen to my objections when they simply told me I would have to use HRT.[6] I attempted on more than one occasion to discuss my understanding of the research and I was literally laughed at! It is a relief to be seen in clinic by someone I can talk to openly.

The importance of having fears taken seriously in the period after treatment cannot be over-estimated. As Kaye put it, after her operations she was

... forever feeling for things. When you find any lumps coming up or any little trauma you get worried.

Although Kaye found that the incessant worry and compulsive urge to feel for lumps died down of its own accord, Ann T found the best way to ensure her peace of mind was to insist on regular check-ups and to watch her diet. Even so, her heightened sensitivity to changes in her health meant that a few years later she rushed into a hysterectomy rather faster than she might have otherwise.

I became very conscious about what I should eat to keep my

---

6. Hormone Replacement Therapy.

calcium levels up for my bones and my cholesterol levels down because there's a lot of heart disease in my father's family. I insist on yearly check-ups and I have six monthly blood tests so I can watch my calcium level, my liver count and my cholesterol. I'm doing everything for my peace of mind so that I can get on with life, and not worry or panic if something crops up. That's what I did a couple of years after the mastectomy when we found that my ovaries were covered with cysts. I was going home to Ireland. Everything was booked, everyone was ready and then six weeks before, I got these awful pains in my stomach. I went to a doctor in Geraldton who did an ultrasound because I wanted to know why the cysts kept coming up. While he was doing the ultrasound he kept saying, 'It's a bit odd, this dark area there. I can't make out what it is.' Gee! That put the wind up me so I said, 'If they're not working, obviously the oestrogen is down and I don't really need them. Take them out.' That was the sorriest thing I've ever done. It was too fast and it was only the fact that I wanted to go home to Ireland and wanted it over with before I left. About three weeks later I got really depressed because it had been too rushed.

Learning to survive entails more than negotiating on-going contact with the medical system or contending with increased susceptibility to health matters. Most treatments for cancer are pretty rigorous and can knock the stuffing out of the strongest of constitutions. For an older person, like Margaret W, two rounds of surgery and the development of secondaries left her physically weakened, although she adapted to the changes this caused with the equanimity which characterised her whole approach to cancer.

When I came out of hospital I had to have a walking frame. Then I went to a stick. I can get about the house without a cane, but I couldn't go out without one. We have got the wheelchair and my son puts that in the car to get me out a bit, but I don't do any of the things I used to do and I don't like going out much any more. It's too inconvenient because even getting dressed tires me. To be honest I feel quite content to do nothing. I feel relaxed. I used to like reading but I can't read any more. I used to love doing crosswords but I can't do a crossword any more. My concentration's gone completely but it might come back. I don't feel ill. I feel exhausted, but I think that might be something to do with the weather. But I can't say that I'm bored or unhappy. I'm quite content. I've got a pleasant room and a nice outlook. That's not a bit like the extremely active lady I used to be, but that's me now. This cancer has changed me considerably.

When treatment managed to catch a cancer before it spread, the challenge became one of regaining physical strength and a sense of 'normality' as fast as possible. Ann T found that physical activity and the realisation that she could look 'perfectly normal' despite her mastectomy helped her get back into life. She also found inspiration from another woman who had survived breast cancer.

I joined AussiSwim[7] until I got too lazy! Actually, I think my arm got a bit sore. I should have kept up with it; I can breast-stroke and I can backstroke but I can't do overarm and I think that was it. I just gave up after a while but I still went to the pool all the time. It didn't worry me. I was told that the lifesaver had a prostheses. She was lovely: about forty-five or fifty, a grandmother, always in a bikini. There's no way I'd ever have known and that's what I wanted to be like. You have to get back to looking perfectly normal. I went to work one morning and forgot my prosthesis. Nobody else knew except me but I couldn't sit there like that because I felt strange. I had to go home and put it back in. It's very seldom I'll leave my prosthesis off,

---

7. AussiSwim is a non-competitive swimming club where you monitor your own progress.

even at home. I didn't wear a bra up to the time I had the mastectomy—well not often—so that was one of the big things for me: having to wear a bra because I had to have the prosthesis. Now of course, they have got new prosthesis that stick on but the price is a bit prohibitive so I don't use them except in my bikini. That gives you great freedom.

Freedom to venture out in a crowd with confidence despite the knowledge that your body has been changed for ever is important for women who have had a mastectomy. But Mara found that living with that knowledge left her very aware of other women's breasts.

My daughter asked me once, 'Do you feel upset when you see us having a shower and see our breasts? How do you feel when you walk in the streets and see a lady's breasts?' I said; 'The funny thing is I only notice if they are lopsided!' You know how usually breasts are not developed the same on both sides and one breast hangs down, the other one up? I notice those things so I must be looking for imperfection in normal people to console myself!

Consolation could also be found in awareness of the number of other women who have had breast cancer. Ann T found that talking with women newly diagnosed with breast cancer helped her to turn her experience into something she could use constructively. At the health insurance office where she worked, many women would come in to make a claim for a prosthesis.

I would always tell them about myself. I never hold back because when you first have it, you like to talk. I don't try to be nosy but I'll ask them if it is recent and will say, 'I've had mine five years. One of my colleagues has had hers seven years but we're fine. If you ever have any questions, just ask and anything I can help you with, I will.' That's how I feel I can

> help. People do want to hear the positive side. I knew that because the fact that my aunt had breast cancer and was still alive helped me a lot. There's enough people will tell you all the negatives.

Although optimism from any source was welcomed, it gained particular significance if it came from someone who had already been through the experience of cancer. Julie remembered that

> ... reassurance was probably the greatest thing I needed. All I wanted to hear was that I'd be OK, even if I knew that they really didn't know. It gave me a good feeling to have positive comments from friends. If someone didn't want to talk about my illness there'd be dumb silence, and I couldn't get out what I wanted to say. I really did want to meet somebody who had gone through the experience of cancer, and was well again because all I could think of was the friends of mine that hadn't made it. In the beginning that was the difficult part. Then I began to feel stronger in myself physically, especially after a friend of mine from work visited me in hospital. She got an awful shock when I said, 'Things aren't all well. They have found cancer.' She looked quite stunned, and then in a very quietly-spoken voice she said, 'Oh, Julie. I got over bowel cancer and you're a much stronger person than I am. I'm sure you'll get over it as well.' I had no idea. Later I thought, 'I am *strong*! I'll be OK.' You really do need to hear somebody being very positive about cancer even though deep down you know that there can be no answers and no assurances.

Kaye also emphasised the need

> ... to try and keep your hopes and spirits up. The way medicine is now, there are so many options. For many people, cancer is not a short term sentence; some people do survive for

quite a few years and if you can see that, it gives you a little bit of hope. But unfortunately, it depends on what type of cancer you have. Sometimes there isn't any hope. All you can do then is try to keep your spirits up because you can get so low.*

These women found many ways of bolstering their spirits, all tailored to their physical and emotional capabilities at different stages of their cancer experience. While getting back to work, resuming physical exercise, taking special care with diet, or getting on with an active social life was appropriate for some women once treatment was over, for others whose treatment regimes were on-going, doing tapestry, sitting in a spa, or having coffee with friends helped. Even when she was very unwell, Tiny found very simple ways to make sure that she 'didn't feel down'.

I look outside and see the sun shining. That is what I like in Australia; every day it is nice weather, and that makes me feel better. There were some times when I was in a room in the hospital with no windows. I hated it because I couldn't see the sun.

Carmen found that during long periods at home alone during chemotherapy, she really needed somebody to boost her system.

It would be really good to go to a movie, or read a book or watch TV together so that you can discuss it. Even going to the beach or going for a walk is good because it really does take your mind off your depression. It takes your mind off your feelings from all the side-effects. The more you think about them, the more you feel them.

Mara considered that her worst period was waiting for the operation. After that she decided she simply had to 'make the best of a bad situation'. Once she had had the double mastectomy she decided that the cancer had been taken out; that was how she 'looked forward'.

> *I look at every day as a bonus. Every day that I live after the operation is like a gift to me, it's a new day and I enjoy every day in a different way. I find if I cannot do something today, I'm not worried. I don't panic if I forget something. What I can do, I do; what I can not do can wait. It won't run away and if I'm not alive the world will still go on.*

She found that, while positive thinking can't help all the time

> *... it is very important for the quality of life, especially if you find you only have a little bit left. Positive thinking can really improve the way you live and survive. It was during the operation that this house was built and my husband used to say, 'If I knew that this was going to happen I would never have built a new house!' But in a way that kept us on the go because we had to order things and select things right after I got out of hospital. The shell was there and the roof, but the interior had to be organised after I got out of hospital and that kept me fairly busy. I had no time to brood.*

Several women found that setting new goals and keeping busy were effective ways of getting on with life. Even while suffering from treatment-induced disinterest in the life going on around her, Carmen realised the importance of planning for her future.

> *Once I'm over my chemo, I've got to set myself goals. I've got to be able to have the willpower to start life again because I've put life on hold at the moment. I've not had interest in anything except for building this new house and now I'm at the stage where I don't know if I'm going to sell it to get rid of*

the terrible debt or keep it, rent it and let people pay it off. If I can survive I need to have some new goals. I am thinking of studying because you've got to have something to keep spurring you on. At my stage of the sickness I've come to a time of my life where I don't know where I am. I don't know what I want, or what I expect out of life any more. So, this is where I need to look into the future, to start my life afresh again, to find a little desire to live because at the moment nothing really interests me any more. I try to think of what I want and there really is nothing because I've lost that interest.

Sometimes, regaining an interest in life meant reassessing priorities, figuring out what things might be accomplished or what aspects of life could be focused upon. At other times, it required shutting down and not thinking too much about anything. Beth did a bit of both, depending upon her physical and emotional resources.

You have to learn to make the most of what you've got. Sometimes I think a lot more about life, the universe and all that. But at other times I won't think at all because what I'm thinking isn't nice and it's safer not to think at all. On those days, I get busy. People say live every day for what it is and at first I was very much like that, I couldn't think too far ahead until the first CT scan showed that the cancer wasn't galloping away. I'm getting back into the old ruts a bit now and I'm thinking of doing a PhD. That means I am thinking five years ahead. I don't want to be one of those people who aims to survive until the end of my PhD and then falls off the perch, so I'll have to have another aim up my sleeve by then.

Planning for a future could be largely contingent upon a hopeful outcome of treatment, as Julie found.

You must get over each hurdle as it comes. The old cliché of

Songs *of* Strength

one day at a time is definitely true. Firstly, you have to get over the operation, then you have to get your strength back, then cope with the chemotherapy, and then take each day as it comes—and you have to think positive the whole way through. In the middle of my chemotherapy sessions I thought the world was going to end because it made me so terribly sick. The only way I could cope was to set goals for myself. I'd think, 'That's one down, so many to go and I'm on the downhill run.' That gave me something to look forward to.

Kaye also learnt to take things a day at a time. This was much easier when she had company—people who kept her busy and tried to keep her mind off cancer. But when she was alone she found that her mind

... was working overtime. I tried to look ahead. I tried to make long-term plans and keep my mind occupied although if I'd had my way I would have curled up in the corner of a dark room and hoped that it was all going to pass me by. That's what I felt like most of the time: blocking it out. I went through quite a long period of depression. That's why I was given antidepressant tablets to calm my nerves down. They just made me sleep. At first that was the way I wanted to be because then I wouldn't have to think about it. Bit by bit I realised that I was sleeping the time away and I thought 'No'. It took a long time—about six months—but I did come back. I tried not to show people too much of that depressive side but inside, when I was by myself, I let go. No-one suggested I go to counselling but then I went through a funny stage where the less I knew, the less I had to worry about. I didn't want to know the gory details. All I wanted to know was whether they had got it all out and would it come back. I didn't want to keep talking about it—it was too raw.

One of her biggest hurdles was getting over her guilt: she believed that she had probably caused her cancer and that she was somehow a failure because of it. Despite reassurance and support from her husband, it took her some time to overcome the depression which accompanied this deep sense of her own accountability.

> *I felt guilty that I was sick because I'd smoked all that time when I shouldn't have. I felt that I had brought it on myself and then put everything on my husband's shoulders, and plonked it on the kids as well. I felt like a failure for getting this thing and for all the trauma it would cause them if I died. That was the way my mind thought. I had the cancer. I must have got it some way. What could I have done that would have stopped me from having it? If it did come through smoking, I'd made myself get it. I went right through this business with my husband, apologising to him for putting all this on him, for being a failure. I felt as though I wasn't a very good mother and I wasn't a very good wife, and I asked him how he put up with me. He just said, 'I love you. You would have done the same for me.' I knew I would do the same, but I didn't think like that in the beginning.*
>
> *Having young children gave me the incentive to try different things. Not that I wouldn't have tried for my husband but it was the children that really kept my mind off it because the less I had to talk about it the less I had to think about it. I suppose I was working things out through them. I know they did help.*

The needs of her children also helped Marinomoana pick up the pieces after an extended period of depression. The worst bouts of depression usually came hard on the heels of the death of friends she had made at the cancer support groups.

> *I used to feel guilty about being alive. That's sad! My*

psychologist helped me work through that. He asked me why I felt guilty and I said, 'Because everyone else is dead.' He said, 'Then you should be jumping for joy! They would be for you.' Such common sense! My husband was apparently telling me the same thing but I couldn't hear him. You don't hear your partners. It was like, 'Shut up, You're not living this!' It was part of the wallowing in self-pity but I didn't know what depression was because I'd never been depressed before.

It took me a long time—about three years after diagnosis—to come out of that. It was hard. You have peaks of highs—mountain-top highs—and you have depths-of-hell lows, and when you're down you take everyone else with you. That's the horrible bit. I didn't have difficulty keeping the very deep lows away from my children because they were really lovely little boys during that time; they were an absolute joy. I remember one day when I was feeling really depressed and I could hear this song coming up the street. I walked out and it was my little boy singing, 'Star of wonder, star of light' at the top of his voice. He'd learnt it at school. They used to bring me out of my depressions very easily. My children made my life worth living—along with my husband's dry sense of humour!

While several women recognised a period of depression after their diagnosis and treatment, only Noelle focused upon the issue of anger.

People kept asking me, 'Aren't you angry about getting cancer?' For a long while I was very confused about that. I'd say, 'No. What can I be angry at?' Cancer wasn't hiding behind a bush going, 'Eeny meeny miny mo. Right! We'll take this one!' I don't feel like a victim and I haven't felt sorry for myself. At times I feel sad and down but it's not pity, it's not 'poor me, why me' because I wouldn't wish this onto anybody else. But these people kept on saying, 'Aren't you angry? I'd be angry!'

Quite often people put doubts in your mind. You feel you're going the right way then somebody says, 'But shouldn't you be doing this?' You think 'No' but then you go away and think 'Maybe'. Then you start doubting yourself. So I started thinking maybe I should be angry but I still couldn't figure out what to be angry at. In the end I thought the only thing I could be angry at is myself and why should I be angry at myself? I mean, this thing is beating up on me! I'm not going to beat up on myself! I did that years ago!

The anger did come, however, just recently—after coming home from my holidays. While I was away I found more lumps so I rang my surgeon and he had made arrangements for me to go into hospital to have them removed a couple of days after my return. It felt like I was on a merry-go-round, and the anger came when I was ringing my family and informing them, again. It had only been a month since the last round and they were still reeling from that lot. I know I was. It was anger about what it does every time I have to tell my family, not so much what it's doing to me. I can see what it's doing to my family.

While Noelle never accepted the 'Why me?' response to cancer, she nevertheless tried to 'find some kind of meaning' in why she got melanoma.

I was talking with a friend the other day about the type of illnesses we get and whether they are a reflection of what has happened in our lives and the emotions we take on board. Why did I get melanoma of all things? Why wasn't it breast cancer or cervical cancer or some other woman's disease? Why not lymphoma? There's plenty of cancers to choose from so why did I get one which means I'm having to have bits cut out of me every month? If you want to really delve deeply, it's a form of mutilation. So that got me thinking, 'Good grief! Why am I mutilating myself?' Nothing comes to mind and I have come to the conclusion that I don't need to justify the reason why I have cancer! It seems to me that is much like asking why I wasn't born in Rwanda, or why I wasn't born intellectually disabled? Why not cancer? Maybe I'm staving off the heart attack with the good diet I'm on because of melanoma!

Several women found that they had to contend with variations of this, particularly when the traumas of treatment seemed insurmountable. Margaret P found herself pondering upon the way

... some people talk about the psychological causes of cancer. Could traumatic events in your life, like a divorce, or finding out that your kid is on drugs, have caused cancer? If you carry that to extremes, you are actually telling a person that they caused their own cancer, and the natural progression of that is if they've caused it, they can cure it. They're always telling us about how important positive attitude is, which is like saying it's up to you whether you live or die. That is bullshit for people with an incurable cancer. You have no chance right at the beginning, so what difference does positive attitude make? I know that there are genetic and environmental links because there's four in my family with low-grade lymphoma.

Psychological problems might add an extra ingredient for some people but you don't cause your own cancer just like nobody asks for their kid to be run down by a bus. I am sure that how you feel can influence the way you respond to treatment because if you are feeling happy and hopeful then it is not so hard to put up with the side-effects of chemo. I've seen that in myself. But your emotions are only an influence, they do not decide how you are.

Julie found that she got through many of her worst times through quiet periods of reflection and prayer.

> *I don't like preaching religion, because I believe each to their own, but I am a very religious person having been to a convent school. I do say silent prayers, and I'll listen to Him and I know my faith strengthened through this experience. I do believe there's a God and I believe that sometimes these things are sent for a reason. Ours is not to question. A lot of people seem to think they're being punished: 'Why me? What did I do? Why did God give me cancer?' That is not what it's about. It's happened and when you do deal with it you definitely come out a stronger person.*

This acceptance that cancer had to be lived with to the best of their ability best sums up the ways in which all of these women have learnt to survive. Noelle likened the whole process to sitting for a test.

> *I don't like tests and this is a test I definitely don't want to take. I was never any good at tests and I just might get this one wrong. But deep down I know that with this test there is no right way or wrong way. You do it your own way and your own way is the right way.*

Annie encapsulated the process of learning to survive in similar terms.

> *Difficult as it might sound, you realise that your life is not going to end today or tomorrow or probably next month. If you are going to die from cancer it's going to take a while, and wouldn't it be a waste to give up? That's not easy to arrive at, and whatever strategy somebody uses—whether it's to get under the doona and lie there for a couple of weeks or to do something mad and go and spend every penny you've got—*

whatever you do is the right way to do it. There are absolutely no rules and no guide-lines for having cancer and whatever you do, you should be patted on the back. There's no right and wrong way of dealing with cancer.

NEW PRIORITIES

It is one of the curiosities of human existence that it can take a crisis like serious illness to stop us in our tracks and make us reassess priorities. Anne K believes that this is because

... we really feel we're invincible otherwise. Everybody else gets cancer except me. You just don't feel it's going to happen to you.

Until it does, there is little cause to do a stocktake. For all of these women, cancer arrived as a shock, a crisis that had to be contended with and the development of new priorities was closely related to the ways in which they learnt how to survive with cancer. New priorities were not always dramatic. They came in a range of guises from the smallest of accomplishments to fresh understandings of the self. While all of the women found that there were ways they could turn the experience into something constructive, several felt ambivalent about being forced into a situation in which they had no choice but to reassess their lives. As Kaye put it

Some people think there are times that you need a shake up in your life, but I can think of better things to shake you up than cancer!

Margaret P was even more emphatic and dubious about the value of the 'lessons' and 'benefits' of cancer.

Some people think that getting cancer and getting over it is a

big benefit to them because they learn a lot. Maybe—but isn't it something you would rather not have learnt? It's not something that anybody would choose to go through. I've met a lot of people because of cancer, people that I never would have met, and I've made heaps of friends, but it's still something that I would give away if I had the choice.

In direct contrast, Noelle came to the conclusion that getting cancer turned her life around.

It has opened up my eyes. There's a saying, 'The teacher arrives when the student is ready.' Everything we need to know is there in front of us but the trouble is we aren't always aware of it. The information is being fed to us in our daily lives but we only take on a certain amount of information. The rest doesn't seem to be important, or we don't recognise it as important. It's not until we get further along the line, when we are ready, that we realise something has been staring us in the face for years. When you are at the coal face you don't see anything else, and it's only when you are given the opportunity to stand back that you reassess things. I made all these mistakes in my life and emotionally I was such a mess that I wasn't recognising anything. Sometimes, it was enough just to get through the day, so if nothing else cancer has meant the scales have dropped from my eyes. It amazes me—every day brings a new experience and I hang onto it and cherish it. Before, the experiences were probably there but they weren't cherished. Now they have more meaning. Before I would do things just to please other people but now it's got to be because I want to do it. That may sound selfish but if I'm going along to keep everybody else sweet, then it is for the wrong reasons. I don't allow myself to be coerced into something I don't want to do any more, and if I really want to do something, then I'll go out and do it.

Songs *of* Strength

In one sweep, Noelle identified two of the most dramatic ways in which cancer changed the ways many of these women looked at, and experienced, the world around them: an increased capacity to treasure the most inconsequential of daily experiences and a heightened value of their own lives. Lynne expressed this kind of reassessment, focusing on the things and people that she wanted in her life.

For me, the most important thing about having cancer is that I've integrated parts of myself that would have been left dangling. I went through a whole lot of stuff about the kinds of relationships that I wanted to have. Lots of people have this tremendous ability to sustain relationships and friendships that aren't satisfying and are actually quite negative. I went through a process of thinking: do I want this kind of mediocrity in my life?

My cancer has made me a bit less compromising. I want to live a life that's really exciting, that's satisfying and that enables me to achieve the sorts of things that really turn me on. I don't want to have a whole lot of mediocre people or situations around me. Part of being uncompromising is being really honest with other people and with myself about my lifestyle and what I want. It's a bullshit-cutting-out experience, it really is, and I'm even more maniacal about those things than I was before!

Margaret P on the other hand doesn't believe that having cancer has had a substantial impact on her values and attitudes, although she does believe that being seriously ill for a long time has been so relentless that it has changed her behaviour and priorities. She has learnt to be more assertive and more selfish, a quality she would have once frowned upon but came to consider essential to her survival because

... you've got to be selective with the energy you've got,

especially when you are on treatment; you have to save your energy, you've got to marshal it for use when you need it and not waste it. This can seem selfish. I have become more assertive and that means I have changed my behaviour. I used to be a real mouse! You emphasise some things more than you did, and de-emphasise others. You see some things as no longer important. You worry about different things. I've quit worrying about shit that doesn't matter. I go to bed at three o'clock and get up at twelve if I feel like it. In the summer I hang around in my nighties all day. I made myself some beautiful full length silk nightgowns, with fitted bodices, and they are cool and comfortable. Sometimes my daughter has a go at me for not getting dressed but I say, 'Why should I?' I do as I like and I don't worry any more, but it's taken me all my life to get to this point. Some people seem to change their priorities early in the piece.

The quality that Margaret P defined as 'selfishness' Mara explained as taking herself 'more seriously'.

I started to put more importance on what I want. Before it was family first, husband first, even my dog and cat first! But after the operation I started thinking of myself as important too. That's one positive change. Now I know how to stand up and say 'no'. Once, if my daughter said, 'Mum, could you baby-sit?' I would have postponed everything and rushed to the baby-sitting job. Now I don't cancel anything because I think it's no good being there for them all the time. I say, 'I'm sorry I have to go out' or 'I have to meet somebody for coffee or a dinner engagement.'

Such reassessment of a woman's role as family nurturer could have constructive spin-offs, both in philosophical and practical terms, as Anne K explained.

Before leukaemia I was the wife at home, helping my husband, planning the kids' futures, planning my own future. I don't do anything at all like that now. It doesn't matter a damn to me. I don't try to plan for the future. It probably makes us nice and comfortable and secure thinking we're planning for a future, but you don't know what it holds. The best of plans can go very badly wrong.

I'm now very focused on my children as individuals. I really enjoy them. I hadn't time to enjoy them before. If they don't turn out to be doctors or lawyers, it's not going to be any big deal. I'm trying to teach them that there's a lot more to life than being academically successful or having lots of material things. I don't have the drive or ambition to make heaps of money like some people have. I think that's crazy. In that respect I think quite differently to the way I used to. I'm just so damned glad to feel so good and I think that's rubbed off on the kids. They've seen how I've been and how I am now and I think they've learned from my experience: it's a good idea to try and enjoy your life and not be so crazy about trying to make heaps of money or trying so hard to be successful, either in the eyes of others or yourself.

Tiny described going through the same kind of reassessment of material things, with similar consequences: a renewed emphasis on family relationships and an enhanced ability to circumnavigate situations which she once would have viewed as problematical.

The most important thing I've learnt is that money is not the first thing that matters. The important thing is that you've got your family. You realise that you need your family more than you did before. Before there were a lot of little things that I would make a lot of. Now I think: it's not worth making a problem for that. And I have seen a lot of people much younger than I who are very sick and on chemo, so I am happy that

I'm older, although it would be better if I was older still! Having older children made it a little easier too because we could discuss everything. I have been more open towards things and talk more openly about things than I did before. I think differently about things than I did before.

Tiny was not the only woman to find that a reappraisal of the value of material possessions spilled over into other aspects of her life. Ann T found that a major consequence of her experience has been a greater ability to control stress. For her that has meant focusing on the present rather than worrying about the future, although that doesn't mean she doesn't dream of things she hopes to do.

I did have new priorities and I've been going through my priorities every time something drastic happens! I've got rid of a lot of the stress. It does come back every now and again, but then I sit back and think, 'Don't worry about it!' That de Silva course I did helped me to get my priorities right. Life is for living now, not for when we retire. What's the point in saving for when you're sixty-five? You mightn't even be here, or you might be too old and decrepit to use it. The way I'm going I'll be fit and healthy and I won't have tuppence! When we started married life we had three years in a caravan before we went up north and when we were up there we spent just about all the money we ever had before we came back down. We had enough to pay for half a house. My idea is that if everything went wrong, we could sell the house and go back in the caravan. I like having money because it is a great feeling to be able to go out and spend something now and then but I wouldn't be devastated if something happened and we had to go back into the simple living in the caravan. My husband's dream is to get a boat and sail around the world. Mine is to get the caravan, tow it all around and meet him. I'll be his woman in every port.

Julie had already learnt the transient nature of material goods when she lived through Cyclone Tracy in Darwin in 1974, and as she knew only too well

> ... *after you've finished that experience and you start picking up the pieces, you begin to want again—I suppose it's human nature.*

Her experience of cancer served to 'refresh her memory' and she found that

> *... material things became less and less important to me after my diagnosis. The important thing was, and still is, my health, and the health of my family. When other people are feeling a bit sorry for themselves, I can always say, 'But you've got your health,' and I make them realise that things could be a lot worse. I think I became more compassionate and the whole experience has given me a lot of new skills dealing with people. I feel comfortable talking to people with all sorts of problems. Some of their problems seem quite minor compared to a cancer diagnosis, but it's a problem to them. It's made me realise that each and every one of us has problems, and they affect each of us differently.*

Julie has found that this more compassionate understanding of the problems people encounter had served her well in her work as a public servant, where she deals with the public on a daily basis. Beth also found that she brought new skills and perspectives to her profession as a nurse educator.

> *Only a week before I found out I needed major surgery I'd been giving a class to nursing students about empowering a patient. I used incidents that the students had brought back from their work in hospitals. One of them was about a lady*

in hospital who'd been told that she had a lump and the doctor said, 'I've got a cancellation for tomorrow so I can fit you in for a lumpectomy and whatever else we need to do. See you then.' I asked the nurses how they would empower that person to ask the right questions so that she could consider the alternatives. After I'd had my initial diagnosis, I thought how hypothetical that was because I realised that all I wanted to do was to get into hospital and get that thing cut out! It made me very aware of what a difference there is between theory and reality!

Now when I give that session I use the same case but when the students jump in and say how they will try to stall things to give the woman more time to make decisions, consider alternative treatments—or to say no to treatment—I react differently from how I used to. I now ask them to consider the woman's emotional as well as rational responses. I guess overall I try to get the students to see things from the patient's perspective more—how she feels, what she wants—and to honour her decisions even if the nurses disagree with it. It is what the patient wants to do—not what the nurses and doctors will do—that is at the centre of this experience.

Beth also found that her diagnosis encouraged her to rationalise her professional activities so that she now focuses her energies on issues which she is passionately interested in.

I dropped so many things that quickly. I'd nearly finished some protocols on elder abuse. They were at the point where I needed to go away for a week to move sentences and rephrase ideas to tighten it up—the kind of work that makes good quality writing—but suddenly it wasn't important any more. I was on a government reference group and a whole pile of committees, and I said no to most of them and only kept the ones that I am really interested in. If I do anything now, I'll do something on women's experience of cancer. I want to look at what it is that keeps women going. What it is that makes women survive the experience. I think women have got to be strong enough to tell people that we're important, strong enough to demand our rights, strong enough to say no to people, strong enough to cry, and to think that it's not a weakness. We need to be strong enough to ask for the help we need.

Annie has no doubts that work has been pivotal in helping her survive the experience of living with cancer, although she has had to reassess how she tackles the job. Along the way she has found some unexpected advantages.

My career was looking good when I was diagnosed and it was looking like I was going to go somewhere. The day I was diagnosed—forget it: I can't go up the career path with incurable cancer! But it's interesting—I think I've done more in my career since I've had cancer than I would have otherwise because I'm no longer scared of what people think. What they think is not going to bother me anyway because I haven't got a career to worry about messing up! I've been quite vocal on a lot of issues just because of that. It has given me the confidence to know that it doesn't matter if I put my foot in my mouth. Cancer doesn't actually get any ticks for that, and let's not mention the word positive! Before cancer, career was a priority. Since then it has become very urgent to travel. I took out my super and spent all that on taking the kids to America. After that I've travelled as much as I could although now I've found out that I can't do any more travelling because it's too painful and just not worth it.

What are my priorities now? Eating nice food. I don't know really. I can't set up new projects. I can't develop a new research area so there's no point worrying about it. In fact I've given away a lot of research topics that I was going to do and it's nice to see them being done. Anything I do now has an immediacy about it—it has to be done within a month or it has to be a project where somebody else can take over whenever I need treatment. Anything I do now has to have an immediate outcome. If I can see that it's not being effective then I drop it because it's not worth spending the energy trying to shift mountains. The committees and projects that I'm involved with now are doing things and they won't fall in a heap if I can't continue my involvement. To an extent I've lost that desire to possess things. In this situation, you divest your ego a bit more because you have to allow other people in to take over if you can't do it. It was very hard doing that! I like being in control and I don't think I could walk away from my two major projects. I'd want to be in the background somewhere, on the phone. I'll probably die with a phone in my hand!

Once Julie had recuperated from treatment, she decided to see how far she could push her physical and mental boundaries.

When I was on chemo my finger and knee joints became very stiff. I've still got a few of these side-effects left and it makes me a bit cross, although it's minor compared to how I was feeling. A few months ago at work they offered a management course called Learning the Ropes and to get through this course I had to abseil down a cliff—it was a self-esteem thing. I'm very frightened of heights, but after four days with a mixture of males and females that I'd never ever met before, I became so confident, so part of this team, that I went down the quarry at Gosnells. I was actually more scared going up because you have to use a rope and you were not actually hooked on. With my knees so stiff it was very painful, but I thought, 'I am going to do this if it kills me.' A lot of people backed out, and they asked who wanted to go first. I thought if I didn't go first,

I'd faint. I've got some photos somewhere and my face is as white as a sheet. Over I went. I felt so good because I'd been so weak after the two operations and the chemo, that to get to the stage at fifty years of age where I could do that was the biggest achievement of my life.

When we went to Phuket in January this year for a holiday, I did a parasail. That was another big achievement. There was no way in the world I would have been doing things like that before but I now think, 'I've been through much worse than this. I can do this.' It's exciting and it's been a really new learning experience. I think my husband worries what I'm going to do next, but I think that if you tackle cancer then you can tackle most things in life.

Julie was three years down the track from treatment when she launched herself off a cliff on the end of a rope and took to the skies. Such methods of extending horizons, even if desirable, were simply not an option when treatment was still being undergone. Carmen made less strenuous, but equally significant, activities part of her new priorities. She also found great pleasure and renewed worth in the smallest of achievements.

I've been going to the movies more frequently than I used to. Even though it's tiring to get there I have found it's terrific to watch a good comedy. I find even a picnic out in the sunshine is really good therapy because I stop and look at God's beautiful creations and appreciate what life's all about. Entertainment is vital because if you don't get up and go out you tuck yourself away in the doldrums. I should go out a little bit more and enjoy myself, but I do tend to hide away because I've got nobody to do these things with.

I've realised that I'm vulnerable and that death can be imminent. This has made me treasure every moment of this earthly life as precious, even though I look forward to the next life. Before it happened, I probably wasted a lot of time. Now, I tend to appreciate every moment and I cherish the faculties I have: to be able to see, hear and walk are things you take for granted until you are restricted by illness. Now, when I've done something, it's such an achievement that I feel really happy, even if I've just dried the dishes! Each thing that I do is really wonderful. I started writing down the things I did each day and some days I had done twenty things. I couldn't believe it and I was so thrilled. I think that's what gives you your sense of worth—knowing that you can do something.

Kaye became aware of her mortality when she first came out of hospital.

I was very aware of all the things I'd never done, so I made a list of all the things that I was going to do, like go to an opera, or go horse riding. I wanted to get out and do things. I didn't want to miss out. We went on a few camping trips, and spent a lot of time with the kids. Life becomes more precious. It's almost like you count every hour of the day. I didn't even want to go to sleep at night because I knew it was a waste of time. But time goes by and I started to calm down and then my priorities started to waver off onto other things. That took around about the same time as the depression—about six months down the track I realised that I hadn't dropped dead and another lump hadn't arrived. By the time I felt better health-wise I never really got around to doing all the things on my list. All these years down the track I don't really have the same sense of preciousness although I still think along those lines occasionally. Back then I was practically thinking about it every day. Then it was every week. Now, I thank God that I'm still here.

Rae also 'thanks God' for her life. Like Kaye, but for different reasons, she does not think that her experience has made a substantial difference to her priorities. She believes that

> *If my cancer had gone any further and I'd had to have chemotherapy then perhaps I would be thinking of things that I would really like to do, but at the moment I'm just enjoying the family growing up, doing things around the retirement village, going out with friends and doing knitting for the family. Easy things. The doctor said, 'Watch what you eat,' so I'm more conscious about food. I take each day as it comes although that's easier said than done. I try not to worry about things but I still do. I don't think I've changed my life. If anyone who hadn't seen me for twelve months saw me now I don't think they would see a change in me. I haven't thought, 'I want to do this and this before I die.'*

Energy and resources can be central to implementing new priorities. Margaret P rejected her then husband's offer to sell up their home and business and take her on a world cruise just after she was diagnosed because she wanted her life to continue as normally as possible. Eight years down the track, divorced and with her lymphoma progressing unrelentingly, she would now like to go around the world but hasn't the money. While there are many things she would like to do but can't because of her deteriorating physical condition, she managed to achieve something she has always wanted to do.

> *I left school at fifteen and I'd always wanted to prove I had a brain. I knew I wasn't that thick so after I was diagnosed with cancer I did my Tertiary Entrance Exam, and then I started uni full-time in 1990. Getting that piece of paper was very important to me and my uni mates have been absolutely brilliant. Now I have a degree in psychology.*

Margaret P may well have got around to doing a degree whether or not she had been diagnosed with an incurable cancer. In the same way, Julie may have combated her fear of heights, Carmen may have decided to start going to the movies or making time for picnics. Annie probably would have made it to the United States—one day. Mara and Noelle may have found other reasons for taking themselves seriously and doing things because they wanted to, while Lynne may have come to the conclusion that she had had enough of mediocrity via another route. And any number of life circumstances can make a person stop and smell the roses. But many of these women found that their diagnosis of cancer promoted a certain urgency. It was a circumstance which propelled them into action and made them want to get on with the business of living. Like all the other women in this group, Marinomoana found her own ways of doing that. In the process of describing these, she also summed up a sentiment shared by all the others who contributed their experiences to this book.

I had a list of things that I wanted to do when I was diagnosed because when you think you've got a short time, you start on down that path to accomplish those things. I wanted to watch the Celtics play basketball; meet Kevin McHale; finish my education. I haven't done the first two and I didn't realise that my education was going to take this long! At first I decided I wanted to get my TEE so I enrolled in some TAFE courses. I just wanted to be able to say, 'I did that. That's something.' I didn't think about university because that was for clever people! But then I was offered a place at university so I thought, 'Oh, all right then!' I didn't realise that ordinary people are at university striving. Now I'm one of them and it's good. I like it!

I think that that's what kept me going, 'cos I was actually at a stage when I was doing nothing besides basketball and looking after the boys. Then university became a priority. I am studying Aboriginal and Intercultural Studies and Women's Studies. It has shown me that it doesn't matter where we are from, or where we live or who we are, women tend to have a lot of the same stories. Although there's lots of differences, we are suffering the same injustices across the board, and I'm always surprised—you'd think after four years of study I wouldn't be! University was a saving grace for me, and it was because of university that I was asked to come to this group. Otherwise it wouldn't have happened and I would have most probably lived out my life in this house, with my kids and not contributed anything. Well, maybe not but this is what I love about this project. This is gonna be effective in so many different women's lives and whether I die tomorrow or in twenty years' time, it doesn't matter. This will be my last hurrah. It's good that it's not going to go unsaid. It's like my legacy.

Conclusion

IN THIS BOOK WE HAVE TRIED TO COVER ASPECTS OF THE CANCER EXPErience which we found were important to us. As you have read, most of us shared common experiences but we came to handle these in many varied ways depending on our backgrounds and current lifestyles, on the support we were given and the particular type of cancer we had. In fact, the way in which we dealt with cancer was, for each of us, a very individual one.

Firstly came the shock of diagnosis which for many of us was totally unexpected. Then the tumultuous weeks which followed when we were forced to find ways of dealing with the pain of confronting what then seemed to be a death sentence, of telling our partners, children, parents and friends, of coping with treatments and finding ways of weaving through too little or too much information. Some of us wanted to find a quiet warm corner to hide away, others wanted to confront cancer head-on. In whichever way we dealt with those first few weeks we all came through this period of confusion determined to return to our 'normal lives' as quickly as possible. What might have seemed to have been dull and routine was now something to be aimed for. For many of us, our work became our goal and a place to escape to and 'forget' that we had or were recovering from cancer. As well, our families, particularly for those women with grandchildren, and friends helped to fill the void of uncertainty.

Another aspect for which we had to find strategies that suited ourselves were the ways in which we dealt with the medical and hospital systems, with our families and friends and with those who may have meant well but became annoyances. We learnt to develop patience, not only with dealing with people who felt particularly uncomfortable with cancer, but also with the inevitable waiting. The days waiting for test results or treatment, the hours spent waiting in doctors rooms or clinics or hospital beds. Trying to maintain a sense of ourselves while undergoing chemotherapy, radiotherapy and surgery was another challenge and one for which we devised our own unique methods.

We have had to face the likelihood of death and dying and make practical arrangements and decisions which were at times painful. And we have lost friends. Throughout the course of writing this book, three of the women in the group have died, one woman has developed secondary cancer and the condition of a few of the women has worsened. Other women have passed the 'five-year' cancer-free period and look back on the experience as one which has inevitably reshaped their lives. However, an aspect common to all of us is that we have discovered that we live until the day we die—the diagnosis of cancer does not mean an instant death. We have found that in order to live to the fullest does not require 'bravery' or 'courage', but a willingness to muster our energies and aim for a 'normality' in our daily lives.

Although none of us would have wished for the cancer experience, through it we have each gained strengths we didn't know we had, and the ability to appreciate what we had previously thought were the mundane and routine things in life. We know that, in your own individual way, you will come through the cancer experience as we did.

THE WOMEN'S CANCER GROUP